THE SKIN AND SYSTEMIC DISEASE

Dedication
In memory of my father, Zachary Lebwohl

THE SKIN AND SYSTEMIC DISEASE

A COLOR ATLAS AND TEXT

SECOND EDITION

Mark G. Lebwohl, M.D.
Sol and Clara Kest Professor and Chairman
Department of Dermatology
The Mount Sinai School of Medicine
New York
USA

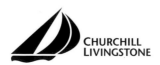

London ■ Edinburgh ■ New York ■ Philadelphia ■ St Louis ■ Sydney ■ Toronto 2004

CHURCHILL LIVINGSTONE
An imprint of Elsevier Limited

First edition 1995
Second edition 2004

ISBN 044306539X

British Library Cataloguing in Publication Data
A catalogue record for this book is available from the British Library

Library of Congress Cataloging in Publication Data
A catalog record for this book is available from the Library of Congress

Note
Medical knowledge is constantly changing. Standard safety precautions must be followed, but as new research and clinical experience broaden our knowledge, changes in treatment and drug therapy may become necessary or appropriate. Readers are advised to check the most current product information provided by the manufacturer of each drug to be administered to verify the recommended dose, the method and duration of administration, and contraindications. It is the responsibility of the practitioner, relying on experience and knowledge of the patient, to determine dosages and the best treatment for each individual patient. Neither the Publisher nor the editors nor contributors assume any liability for any injury and/or damage to persons or property arising from this publication.
The Publisher

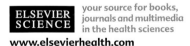
your source for books, journals and multimedia in the health sciences
www.elsevierhealth.com

Printed in China

The publisher's policy is to use paper manufactured from sustainable forests

Commissioning Editor: Sue Hodgson
Project Development Manager: Belinda Henry
Project Manager: Glenys Norquay
Design Manager: Jayne Jones

Contents

Preface

This book, like its predecessor, comprehensively reviews the cutaneous manifestations of systemic diseases in an atlas format with substantial text. This edition differs from the earlier version in that numerous clinically useful tables have been added. For example, the first chapter includes tables listing the causes of Raynaud's phenomenon, the incidence of antinuclear antibodies in different connective tissue diseases, antinuclear antibody immunofluorescent staining patterns, and features that distinguish psoriatic arthritis from rheumatoid arthritis. Diagnostic approaches to the work up of patients with chronic urticaria and to the work up of patients with septal panniculitis are also presented in tables, as are criteria for the diagnosis of Kawasaki disease or rheumatic fever.

Perhaps the most useful tables deal with an organized approach to the diagnosis of fever and rash in the chapter on infectious diseases. This approach was first developed by Tom Fitzpatrick, whose student, Michael Fisher, described the differential diagnosis of fever and rash with Susan Katz in a chapter they wrote together for my first book, *Difficult Diagnoses in Dermatology*. In that chapter they simplified the diagnosis of fever and rash by basing the differential diagnosis on morphology of the lesion. By dividing the differential diagnosis into vesicopustular eruptions, purpuric eruptions or erythematous eruptions, the list of possible diagnoses is narrowed down to a smaller, more manageable list of possibilities, which can then be addressed in a methodical manner.

Based on their beautifully written chapter, I added tables listing the clinical features and laboratory tests that distinguish each of the possible diagnoses on the list of vesicopustular eruptions, purpuric eruptions, or erythematous eruptions. Those tables which were added to the original chapter now constitute tables 9-2, 9-3 and 9-4 of this book.

This edition also makes substantial use of acronyms such as 'ANTINUCLEAR,' which identifies criteria for the diagnosis of systemic lupus erythematosus or 'ACCNE' for criteria for the diagnosis of rheumatic fever. The differential diagnosis of causes of leukocytoclastic vasculitis ('MSHC' for Mount Sinai Hospital Center) or causes of erythema nodosum ('BED REST') are also included, as are *L's* for lymphocytic infiltrates, *P's* for lichen planus and *D's* for features of pellagra. As I have lectured around the country, it has been rewarding to hear students quote mnemonics that first appeared in the original edition of *Atlas of the Skin and Systemic Disease*. The mnemonic for the diagnostic criteria for lupus was used as an example of the teaching value of acronyms in an article published in the *International Journal of Dermatology* (K Al Aboud et al. Mnemonics in dermatology; an appraisal. *Int J Dermatol* 2002;41:594-95). That acronym, ANTINUCLEAR, was written for the first *Atlas of the Skin and Systemic Disease*. Although the source of the acronym was not credited in the article, there is no greater reward than the knowledge that information published in my book is being used by dermatologists to help care for their patients.

Many new figures have been added to this edition of *The Skin and Systemic Disease*, while the best photos of the first edition have been retained. Thanks to photography equipment, software, and lots of free advice from Canfield Clinical Systems' (Fairfield, NJ), many distractions in early photos have been removed without altering the integrity of our clinical pictures. For example, cyanosis of the digits in Figure 5-2 was apparent in the first edition, despite the wildly colored tie in the background of the photograph. Thanks to the Canfield software, the tie is now white, and the photograph superior even though we have not altered the fingers or their color at all. Since publication of the first *Atlas*, conditions such as paraneoplastic pemphigus and the cutaneous side effects of medications such as protease inhibitors have been described. Bioterrorism is a new word, and the cutaneous manifestations of anthrax, vaccinia and smallpox were not considered in the first edition of *The Atlas of the Skin and Systemic Disease*. All of these conditions and many others have been added to the current edition. It is my hope that medical dermatology will progress so quickly that future editions of *The Skin and Systemic Disease* will require even more change.

Credits

The following people contributed photographs for use in *The Skin and Systemic Disease*: Blanche Alter, Ernest Ast, Fabio Barbosa, Burton Belknap, Vincent Beltrani, Brian Berman, Jeffrey Bernhard, Sally Bishop, Edward Bottone, Martin Brownstein, Walter Burgdorf, Vincent Cipollaro, Steven Cohen, Stephen Comite, Gregory Cox, Renata Dische, Stuart Eichenfield, Raul Fleischmajer, Glenn Fuchs, Wayne Fuchs, Walter Futterweit, Charles Gerson, Robert Gilgor, Fredda Ginsberg-Fellner, Neil Goldberg, Marsha Gordon, Marc Grossman, Jeffrey Gumprecht, Alejandra Gurtman, Martha Guttenberg, Suhail Hadi, James F. Holland, Brad Katchen, Hirschel Kahn, Rhona Keller, Francisco Kerdel, Leslie Kerr, Ezra Kest, Michael Klein, Peter Koblenzer, Ronni Lieberman, Burt Meyers, Kenneth Neldner, Juan Orellana, Robert Phelps, Daniel Present, Sharon Raimer, E. Chester Ridgeway, Donald Rudikoff, Malcolm Rustin, Neil Sadick, Lilianna Sauter, Neal Schultz, Ronald Shelton, David Silvers, Robert Schwartz, Deborah Shapiro, Harry Spiera, Leonard Steinfeld, Mark Swartz, Maria Chanco-Turner, Steve Tyring, and Richard Warner.

Figs 1-1, 3-1A, 4-1, and 4-2 from the Rare Book Collection, New York Academy of Medicine, New York, with permission.

Figs 1-3, 5-21, 6-33, and 6-34 from the American College of Rheumatology, Atlanta, GA, with permission.

Figs 1-17, 1-27, 1-32, 1-39, 1-45, 3-25, 4-112, 6-24, 6-25, 9-34, and 11-99 from Lebwohl M (ed). *Difficult Diagnoses in Dermatology*. New York: Churchill Livingstone; 1988, with permission.

Fig. 1-24 from Lebwohl M. Cutaneous manifestations of internal malignancy. *J Fam Med* 1983; 8, with permission.

Figs 1-75B, 1-79, 8-20, 8-21, and 9-83 from the Bronx Veterans Administration Medical Center, Bronx, New York, with permission.

Figs 2-31, 2-35, 2-36, and 3-22 from Fleischmajer R. *The Dyslipidoses*. Springfield: Charles C Thomas; 1960, with permission.

Fig. 2-42 from Lebwohl M, Schwartz E, Jacobs L et al. Abnormalities of fibrillin in acquired cutis laxa. *J Am Acad Dermatol* 1994; 30:950, with permission.

Figs 3-10, 3-12, 3-16, and 3-21 from Fleischmajer R, Dowlati Y, Reeves JRT. Familial hyperlipidemias. *Arch Dermatol* 1974; 110:46, with permission.

Fig. 3-13 from Fleischmajer R, Tint S, Bennett HD. Normolipemic tendon and tuberous xanthomas. *J Am Acad Dermatol* 1981; 5:291, with permission.

Figs 3-43 and 3-46 from Fleischmajer R, Nedwick A. Progeria. *Arch Dermatol* 1973; 107:254, with permission.

Fig. 4-54 from Lebwohl M, Fleischmajer R, Janowitz H et al: Metastatic Crohn's disease. *J Am Acad Dermatol* 1984; 10:33, with permission.

Figs 4-67 and 4-68 from Mock WH, Weiss RS. Pellagra. *Arch Dermatol Syphilol* 1925; 12:653, with permission.

Figs 7-7A and 7-7B from Wood L, Cooper D, Ridgeway EC. *Your Thyroid*. Boston: Houghton Mifflin; 1982, with permission.

Fig. 8-1 from Riccardi VM, Mulvihill JJ, Wade WM (eds). Neurofibromatosis (von Recklinghausen Disease): Genetics, Cell Biology, and Biochemistry. *Advances in Neurology*. Vol. 29. New York: Raven Press; 1981, with permission.

Fig. 8-8 from Bruckner HW, Borbaty M, Lipsztein R et al. Treatment of a large high-grade neurofibrosarcoma with concomitant vinblastine, doxorubicin, and radiotherapy. *Mt Sinai J Med* 1992; 59:429, with permission.

Fig. 9-11 from Fitzpatrick T. *Color Atlas and Synopsis of Clinical Dermatology*. New York: McGraw-Hill; 1992, with permission.

Fig. 11-17 from Lebwohl M, Contard P. Interferon and condylomata acuminata. *Int J Dermatol* 1990; 29:699, with permission.

Figs 9-99 and 9-100 from the World Health Organization, with permission.

Fig. 9-101 from Tyring S (ed). *Mucocutaneous Manifestations of Viral Diseases*. New York: Marcel Dekker; 2002, with permission.

Acknowledgments

When the first edition of *Atlas of the Skin and Systemic Disease* was published in 1995, I acknowledged several outstanding books that served as references, including Braverman's *Skin Signs of Systemic Disease*, *Dermatologic Signs of Internal Disease* by Callen, Jorizzo et al., *Dermatology in General Medicine* by Fitzpatrick et al., and Moschella and Hurley's *Dermatology*. I also acknowledged pediatric atlases and texts including Prose and Weinberg's *Color Atlas of Pediatric Dermatology* and Schachner and Hansen's *Pediatric Dermatology*. Since that time, online access to medical journals has improved dramatically, and information can be obtained easily from original sources at a moment's notice. Nevertheless, I have borrowed significantly from *Difficult Diagnoses in Dermatology*, a textbook that I edited in 1988.

I had been asked to edit a second edition of *Difficult Diagnoses in Dermatology*, but instead I preferred to borrow the most useful tables for this new edition of *The Skin and Systemic Disease*. In particular, I am grateful to Michael Fisher and Susan Katz, who wrote a superb chapter on 'Fever and Rash' for *Difficult Diagnoses in Dermatology*. Table 9-1 is taken directly from their chapter, as are Tables 9-2, 9-3, and 9-4. I helped put together the latter three tables in the original chapter based on the superb material Drs Fisher and Katz provided.

I have to thank my teachers and colleagues without whom this book could not have been written. Dr Raul Fleischmajer, my predecessor as chairman of the Department of Dermatology at Mount Sinai, not only provided me with many of the photographs in the first edition of *Atlas of the Skin and Systemic Disease*, but has continued to teach me about connective tissue diseases. Many of the original photos, and some of the new ones, were provided by Dr James F. Holland, one of the world's leading oncologists and outstanding teachers. I have been fortunate to learn from him every time we see a patient together. Dr Robert G. Phelps continues to provide me with clinical and histologic slides and beautiful photomicrographs. I value the clinical excellence he brings to the care of my patients, his dedication to teaching and his friendship. The same must be said of Drs Steven R. Cohen, Marsha L. Gordon, Suhail Hadi, Irwin Kantor, Donald Rudikoff and James M. Spencer. All are outstanding clinicians, superb teachers and good friends without whom I could not have run the Dermatology Department at Mount Sinai, and all have contributed photographs to this book. Many of the photos in the first edition came from the collections of Fabio Barbosa, Vincent Cipollaro and the rare book section of the New York Academy of Medicine, and I have kept the best of those photos in this second edition.

I am especially grateful to my patients who willingly posed for the photographs in this book. I am also grateful to the residents, fellows and staff of the Dermatology Department at Mount Sinai who have provided many of the photographs used in the original *Atlas of the Skin and Systemic Disease* and in this second edition. I must thank Victoria White for her devoted work and many hours of typing and preparing each of the chapters. Special appreciation goes to Marion Rodriguez for typing, copying, answering e-mails, tracking down figures, orchestrating my schedule and doing all of the things necessary to make sure this book was successfully completed.

This second edition of *The Skin and Systemic Disease* would never have been written without friendly and persistent encouragement from Sue Hodgson, my publisher at Elsevier. Sue's persistence with remarkable good humor despite my having missed many deadlines should be recorded in *The Guinness Book of World Records* under the heading of *patience*. Finally, and most importantly, my wife, Madeleine, and my children, Andy and Eve, deserve my greatest thanks. They put up with my incessant writing and rewriting. They always help me maintain my spirit and teach me all the computer skills I know. Their constant support enabled me to write this book and much more.

Mark G. Lebwohl, M.D.

1 Rheumatologic diseases

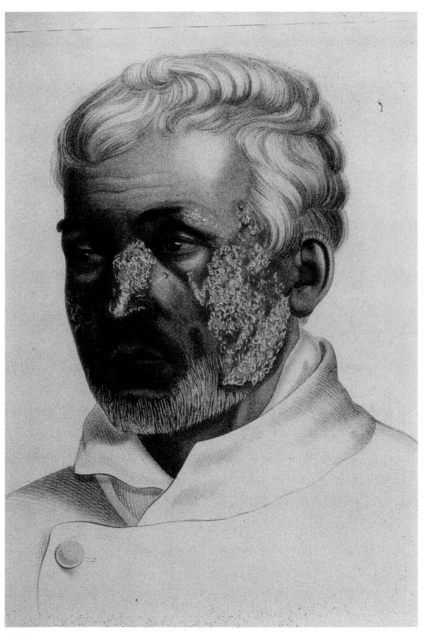

Figure 1-1

Lupus erythemateux by Pierre Louis Alphée Cazenave.
From Cazenave PLA. Lecons sur les Maladies de la Peau. Paris: Labé; 1856. With permission from the New York Academy of Medicine.

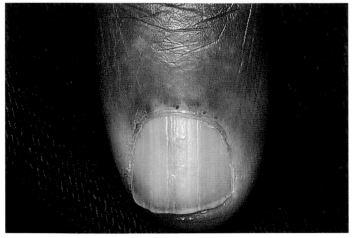

Figure 1-2

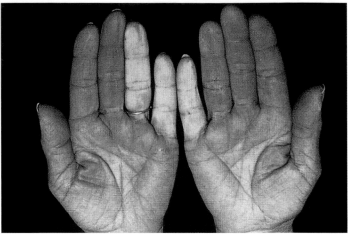

Figure 1-3

Cutaneous symptoms are so intimately associated with rheumatic diseases that they feature prominently in the criteria for the diagnosis of a number of disorders including lupus, scleroderma, and dermatomyositis.

Several skin lesions, such as **periungual telangiectasia**, are nonspecifically associated with rheumatic diseases, although they also occur with other conditions or in the absence of systemic disease. Cuticular telangiectasia is seen in lupus, dermatomyositis, scleroderma, and a small proportion of rheumatoid arthritis patients. On visual examination, telangiectasia can appear as pinpoint red macules or as

diffuse erythema. The patient in Figure 1-2 presented with joint pain and periungual telangiectasia months before developing the more specific features of systemic lupus erythematosus.

The **Raynaud phenomenon** is another condition commonly associated with rheumatic diseases. It is characterized by episodic vasospasm resulting in ischemia of the digits. The hands, feet, ear lobes, nose, forehead, knees, and elbows can be affected, and episodes are generally triggered by exposure to cold or emotional stress. The characteristic color changes of white, blue, and red represent initial pallor (Fig. 1-3) caused by arterial vasoconstriction, followed by cyanosis due

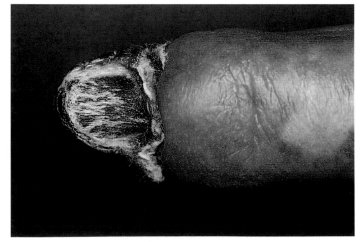

Figure 1-4

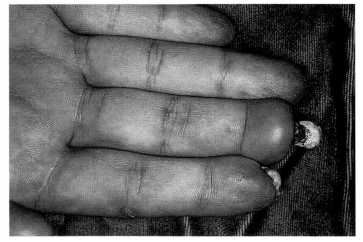

Figure 1-5

to stagnant blood flow and, finally, erythema resulting from reactive hyperemia. The color changes are associated with pain, tingling, burning, and occasionally swelling. In severe cases, necrosis of the digits can result (Fig. 1-4). Raynaud phenomenon is quite common, affecting up to 10% of otherwise healthy women. Women are affected almost eight times more than men.

Over 90% of cases of Raynaud phenomenon are not associated with an underlying cause. These patients have a more benign course and their condition is termed **Raynaud disease**. The Raynaud phenomenon, however, can occur in conjunction with a number of disorders, par-

ticularly connective tissue diseases (Table 1-1). Raynaud phenomenon develops so frequently in lupus that it once was a criterion for the diagnosis of that disorder, and it is a cardinal feature of scleroderma. Treatment with β-adrenergic blocking agents such as propranolol can exacerbate the condition. Other medications, including bleomycin, have also been associated with Raynaud phenomenon, as has exposure to polyvinyl chloride, and use of a pneumatic hammer. Figure 1-5 shows the hand of a hammer operator with severe Raynaud phenomenon that resulted in ischemia, necrosis, and loss of the distal tips of two digits.

Table 1-1. Secondary Causes of the Raynaud Phenomenon

Connective tissue diseases
 Scleroderma
 Systemic lupus erythematosus
 Rheumatoid arthritis
 Dermatomyositis
 Polymyositis
 Mixed connective tissue disease
 Sjögren syndrome
 Necrotizing agents
Occlusive arterial disease
 Arteriosclerosis obliterans
 Thromboangiitis obliterans
 Thromboembolism
Drug-induced
 Ergot alkaloids, methysergide
 β-adrenergic antagonists
 Clonidine
 Bleomycin
 Sulfasalazine
Neurologic disorders
 Cerebrovascular accident
 Poliomyelitis
 Carpal tunnel syndrome
 Intervertebral disc compression
 Thoracic outlet compression syndromes
 Syringomyelia
 Shoulder girdle compression syndromes
 Reflex sympathetic dystrophy
Blood dyscrasias
 Cryoglobulinemia
 Macroglobulinemia
 Cryofibrinogenemia
 Polycythemia vera
 Paroxysmal hemoglobinuria
 Cold hemolysis
Hepatitis B antigenemia
Neoplastic
 Multiple myeloma
 Occult carcinoma
 Pheochromocytoma
Occupational or environmental exposure
 Occupational acroosteolysis
 Pneumatic hammer disease (vibration)
 Sequelae of blunt trauma
 Sequelae of cold injury
 Vinyl-chloride manufacture
Miscellaneous
 Mitral valve prolapse
 Myxedema
 Primary pulmonary hypertension
 Fabry disease
 Heavy metals (lead, arsenic)

Reprinted from Halpern J. Raynaud's phenomenon. In: Lebwohl M, ed. Difficult diagnoses in dermatology. New York: Churchill Livingstone; 1988:47.

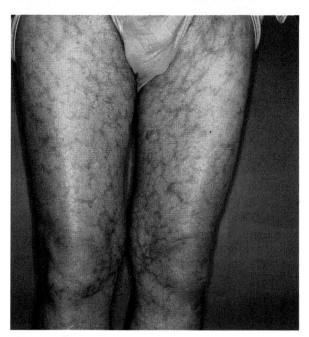

Figure 1-6

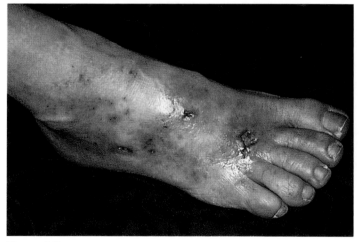

Figure 1-7

exposed to cold, but livedo reticularis occurs at any temperature. Patients with livedo reticularis should be investigated for SLE and periarteritis nodosa. The extensive livedo reticularis shown in Figure 1-6 occurred in a patient who developed a scleroderma-like syndrome following therapy with bleomycin. Rheumatoid arthritis, cryoglobulinemia, and other conditions have rarely been associated with livedo reticularis. In many patients, the association between livedo reticularis and an underlying disorder is not apparent at the time of presentation, but a disorder may develop ultimately in patients who are followed for long enough.

Livedoid vasculitis is also known as atrophie blanche (Fig. 1-7). It occurs in some women with persistent deep purple livedo reticularis. Painful recurrent ulcers develop over the lower leg and ankle, and the ulcers heal slowly with characteristic white sclerotic scars and overlying telangiectases. This condition is occasionally associated with lupus, and some patients have circulating anticardiolipin antibodies.

Livedo reticularis is a third cutaneous pattern associated with connective tissue diseases. It is characterized by reticulated erythema, which is purplish at times, and most commonly affects the lower extremities, although the upper extremities and trunk can be involved. The cutaneous mottling resembles cutis marmorata seen in infants

Table 1-2. Incidence of Antinuclear Antibodies in Connective Tissue Disease

Disease	Antinuclear Antibodies	Incidence
Systemic lupus erythematosus	ANA	95–99%
	dsDNA	50–55%
	Histones	80%
	RNP	35–45%
	Sm[a]	30–40%
	SS-A (Ro)	30–40%
	SS-B (La)	10–15%
	PCNA/cyclin	3–10%
Drug-induced disease	ANA[b]	95–100%
	Histones	95–100%
Mixed connective tissue disease	ANA[b]	100%
	RNP	95–100%
Scleroderma	ANA[b]	96%
	Scl-70[a]	30–70%
CREST syndrome	Centromere[a]	70–90%
Localized scleroderma	Scl-70	44%
	ANA	46%
	Antisense DNA	50%
Sjögren syndrome	ANA[b]	55%
	SS-A (Ro)	60–70%
	SS-B (La)	40–60%
Polymyositis	ANA[b]	86%
	Jo-1[a]	25–37%
Polymyositis/scleroderma overlap	PM-Scl	60–80%
	Ku	10–38%
Dermatomyositis	ANA[b]	40–80%
	PM-Scl	8%
	Mi-2[a]	0–5%
Rheumatoid arthritis	ANA[b]	20–50%
	Histones	15–20%
	RANA	90–95%

[a] Disease specific marker
[b] Connective tissue screen

Antinuclear antibodies are found in nearly all patients with lupus, but are not specific for this disease. Table 1-2 shows the incidence of different antinuclear antibodies in various connective tissue diseases.

Systemic lupus erythematosus (SLE) is an autoimmune disorder associated with a wide array of manifestations, many of which involve the skin. Diagnosis depends on a combination of clinical and laboratory criteria. Eleven criteria have been proposed (Table 1-4), and a diagnosis of SLE is established by determining that four of the criteria are present. Not surprisingly, cutaneous findings figure prominently in the diagnostic criteria.

Malar erythema, the so-called butterfly rash (Figs 1-8 and 1-9), is often abrupt in onset and frequently accompanies flares of active systemic SLE. Nonscarring erythema and edema can last hours or days, occasionally longer. Malar areas are most typically affected, but diffuse facial involvement can occur. Erythema of sun-exposed and sun-protected areas of the trunk and extremities also occurs, often with exacerbation of systemic symptoms. Treatment of the systemic disease will result in the resolution of cutaneous symptoms. Postinflammatory hyperpigmentation frequently remains in dark-skinned individuals.

Discoid lupus erythematosus (DLE) is most commonly seen in patients with a form of lupus that has been termed chronic cutaneous lupus erythematosus. Unlike malar erythema, which is associated with acute lupus erythematosus, patients with DLE usually have a more benign course, without the internal organ involvement of SLE. Lesions are typically erythematous papules, patches, or plaques with characteristic follicular plugging (i.e. dilated hair follicles filled with hyperkeratotic plugs, as shown in the ear in Fig. 1-10. The patches and plaques are often round with a border of hyperpigmentation that can expand. Individual lesions can become crusted, and heal with scarring and central depigmentation (Fig. 1-11). DLE generally affects the face, scalp, and ears. The term "generalized" DLE is used for patients who have cutaneous involvement of the trunk and extremities, as well as involvement above the neck. It has been suggested that patients with generalized DLE may be more prone to develop symptoms of SLE.

Approximately 25% of patients with SLE have discoid skin lesions, but only a small percentage of patients who only have discoid skin lesions will go on to develop SLE. Nevertheless, patients with long-standing chronic cutaneous lupus erythematosus rarely develop systemic disease.

Table 1-3. Immunofluorescent Antinuclear Antibodies Staining Patterns on HEp-2 Cell Substrate

Pattern	Associated Specificity	Disease
Homogeneous	dsDNA, histone	SLE, drug-induced SLE, nonspecific connective tissue disease
Peripheral	dsDNA, lamin	SLE
Speckled	Sm, RNP, SS-A(Ro), SS-B(La)	Scleroderma
Centromere	Centromere	CREST
Cytoplasmic	Various	Polymyositis/dermatomyositis

Antinuclear antibodies can be detected on cultured mitotic human epitheliod cells (HEp-2) or other tissues by indirect immunofluorescence. The pattern of fluorescence may aid in identifying the disease (Table 1-3).

Table 1-4. Modified Criteria for the Diagnosis of Systemic Lupus Erythematosus (four criteria are required to establish the diagnosis) using the ANTINUCLEAR Acronym

Antinuclear antibody
Neurologic disorder—seizures or psychosis
Thrombocytopenia or lymphopenia or leukopenia or hemolytic anemia
Immunologic disorder—positive lupus erythematosus cell preparation, or anti-double-stranded DNA, or anti-sm antibodies, or false-positive test for syphilis
Nasopharyngeal or oral ulcers
Urinary abnormalities—proteinuria or casts
Cutaneous discoid rash
Light sensitivity
Effusions—pleuritis or pericarditis
Arthritis of two or more joints
Rash in malar area

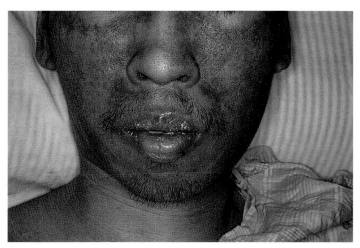

Figure 1-8

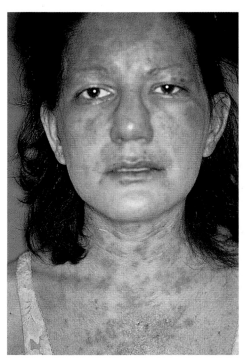

Figure 1-9

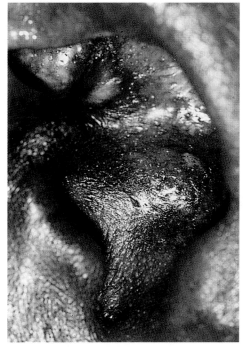

Figure 1-10

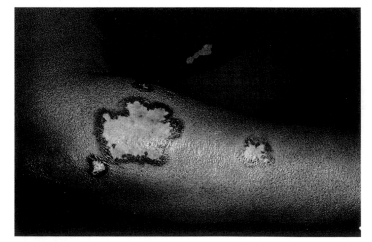

Figure 1-11

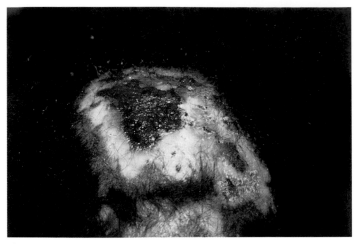

Figure 1-12

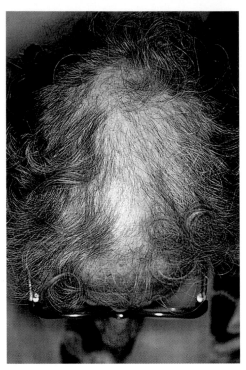

Figure 1-13

A **scarring alopecia** can occur as a result of DLE (Fig. 1-12). This is distinct from the nonscarring **telogen effluvium** that is seen in SLE (Fig. 1-13). The latter type of hair loss is caused by an abnormality of the hair cycle that is generalized and reversible. Patients complain that they are losing large quantities of white-tipped hairs, so-called telogen hairs.

Diagnosis of DLE can be made with skin biopsy and routine light microscopy. Often the clinical appearance is sufficiently characteristic

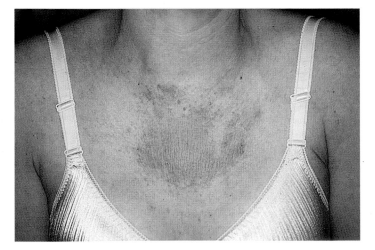

Figure 1-14

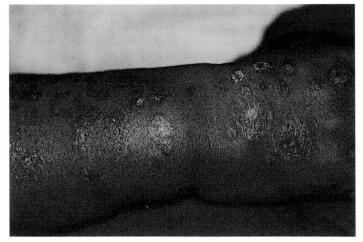

Figure 1-15

that biopsy is not essential, especially when DLE occurs in people with SLE.

Photosensitivity, a third cutaneous criterion for the diagnosis of SLE, has been shown to occur as a result of exposure to ultraviolet light. Patients must therefore be counseled on the use of broad-spectrum sunscreens as well as avoidance of sun exposure. The face, the "V" of the neck and chest (Fig. 1-14), and sun-exposed areas of the arms and legs are characteristically affected. Psoriasiform, erythematous, polycyclic, and discoid lesions have been described.

A subset of lupus known as **subacute cutaneous lupus erythematosus** (SCLE) is characterized by prominent photosensitivity, rash, arthritis, fever, pleuritis, and Raynaud phenomenon. Erythematous scaling papules and patches that have been described as "psoriasiform" or annular are characteristic (Fig. 1-15). Patients with this condition have a more benign prognosis, and the incidence of renal and central nervous system involvement is low. This form of lupus erythematosus can be distinguished serologically because patients have a high incidence of antibodies to SSA (Ro). Antinuclear antibodies

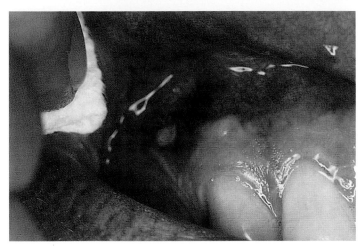

Figure 1-16

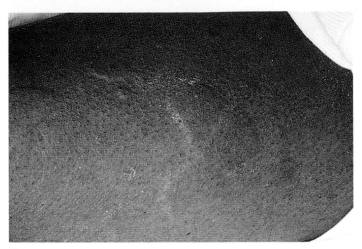

Figure 1-17

(ANAs) can be negative in patients with subacute lupus erythematosus, especially if the ANA assay uses a rodent kidney or liver substrate. Antibodies to double-stranded DNA are only positive in 15–20% of patients with this form of lupus.

Oral ulcers (Fig. 1-16) constitute a fourth cutaneous criterion for the diagnosis of SLE. These oral or nasopharyngeal ulcerations are typically painless, but in addition to ulcerations various mucous membrane lesions have been described, including petechiae, purpura, and erosions. These lesions, which often show the histopathology of lupus

erythematosus, can involve the buccal mucosa, the hard and soft palates, gingiva, tongue, vaginal mucosa, nasal mucosa, and probably any mucous membrane.

A number of nonspecific cutaneous manifestations can also occur with SLE. Urticarial wheals, which on biopsy show the histopathology of a **leukocytoclastic vasculitis,** are frequently reported (Fig. 1-17). Symmetric palpable purpura of the lower extremities can also be seen in patients with a lupus-associated vasculitis. Ischemic infarcts and frank gangrene can occur.

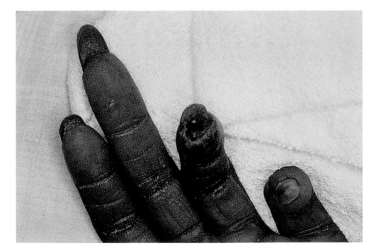

Figure 1-18

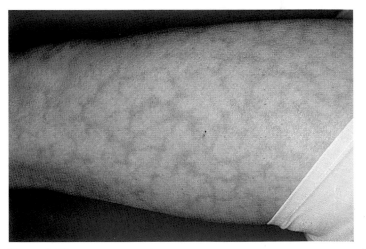

Figure 1-19

Raynaud phenomenon used to be one of the diagnostic criteria for SLE, but because it is not specific for this disorder it is no longer used. Nevertheless, it is a common occurrence in people with SLE, affecting approximately 30% of them, but rarely results in gangrene of the digits. The patient in Figure 1-18 developed Raynaud phenomenon, and the vasospasm sufficiently compromised circulation to the digits so the tip of one of her fingers became gangrenous. Interestingly, Raynaud phenomenon may precede other symptoms of lupus by months or years.

Recurrent thrombophlebitis affects some lupus patients, particularly those with a circulating anticoagulant and false-positive serologic tests for syphilis. Both superficial vessels and deep vessels may be affected. There are recurrent arterial and venous thromboses of the heart, kidneys, brain, and other organs. Repeated miscarriages are common in affected women. Many of these individuals have been found to have anticardiolipin antibodies. Extensive **livedo reticularis** (Fig. 1-19) involving the arms, legs, and trunk is common in people with the **anti-cardiolipin antibody syndrome.**

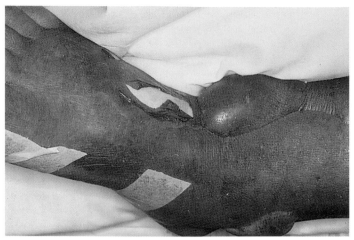

Figure 1-20

Figure 1-21

Several types of bullous lesion have been reported in patients with SLE. Occasionally they arise from urticarial bases or they resemble erythema multiforme. The level of separation is usually subepidermal and direct immunofluorescence reveals immune deposits at the dermal–epidermal junction. Patients with **bullous lupus erythematosus** can become acutely ill. The extent of bullous lesions may parallel the severity of systemic symptoms. The patient in Figure 1-20 developed extensive bullae in association with fever, arthritis, pleuritis, and other symptoms of SLE.

The **lupus band test** involves direct immunofluorescence of skin biopsies taken from patients suspected of having SLE. This test is most specific if the biopsy specimen is taken from uninvolved, sun-protected sites such as the buttocks or the volar aspect of the forearm. In a positive test, immunoglobulins (such as IgG and IgM) and complement are found in a continuous granular band along the dermal–epidermal junction (Fig. 1-21). Over 80% of patients with systemic and renal involvement have a positive lupus band test as compared to only 20% of patients without renal involvement. When lesional skin is tested, IgG, IgM, and complement are found in over 90% of specimens.

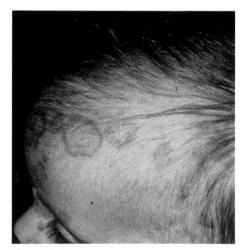

Figure 1-22

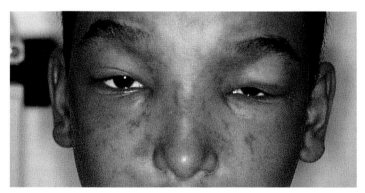

Figure 1-23

Neonatal lupus has been attributed to passage of anti-Ro IgG antibodies (sometimes anti-La IgG antibodies) across the placenta. Some of the infants' mothers have lupus erythematosus or Sjögren syndrome, and others are asymptomatic but can subsequently develop symptoms of connective tissue disease. Infants develop annular erythematous macules and papules, often on the face (Fig. 1-22). The lesions are present at birth or develop shortly thereafter. Congenital heart block due to fibrosis of the cardiac conduction system can occur with or without skin involvement. The condition resolves in a few months, but cardiac conduction defects are occasionally irreversible and may require placement of a permanent pacemaker.

Dermatomyositis is an inflammatory process of striated muscle and skin that results in muscle weakness, particularly involving proximal muscles. In approximately 50% of cases, muscle involvement occurs in the absence of skin lesions, and the condition is then called polymyositis. Patients complain of difficulty with brushing their hair and an inability to climb stairs or to rise from low seats. Muscle tenderness occasionally occurs. Serum muscle enzymes, including creatinine phosphokinase and aldolase, are elevated, and myoglobin is found in the urine when extensive muscle damage has occurred. Electromyograms can support a diagnosis of dermatomyositis, but the results will be normal for around 20% of those affected. Even muscle biopsy can yield false-negative results in approximately a quarter of patients. For greater sensitivity, weak or tender proximal muscles should be selected for biopsy.

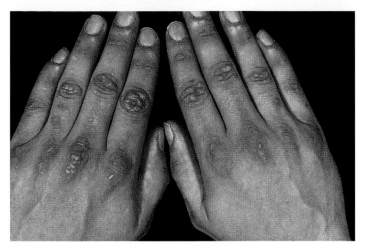

Figure 1-24

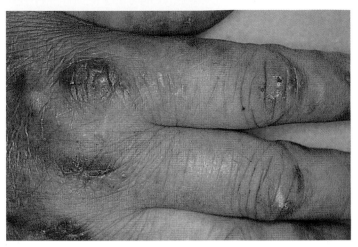

Figure 1-25

In a third of patients, cutaneous symptoms precede muscle involvement. One of the most characteristic findings is periorbital erythema and edema called **heliotrope** (Fig. 1-23). This is often associated with a butterfly rash that simulates lupus. **Gottron papules** constitute a second characteristic sign of dermatomyositis (Fig. 1-24). These consist of erythematous macules and papules on the knuckles (Fig. 1-25), and although they are said to be pathognomonic of dermatomyositis, they can occasionally be seen in other connective tissue diseases including lupus.

Dermatomyositis has long been considered a sign of underlying malignancy. This association stems, in part, from a few well-documented cases in which dermatomyositis disappeared upon treatment of a tumor, and subsequently reappeared when the tumor recurred. Malignancies in adults with dermatomyositis occur in somewhere between 15 and 50% of cases reported. Most of the associated tumors are detectable by history, physical examination, and routine laboratory tests, including chest x-ray, urinalysis, and stool examination for occult blood. Blind, expensive searches for malignancy are seldom fruitful.

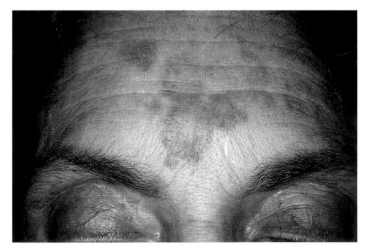

Figure 1-26

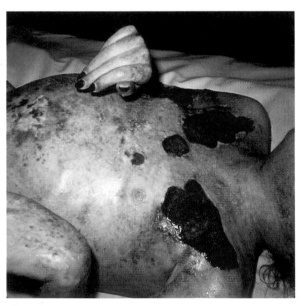

Figure 1-27

Patients with **dermatomyositis** will occasionally develop erythema with scaling, telangiectasia, and atrophy, primarily involving the face (Fig. 1-26) and the "V" of the neck and chest. The rash can be exacerbated by sun exposure. Extensor surfaces of the extremities, including the elbows and knees, are also involved, as can be the torso. Other cutaneous signs of dermatomyositis include Raynaud phenomenon, periungual telangiectasia, erythema, and—rarely—sclerodactyly (i.e. induration of the skin of the digits).

Childhood dermatomyositis is similar to that of adults, and has a number of important features. Calcification of skin or muscle, or both, occurs in approximately two-thirds of cases of juvenile dermatomyositis. Calcinosis may become extensive, and there is no effective treatment. A vasculitic form of juvenile dermatomyositis can involve the gastrointestinal tract and result in abdominal pain, hematemesis, melena, gastrointestinal ulceration, perforation, or death. Cutaneous vasculitis can result in nodules and infarcts with extensive ulcerations (Fig. 1-27). Mortality is very high in the vasculitic form of juvenile dermatomyositis, but the prognosis is good in children without vasculitis.

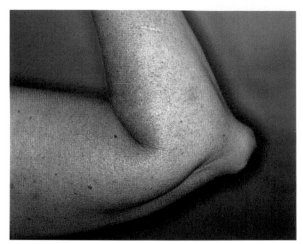

Figure 1-28

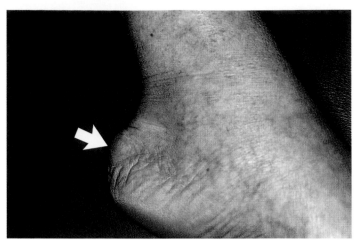

Figure 1-29

Cutaneous lesions are common in **rheumatoid arthritis**. Diagnosis of this disabling disease is established by a combination of criteria that include morning stiffness, joint tenderness or pain on motion, joint swelling, subcutaneous nodules, radiographic changes typical of rheumatoid arthritis, positive rheumatoid factor, and characteristic synovial fluid and pathology. **Rheumatoid nodules** are present in 20–25% of patients and have been associated with seropositivity (of rheumatoid factor) and more severe arthritis. Periarticular sites and areas subjected to mechanical pressure are the most commonly involved, especially the areas around the elbows (Fig. 1-28).

The extensor surfaces of the forearms, the Achilles tendon (Fig. 1-29), metacarpophalangeal and interphalangeal joints, ischial tuberosity, and sacrum can also develop rheumatoid nodules. The nodules are firm and range in size from 5 mm to several centimeters in diameter. They are usually asymptomatic but can occasionally become infected or break down. Rheumatoid nodules are misdiagnosed as gouty tophi, xanthomata, epidermoid cysts, or enlarged lymph nodes.

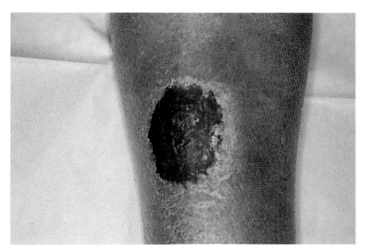

Figure 1-30

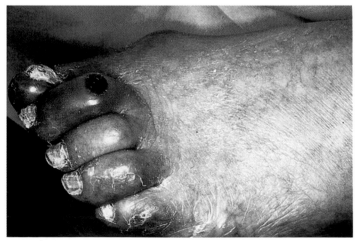

Figure 1-31

Rheumatoid vasculitis, caused by necrotizing arteritis of small and medium-sized arteries, may be indistinguishable from polyarteritis nodosa. Onset can be abrupt, resulting in skin necrosis and ulceration (Fig. 1-30), digital infarcts and gangrene, sensorimotor neuropathy, and visceral infarction. Coronary arteritis and cerebral vasculitis can also occur. Fever and polymorphonuclear leukocytosis often develop in affected patients. Fulminant forms of rheumatoid vasculitis are usually associated with high titers of rheumatoid factor and severe arthritis.

Fortunately, however, fulminant forms of rheumatoid vasculitis are rare. Smaller vessel involvement can occur more insidiously, resulting in palpable purpura, hemorrhagic bullae, urticaria, and vasculitic ulcers. The ulcers are sharply demarcated, deep, painful, and heal slowly. They are often associated with the Felty syndrome, which is characterized by chronic rheumatoid arthritis associated with splenomegaly and neutropenia. More commonly, ulcerations are caused by pressure over extensor surfaces of affected joints (Fig. 1-31).

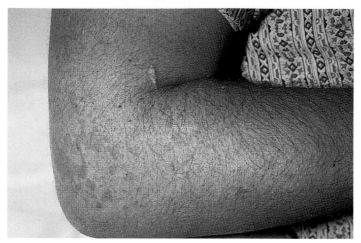

Figure 1-32

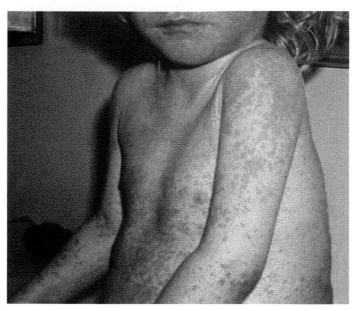

Figure 1-33

Juvenile rheumatoid arthritis (Still disease) is a disease of children under the age of 16 years. Several distinct forms of the disease occur, including polyarthritis that follows a syndrome consisting of high fevers, myalgias, pericarditis, pleuritis, peritonitis, hepatosplenomegaly, and lymphadenopathy. Approximately 30–50% of patients develop an evanescent rash that occurs with fever during the late afternoon or early evening. The eruption is not pruritic and consists of salmon-colored macules and papules on the trunk, face, and extremities. The papules are occasionally described as urticarial, but more commonly they are quite faint, as shown in the patients in Figures 1-32 and 1-33.

Subcutaneous nodules similar to rheumatoid nodules have been described. The course of the condition is variable with the rash lasting anywhere from days to years. The arthritis may resolve spontaneously or may result in progressive deformity of the joints. A distinct polyarticular form without systemic symptoms and a pauciarticular form exist, but these do not have prominent skin manifestations.

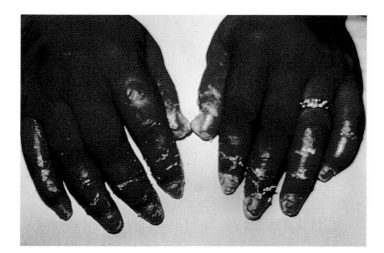

Figure 1-34

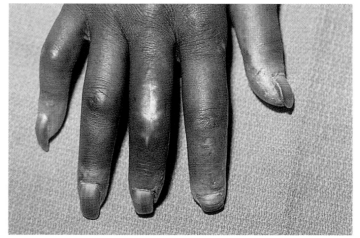

Figure 1-35

Scleroderma, also known as progressive systemic sclerosis, is a connective tissue disease characterized by cutaneous induration and thickening. Systemic scleroderma can be classified as two distinct entities, namely the **CREST syndrome** and **diffuse scleroderma**. The CREST syndrome (*c*alcinosis, *R*aynaud phenomenon, *e*sophageal dysmotility, *s*clerodactyly, and *t*elangiectasia) is more slowly progressive and therefore carries a more benign prognosis. It is distinguished by the presence of anticentromere antibodies. Although cases of scleroderma

without skin involvement (scleroderma sine scleroderma) have been described, cutaneous symptoms are so common that a subcommittee of the American Rheumatism Association found that only one symptom—proximal scleroderma—is needed for diagnosis of systemic sclerosis. Skin involvement often begins with an inflammatory stage consisting of erythema and edema of the hands (Fig. 1-34). This progresses to severe induration of the skin of the digits (**sclerodactyly**) (Fig. 1-35).

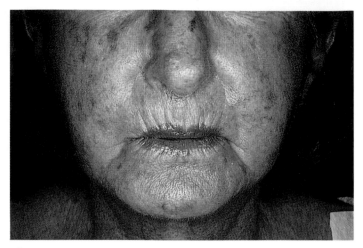

Figure 1-36

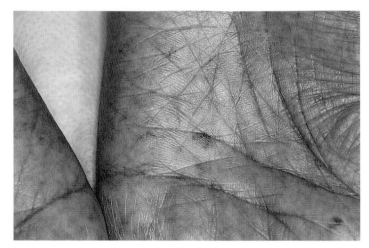

Figure 1-37

Involvement of the face and trunk can occur as well. Patients often present with typical facies, characterized by pursed lips and bound-down skin at the nose, creating a beak-like appearance (Fig. 1-36). **Telangiectases** are also commonly seen, particularly in the CREST syndrome. The face and trunk are often affected, but telangiectases can also be seen on the mucosal surfaces of the oropharynx and gastro-intestinal tract. Gastrointestinal bleeding is nevertheless an uncommon occurrence. Telangiectasia are evident on the face of the patient in Figure 1-36 and on the palm of the patient in Figure 1-37.

Numerous systemic manifestations occur, the most common being esophageal involvement. Dysphagia due to diminished esophageal peristalsis is detected most accurately by esophageal manometry. A barium swallow with fluoroscopic examination may not be sufficiently sensitive, but a cine-esophagram may reveal esophageal hypomotility. An incompetent lower esophageal sphincter results in reflux esophagitis and heartburn. Continued gastric fluid reflux ultimately may cause stricture of the esophagus. Intestinal hypomotility may underlie complaints of constipation, diarrhea, and bowel distention. Over-growth of bacteria results in malabsorption and steatorrhea, both of which are easily treated with tetracycline.

Pulmonary involvement in **scleroderma** is manifested by dyspnea and is caused by localized or diffuse interstitial fibrosis. Chest x-rays

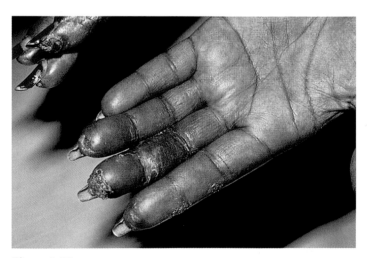

Figure 1-38

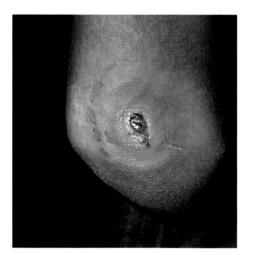

Figure 1-39A

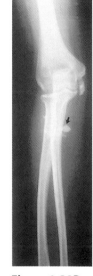

Figure 1-39B

reveal variable changes frequently affecting the lower third of both lungs. Small airway disease and reduced carbon monoxide diffusing capacity occur. Pulmonary arterial hypertension can develop, par-ticularly in the CREST syndrome (50% of patients) and diffuse scleroderma (33%), and right-sided heart failure eventually ensues. Myocardial fibrosis results in cardiac conduction defects on electro-cardiogram, or in cardiac arrhythmias. Pericarditis with pericardial effusion has also been reported. The abrupt onset of renal failure is

common in diffuse scleroderma and is often associated with malignant hypertension.

Raynaud phenomenon occurs in 95% of patients and may be so severe that ischemia and loss of digits can occur (Fig. 1-38). **Calcinosis cutis** occurs in 10% of patients and can result in ulceration (Fig. 1-39A) or serve as a focus for infection. Cutaneous deposition of calcium is seen radiographically (Fig. 1-39B) and often occurs over the extensor surfaces of the elbows. Other radiographic findings include flexion contraction

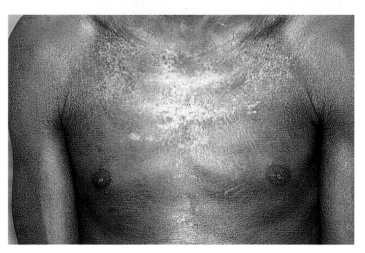

Figure 1-40

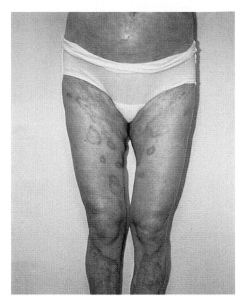

Figure 1-41

of affected joints and digital tuft resorption. Another cutaneous feature is the presence of hypo- and hyperpigmentation in areas of indurated skin (Fig. 1-40).

Sjögren syndrome, also known as the sicca syndrome, is commonly associated with scleroderma and is characterized by dry eyes, dry mouth, and parotid gland enlargement. The Schirmer test shows a reduction in tear production; lip biopsy reveals lymphocytic infiltration of the salivary glands; and there is a high incidence of circulating antibodies to SSA (Ro) and SSB (La). Sjögren syndrome can also be seen in association with other autoimmune diseases including lupus and rheumatoid arthritis.

Localized forms of scleroderma known as **morphea** are not associated with systemic symptoms and are characterized by localized plaques of indurated skin often surrounded by a violaceous halo (Fig. 1-41). A generalized form of morphea can occur but it can be distinguished from systemic scleroderma by the absence of Raynaud phenomenon, sclerodactyly, and internal organ involvement.

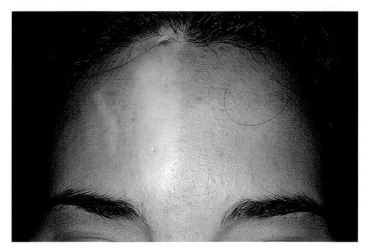

Figure 1-42

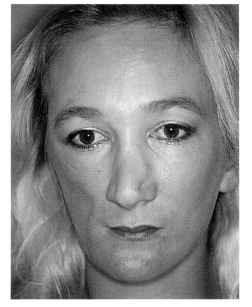

Figure 1-43

Occasionally a linear form of localized scleroderma, termed linear morphea, occurs. Distinctive deformities can result, including a vertical scar-like lesion which has been called **coup de sabre** (Fig. 1-42), and facial hemiatrophy—the so-called **Parry–Romberg syndrome** (Fig. 1-43). The Parry–Romberg syndrome has also been associated with

other autoimmune diseases, and ANAs are often present. Infection with *Borrelia burgdorferi*, the organism that causes Lyme disease, has been associated with some cases of Parry–Romberg syndrome. It has also been suggested that *Borrelia* infection causes some forms of scleroderma, but evidence of this infection is lacking in most patients.

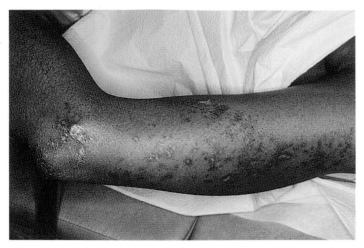

Figure 1-44

Mixed connective tissue disease is a controversial entity that combines features of scleroderma, lupus, and dermatomyositis. Raynaud phenomenon, arthralgias, persistent digital swelling resulting in "sausage fingers", and sclerodactyly are typical features. Esophageal hypomotility, proximal myositis, and pulmonary disease can occur. Malar erythema, lesions similar to those seen in subacute cutaneous lupus, and lesions resembling discoid lupus are occasionally seen in mixed connective tissue disease (Fig. 1-44). This has led some to hypothesize that this disorder is merely a form of SLE, but the presence of high titer antinuclear ribonucleoprotein antibodies serves as a distinguishing marker for mixed connective tissue disease.

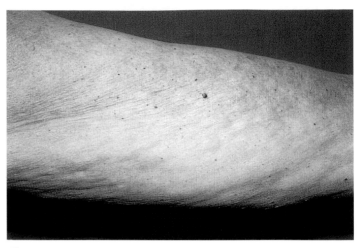

Figure 1-45

Eosinophilic fasciitis is a syndrome with scleroderma-like induration of the skin and marked eosinophilia. Extreme physical exertion or trauma often precedes the condition, which usually begins with painful swelling of the extremities. The skin has a characteristic "puckered" appearance (Fig. 1-45). Although the cutaneous induration of eosinophilic fasciitis can become generalized, it is easily distinguished from systemic scleroderma by the absence of Raynaud phenomenon. ANAs are usually negative in contrast to scleroderma. Several patients with eosinophilic fasciitis have developed hematologic abnormalities, including aplastic anemia, thrombocytopenia, myeloproliferative disorders, Hodgkin disease, and leukemia.

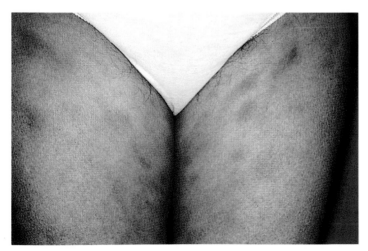

Figure 1-46

Individuals ingesting oral L-tryptophan have developed a condition called the **eosinophilia–myalgia syndrome**. This condition is characterized by severe muscle pain, muscle weakness, oral ulcers, fever, abdominal pain, dyspnea, eosinophilia, and cutaneous erythema or swelling that is painful in some patients. The eruption eventuates in cutaneous induration identical to that seen in eosinophilic fasciitis. The indurated plaques occasionally appear hyperpigmented (Fig. 1-46). A review of some patients diagnosed as having eosinophilic fasciitis

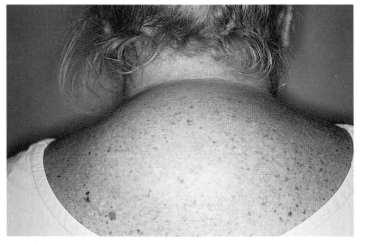

Figure 1-47

revealed that many had been taking oral L-tryptophan, suggesting that the two conditions have many common features and are frequently mistaken for one another.

Scleredema is a scleroderma-like condition that follows a viral or bacterial infection in some patients and is associated with diabetes mellitus in others. Cutaneous induration is symmetrical and usually occurs on the back of the neck and the adjacent upper back (Fig. 1-47). Occasionally it can spread to the face, trunk, and extremities, but the

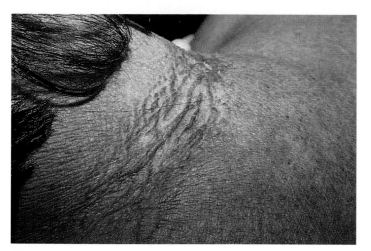

Figure 1-48

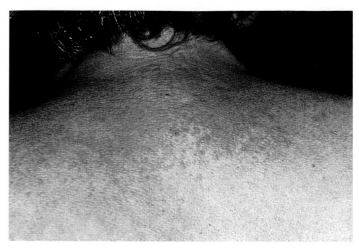

Figure 1-49

hands and feet are usually spared. Raynaud phenomenon does not occur. Affected areas of skin are bound down to underlying structures, and it is often difficult to pinch the skin. Affected areas can feel as hard as stone, and skin markings are lost. Accentuation of skinfolds occasionally occurs where the posterior neck meets the back (Fig. 1-48). In patients in whom scleredema follows infection, the condition is usually benign and self-limiting, resolving spontaneously after 6 months to 2 years. The form of scleredema associated with diabetes usually occurs in obese patients with severe diabetes and a high incidence of cardio-

vascular disease. Scleredema has also been associated with a benign monoclonal gammopathy of the IgG type. It has not been associated with multiple myeloma.

Scleromyxedema, also called lichen myxedematosus, is a rare disease associated with cutaneous sclerosis. Skin changes have been described as fibrous, sclerotic, or wood-like. The skin is diffusely infiltrated and covered with papules or nodules. Involvement of the upper back can simulate scleredema (Fig. 1-49). Histologically, there is increased deposition of mucopolysaccharides in the skin.

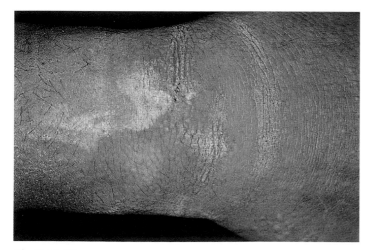

Figure 1-50

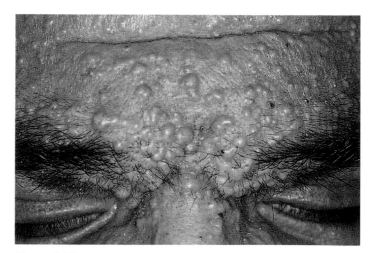

Figure 1-51

Patients with **scleromyxedema** develop skin-colored or red, dome-shaped papules up to 4 mm in diameter over indurated plaques on the face, trunk, or extremities. The papules coalesce from confluent plaques

on the hands, axillary folds, and extensor surfaces of the legs and arms (Fig. 1-50). Coalescence of papules and nodules, particularly on the face, can give rise to a leonine appearance (Fig. 1-51), and marked infiltration

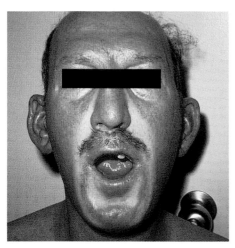

Figure 1-52

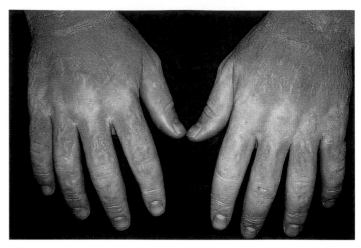

Figure 1-53

of the skin can cause blanching with facial movements (Fig. 1-52). Diffuse infiltration of the skin can result in sclerotic changes that may impede hand movements (Fig. 1-53) or mobility of the extremities. While mucosal lesions do not occur, involvement of the gastrointestinal tract can develop with infiltration of the stomach, intestines, or esophagus. Dysphagia is the most common manifestation of esophageal involvement. Restrictive or obstructive pulmonary disease can occur with involvement of the lungs, and inflammatory myopathy results in proximal muscle weakness. Other manifestations include peripheral neuropathy and carpal tunnel syndrome. A benign monoclonal gammopathy occurs, usually of the IgG lambda type, and there have been instances of multiple myeloma developing in patients with scleromyxedema.

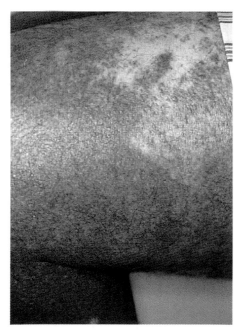

Figure 1-54

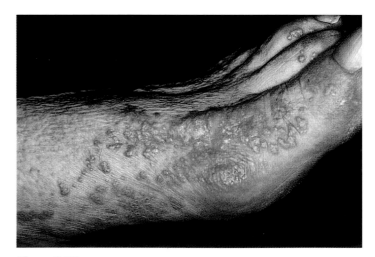

Figure 1-55

Graft-versus-host disease (GvH) is a condition that usually develops following bone marrow transplantation but has rarely occurred from transfusion of blood or blood products. It is not surprising that this condition has features in common with autoimmune disorders, since donor cells mount an immunologic attack against immunocompromised patients who receive the cells. Both acute and chronic forms of graft-versus-host disease exist, and each has distinctive manifestations. **Acute GvH disease** develops approximately 10–40 days after transplantation. It is characterized by a pruritic macular and papular rash (Fig. 1-54) that often begins on the neck, face, upper trunk, hands, and feet and can be associated with tenderness of the palms and soles. This eruption can be indistinguishable from a drug reaction or viral rash.

Fever, hepatomegaly, and lymphadenopathy are often associated. Gastrointestinal symptoms such as abdominal pain, nausea, and diarrhea frequently develop. Hepatitis with elevation of transaminases, alkaline phosphatase, and bilirubin can occur, as can eosinophilia. Occasionally patients with acute graft-versus-host disease develop extensive areas of bulla formation that clinically and histologically resemble toxic epidermal necrolysis.

Three months following transplantation, patients may develop **chronic GvH disease**, which may or may not have been preceded by the acute form of the disease. At the onset of chronic GvH disease, patients may develop **lichen planus-like** papules (Fig. 1-55) that are violaceous and often involve the distal extremities, including the palms and soles.

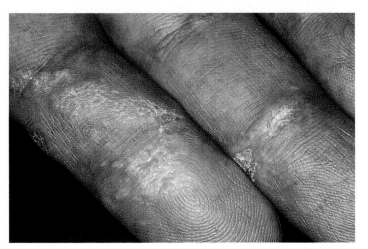

Figure 1-56

A white reticulate pattern similar to that seen on the buccal mucosa of patients with lichen planus can also develop. In some cases, chronic graft-versus-host disease of the hands mimics warts (Fig. 1-56).

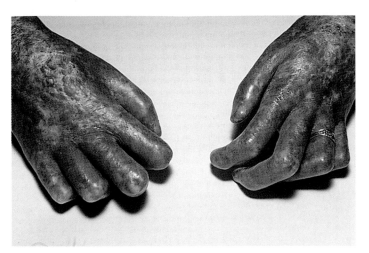

Figure 1-57

With or without lichen planus-like changes, some patients later develop striking **sclerodermatous skin changes** that prominently affect the joints and result in severe flexion contractures of the hands, feet, and knees (Fig. 1-57). The upper trunk is commonly involved.

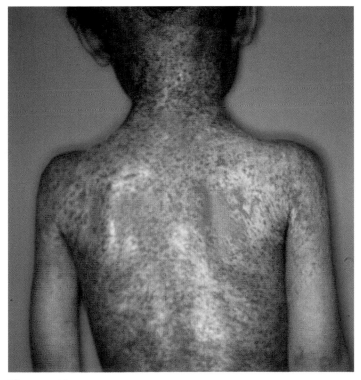

Figure 1-58

Scleroderma-like changes are often accompanied by telangiectases and reticulated hyperpigmentation (Fig. 1-58). Diffuse hair loss and diminished sweating also occur. Chronic diarrhea, lymphadenopathy, arthralgias, pleural and pericardial effusions, and hepatitis can develop. Hepatic transaminases are elevated early in chronic GvH disease, but the

Table 1-5. Causes of Vasculitis using the Mount Sinai Hospital Center (MSHC) Acronym	
Medication	**M**alignancies
Serum sickness	**S**treptococcus, and other infections
Henoch–Schönlein purpura	**H**epatitis C
Connective tissue disease	**C**ryoglobulinemia

alkaline phosphatase becomes elevated later. Sjögren syndrome often occurs and ANAs are common, further indicating the autoimmune nature of this condition.

Leukocytoclastic vasculitis, also known as hypersensitivity angiitis or allergic vasculitis, has characteristic clinical and histologic features despite its diverse etiologies. The first letters of Mount Sinai Hospital Center (MSHC) are helpful in remembering the various causes of vasculitis (Table 1-5).

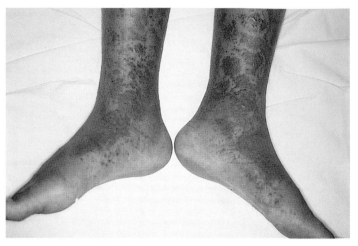

Figure 1-59

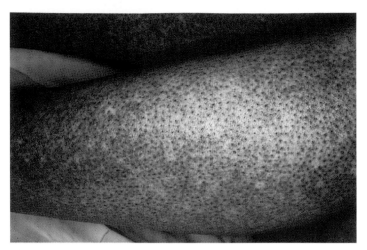

Figure 1-60

Leukocytoclastic vasculitis develops 1–3 weeks following exposure to an infection or medication. Patients develop antibodies that form immune complexes, and these complexes are deposited in the walls of postcapillary venules, initiating the sequence of events that leads to the clinical features of vasculitis. The most characteristic clinical presentation is symmetrical palpable purpura of the lower extremities (Fig. 1-59). Petechiae and nonpalpable purpuric patches can occur as well (Fig. 1-60), and occasionally the arms and torso are involved. Hemorrhagic blisters and ulcers can develop in severely affected

patients. Extensive infiltration by neutrophils can also lead to the development of pustules, which happened to the patient shown in Figure 1-61.

Frequently, systemic symptoms are minor or absent in patients with a cutaneous vasculitis. When present, systemic manifestations can include fever, arthralgias and arthritis; proteinuria and hematuria with renal involvement; abdominal pain or melena with gastrointestinal involvement; and peripheral neuropathy. The course of an episode of vasculitis is variable. Lesions arise in crops that last 1–4 weeks and

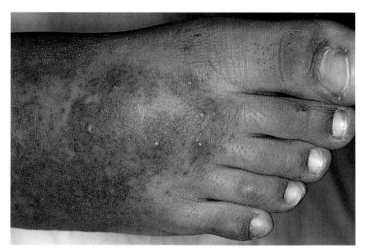

Figure 1-61

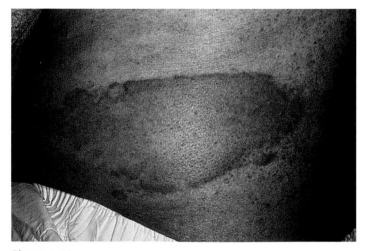

Figure 1-62

usually resolve completely, even when untreated. A single episode usually lasts a few weeks. Depending on the underlying etiology, episodes of vasculitis may or may not recur.

Diagnosis is often easily made on clinical grounds but, when in doubt, skin biopsy can be useful in confirming the diagnosis. If necessary, skin biopsy should be performed on lesions that are 18–36 hours old, because the typical neutrophilic infiltrate may otherwise not be found. Biopsy for immunofluorescence is optimally performed on lesions less than 6 hours old since most immunoreactants are rapidly removed, and very few are present beyond 24 hours. Immunofluorescent examination of biopsy specimens is seldom needed, however.

Hypocomplementemic vasculitis, also called urticarial vasculitis, presents with urticarial plaques (Fig. 1-62) that persist for more than 24 hours and are thus easily distinguishable from allergic urticaria. In addition, patients often complain of burning, rather than the itching associated with allergic urticaria. Fever, nephritis, and other systemic manifestations of vasculitis can occur. Serum sickness is a form of vasculitis that was originally described after injection of horse serum, but it is much more commonly caused by drugs, especially penicillin. It is characterized by lymphadenopathy, arthritis, urticarial wheals, and fever. Rheumatic vasculitis can occur in association with connective tissue diseases, especially SLE and rheumatoid arthritis.

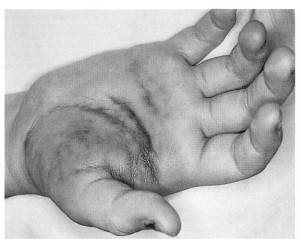

Figure 1-63

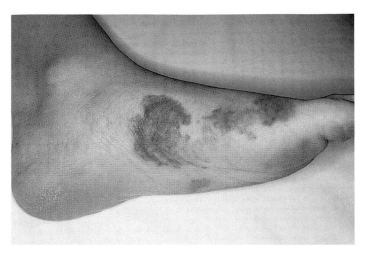

Figure 1-64

Henoch–Schönlein purpura is a form of vasculitis that most commonly occurs in children and young adults. Gastrointestinal symptoms, such as abdominal pain, hematemesis, and melena, can dominate the clinical picture. Other features of this vasculitis include arthralgias and arthritis, symmetrical palpable purpura of the lower extremities, and renal involvement as manifested by hematuria and proteinuria. Figure 1-63 shows acute arthritis of the hand with purpura in a 14-year-old girl who developed repeated episodes of Henoch–Schönlein purpura. At least some cases of this disorder are triggered by streptococcal infection. Henoch–Schönlein purpura differs from other

causes of vasculitis in that biopsy for immunofluorescence reveals IgA in and around cutaneous vessel walls.

Essential mixed cryoglobulinemia is characterized by skin lesions, arthralgias, and glomerulonephritis. The cryoglobulins consist of IgM bound to IgG and thus have rheumatoid factor activity. In one series, 74% of mixed cryoglobulins contained hepatitis B antigen, thus indicating that this condition occurs as a result of infection in many patients. Most recently, hepatitis C has been implicated in the pathology of many cases of cryoglobulinemia. Recurrent palpable purpura is the most common cutaneous manifestation of this disorder (Fig. 1-64).

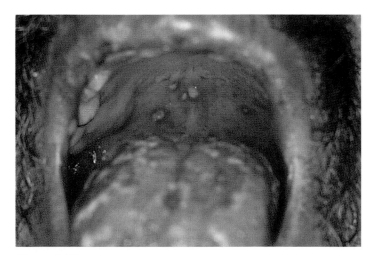

Figure 1-65

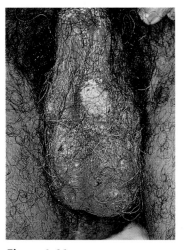

Figure 1-66

Behçet disease consists of a triad of oral, genital, and ocular lesions. Individuals of Mediterranean or Japanese origin appear to be affected more frequently, but the condition has been reported worldwide. Affected males outnumber females by as much as five to one, and the condition occurs most frequently in the third decade, although there have been descriptions of the condition in patients aged 6–72 years.

Different diagnostic criteria have been suggested for Behçet disease, but all include recurrent oral aphthous ulcerations. Oral ulcers or erosions (Fig. 1-65) are painful, sharply demarcated, and heal in 1–3 weeks without scarring. The lips, gums, buccal mucosa, tongue, palate, or larynx can be affected, and ulcerations can be single or, more commonly, multiple. Oral ulcerations occur in virtually all patients with

Behçet disease and can be the first manifestation of the disease. In the absence of other symptoms, the ulcers can be indistinguishable from recurrent canker sores. Other causes of recurrent oral ulcerations, such as inflammatory bowel disease or herpes simplex infection, must be excluded. Nevertheless, a diagnosis of Behçet disease should be considered in anyone with almost constant multiple oral aphthae or with recurrent genital ulcerations.

Recurrent genital ulcers occur in approximately 80% of patients with Behçet disease and affect the vulva, vagina, penis, scrotum (Fig. 1-66), and perianal area. They are more painful for males and can be asymptomatic in females. Genital ulcers occur less frequently than oral aphthae and heal with scarring. Urethritis does not occur.

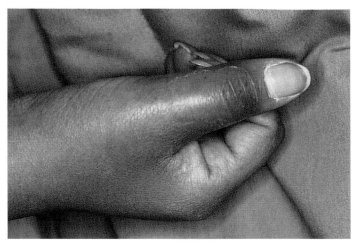

Figure 1-67

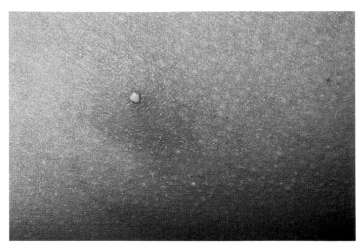

Figure 1-68

Mild nondeforming migratory **arthritis** occurs in approximately 50% of patients with Behçet disease. Figure 1-67 shows acute monarthritis of the first digit in a patient with Behçet disease. Recurrent self-limiting attacks affecting one or a few joints most commonly involve the knees, wrists, elbows, or ankles. Synovial fluid cell counts reveal 5 000–10 000 white blood cells/mm³ consisting mostly of polymorphonuclear leukocytes.

Bilateral and recurrent uveitis affects approximately two-thirds of patients. It usually develops several years after the onset of other symptoms. Patients complain of blurred vision or, in some cases, severe ocular pain. Retinal vasculitis can result in blindness.

Cutaneous lesions have been reported in a majority of patients with Behçet disease, and the appearance of the lesion can vary. Tender erythematous nodules resembling erythema nodosum clinically, but not histologically, are frequently reported. Most specific is a phenomenon known as **pathergy** that frequently appears at sites of venipuncture or intravenous administration. This phenomenon begins at sites of cutaneous trauma as a sterile pustule with surrounding erythema. The pathergy reaction can be useful diagnostically. Intradermal injection of sterile saline can result in the development of erythema or formation of a pustule within 1–2 days (Fig. 1-68).

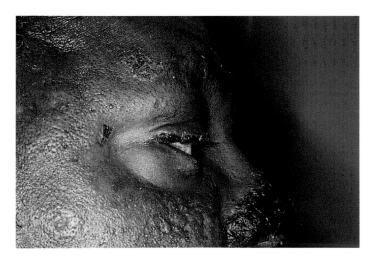

Figure 1-69

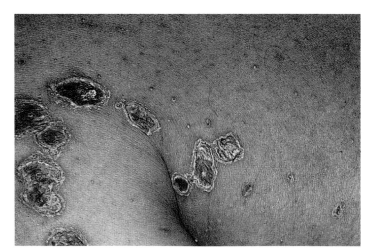

Figure 1-70

Thrombophlebitis, venous occlusions, and arterial occlusions can occur, resulting in cutaneous necrosis and a wide array of signs and symptoms depending on the vessel involved. In the patient shown in Figure 1-69, necrosis of the nasal tip occurred. Less specific pustular, vesicular, acneiform, or pyodermatous lesions have been described as well. The patient in Figure 1-70 developed pustules on the buttocks that rapidly evolved into ulcers and erosions on the arm, chest, and back.

Approximately 20% of patients develop episodes of meningoencephalitis characterized by fever, headache, and stiff neck. Neurologic

symptoms can be focal or diffuse, central or peripheral, and generally develop approximately 2–5 years after the onset of the disease. Other organ systems are affected as well—pericarditis, endocarditis, and cardiac conduction defects have been described. Ulcerations similar to those that develop in the mouth can occur in the esophagus, stomach, intestines, and anus, and perforations can occur. Intestinal lesions can be associated with symptoms that mimic inflammatory bowel disease.

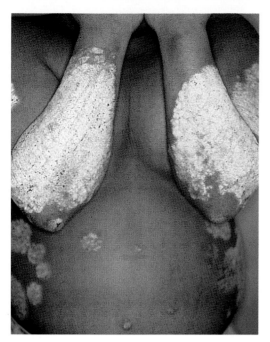

Figure 1-71

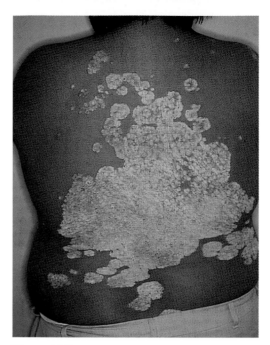

Figure 1-72

Psoriasis is a common skin disorder with a prevalence of 1.0–2.6% of the general population. The average age of onset is between 20 and 30 years. Patients are rarely born with the disorder, and some individuals do not develop signs of psoriasis until after the age of 70. At least one out of three psoriasis patients has a family history of the disorder, suggesting either a multifactorial inheritance pattern or autosomal dominant inheritance with incomplete penetrance.

Several distinct cutaneous reaction patterns have been described. **Plaque psoriasis** is characterized by sharply demarcated erythematous scaling plaques (Fig. 1-71). The elbows and knees are typically involved, as are the scalp, intergluteal cleft, palms, soles, and genitals. Nonetheless, any part of the body can be affected, and in some patients the condition covers large portions of the trunk and the extremities (Fig. 1-72).

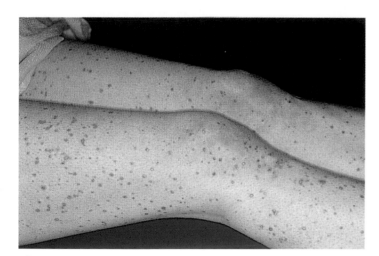

Figure 1-73

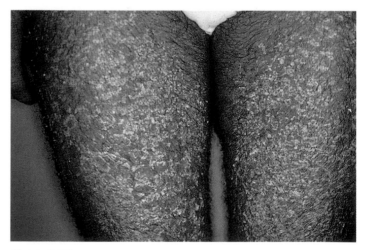

Figure 1-74

Guttate psoriasis occasionally develops after streptococcal pharyngitis or another upper respiratory infection. Skin lesions are erythematous scaling macules and papules (Fig. 1-73) that can become confluent to form plaque psoriasis. Plaque and guttate psoriasis are the most commonly encountered forms of this disorder.

A third cutaneous reaction pattern, **psoriatic erythroderma**, can be life threatening. The patient's entire skin becomes red and scaly

(Fig. 1-74). The protective functions of the skin are impaired, resulting in infection and loss of temperature control. Both high and low temperatures can occur. Percutaneous loss of fluids can lead to hypotension and renal failure, and continued exfoliation of scales may result in substantial loss of protein. Iron-deficiency anemia is common, and leukocytosis frequently occurs because of increased cutaneous blood flow. High output cardiac failure may also occur.

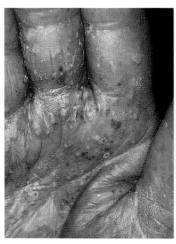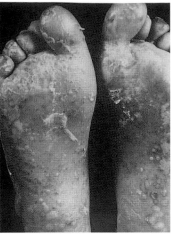

Figure 1-75A   **Figure 1-75B**

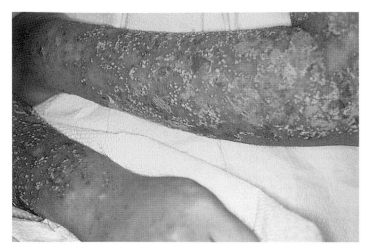

Figure 1-76

Pustular psoriasis, a fourth cutaneous reaction pattern of psoriasis, is characterized by the development of sterile pustules either in psoriatic plaques or in previously uninvolved skin. Pustular psoriasis can be localized, often to the palms and soles (Fig. 1-75) or generalized (Fig. 1-76). Pustular psoriasis of von Zumbusch is a medical emergency characterized by abrupt onset of generalized pustules associated with fever and leukocytosis. Large numbers of sterile pustules appear over a period of hours, quickly becoming confluent and forming lakes of pus. Nail involvement is common, and separation of the nail plate from the nail bed often occurs. Loss of fluid through the skin leads to dehydration. Electrolyte imbalance, hypocalcemia, hypoalbuminemia, and septicemia complicate the clinical picture.

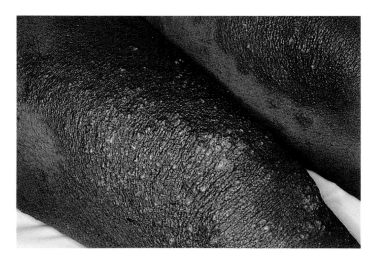

Figure 1-77

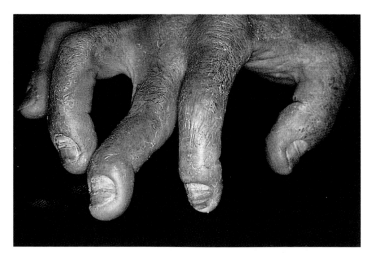

Figure 1-78

Any of the cutaneous patterns of psoriasis can arise *de novo* or can develop in a patient with another preexisting form of psoriasis. Pustular psoriasis of von Zumbusch frequently occurs after withdrawal of systemic steroids in patients with preexisting psoriasis, but it can also arise in those without preexisting psoriasis. **Impetigo herpetiformis** is a generalized pustular eruption that has been described in pregnant women (Fig. 1-77). It is thought to be a form of generalized pustular psoriasis, and it too has severe constitutional symptoms including dehydration, hypotension, renal failure, electrolyte imbalance, and hypocalcemia. In severe cases abortion or death of the mother may result.

Nail involvement occurs in 80% of patients with psoriatic arthritis compared to 30% of psoriasis patients without arthritis (Fig. 1-78). When distal joints of the digits are involved, adjacent nail changes frequently occur. Nail involvement is thus a helpful finding when the diagnosis of psoriatic arthritis is in question. Because hyperuricemia often occurs in patients with psoriasis, and psoriatic arthritis can present as acute monoarthritis, differentiation from gout may be necessary. Fortunately, the two conditions can easily be distinguished by the absence of crystals in the synovial fluid in psoriatic arthritis.

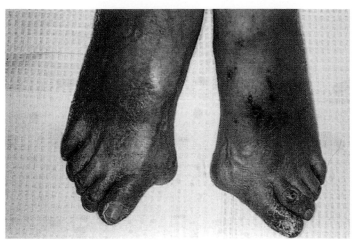

Figure 1-79

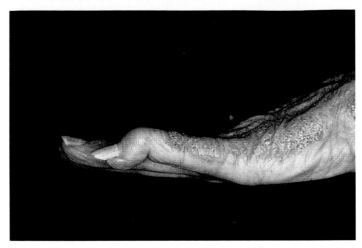

Figure 1-80

Approximately 7% of psoriasis patients have an inflammatory disorder of the joints. Five types of **psoriatic arthritis** have been described. The most common form is asymmetric arthritis involving only two or three joints at a time, especially the joints of the fingers or toes. This pattern occurs in approximately 70% of patients with psoriatic arthritis. Approximately 15% of patients develop a second type of psoriatic arthritis characterized by symmetrical polyarthritis that is clinically indistinguishable from rheumatoid arthritis. Table 1-6 addresses features that support a diagnosis of psoriatic arthritis over rheumatoid arthritis. Ulnar and fibular deviation (Fig. 1-79) and joint deformities identical to those seen in rheumatoid arthritis occur (Fig. 1-80), but rheumatoid factor is not found in the blood of these patients. Classical psoriatic arthritis is a third type that refers to distal interphalangeal joint involvement, but this affects only 16% of

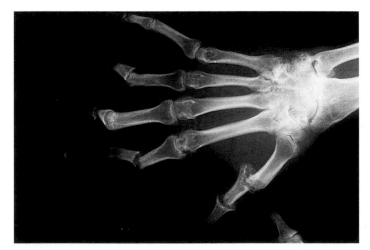

Figure 1-81

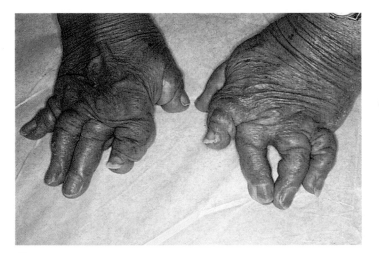

Figure 1-82

patients. Radiographically, there is erosion of the middle phalanx and expansion of the base of the terminal phalanx, creating a "**pencil-in-cup**" **deformity**. In Figure 1-81 similar changes can also be seen in the proximal interphalangeal joints of a patient with psoriatic arthritis. The metacarpal phalangeal and metatarsal phalangeal joints are relatively spared. The most deforming type of psoriatic arthritis has been called **arthritis mutilans**. In severe cases the phalanges are entirely destroyed, resulting in telescoping of the digits, the so-called "**opera-glass deformity**" (Fig. 1-82). This severely deforming condition fortunately affects only 5% of patients with psoriatic arthritis. Finally, 5% of patients have ankylosing spondylitis. As in idiopathic ankylosing spondylitis, human leukocyte antigen-B27 (HLA-B27) is increased, and iritis can occur. There is radiographic evidence of asymmetrical sacroiliitis in some patients. In other patients, asymmetrical syndesmophytes are found in the absence of sacroiliitis. Psoriatic spondylitis can affect any part of the spine, and atlantoaxial subluxation with neurologic sequelae can occur.

In patients with psoriatic arthritis, skin disease is often more severe. Pustular psoriasis, for example, occurs in approximately 25% of patients with severe psoriatic arthritis, but in only 4% of other psoriasis patients. Skin changes precede psoriatic arthritis in most patients, but a small percentage of patients will note joint pain before developing cutaneous lesions.

Table 1-6. Features That Favor the Diagnosis of Psoriatic Arthritis Over Rheumatoid Arthritis

Negative rheumatoid factor
HLA-B27/asymmetrical sacroiliitis
"Pencil-in-cup" deformity (arthritis mutilans)
Erosion of terminal phalangeal tufts
Bony ankylosis
Metatarsal osteolysis
DIP and PIP joint involvement with sparing of MCP and MTP joints
Family history of psoriasis
Enthesopathy/asymmetric joint disease

HLA: human leukocyte antigen; DIP: distal interphalangeal; MCP: metacarpophalangeal; MTP: metatarsophalangeal; PIP: proximal interphalangeal.

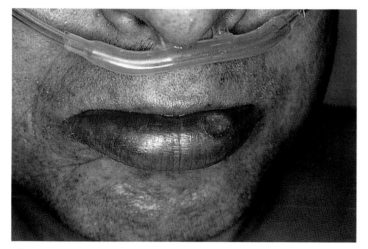

Figure 1-83

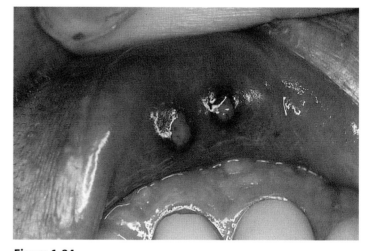

Figure 1-84

Most cases of **Reiter syndrome** have been reported following venereal exposure, although postdysenteric forms also occur, especially after infection with *Shigella flexneri* and occasionally after salmonella or *Yersinia* infections. Males with HLA-B27 are most commonly affected. Distinguishing features include conjunctivitis, urethritis, and the mucosal lesions. Recurrent oral ulcers are common and can develop on the buccal mucosa, palate, tongue, or pharynx (Figs 1-83 and 1-84).

Reiter syndrome frequently begins with symptoms of urethritis. Frequency, dysuria, and urethral discharge can occur. *Chlamydia trachomatis* can be cultured from urethral secretions of some patients, which has led to the hypothesis that infection with a number of organisms can trigger the development of Reiter syndrome in susceptible males.

Conjunctivitis is usually mild and lasts only a day or two, although it may recur or last up to several weeks. It is usually bilateral. A variety of other ocular abnormalities can occur less frequently, including anterior uveitis (iridocyclitis), superficial punctate keratitis, corneal ulcerations, episcleritis, optic and retrobulbar neuritis, and panophthalmitis, which rarely can result in irreversible destruction of the eye.

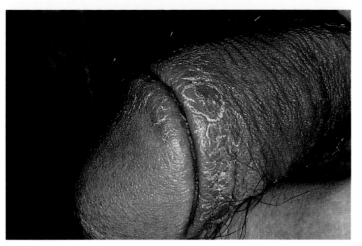

Figure 1-85

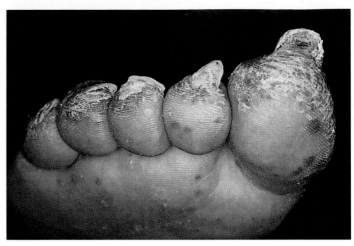

Figure 1-86

Many of the skin changes of **Reiter syndrome** are identical to those seen in psoriasis both clinically and histologically. **Balanitis circinata** refers to scaling, erythematous, psoriasis-like papules on the penis that coalesce into a circinate pattern (Fig. 1-85). The severity of this rash is not correlated with the presence or severity of urethritis. Nail

involvement is common and is characterized by thick, yellow nails with subungual hyperkeratosis (Fig. 1-86).

Keratoderma blenorrhagicum occurs approximately 4–6 weeks after the onset of urethritis and affects 10–30% of patients with Reiter syndrome. It begins as a pustular eruption on the palms and soles and

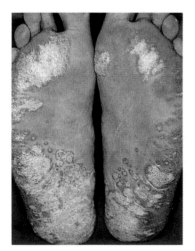

Figure 1-87

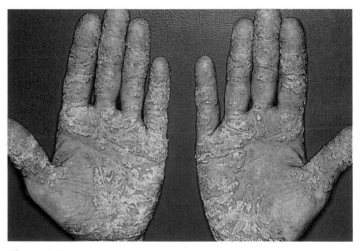

Figure 1-88

may be indistinguishable from pustular psoriasis both clinically and histologically. The pustules are eventually replaced by thick, psoriasis-like scales (Figs 1-87 and 1-88). Other areas of the body may also develop pustular or scaling lesions. Thick scaling of the scalp, similar to psoriasis, has been reported, and a number of patients whose condition eventuated in frank psoriasis have been described. Arthritis begins abruptly and most commonly affects the knees and ankles, but any joint may be involved. The arthritis usually affects only a few joints and is asymmetrical. Sacroiliitis with back pain is common.

Flares of Reiter syndrome are self-limiting, but recurrent. Individual bouts of arthritis may last from a few weeks to several years, and although complete recovery occurs after each episode, new episodes can occur after intervals of weeks to years.

Other systemic complications of Reiter syndrome have been reported including, pericarditis and myocarditis, which result in pericardial friction rubs and heart block. Dilatation of the aortic root has resulted in aortic insufficiency in a small number of patients. Peripheral neuropathy, transient hemiplegia, meningoencephalitis, and cranial nerve palsies have been occasionally reported as well.

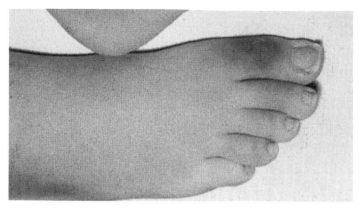

Figure 1-89

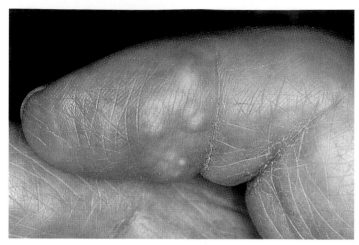

Figure 1-90

Gout is a common cause of acute monarthritis and results from deposition of uric acid crystals in the joint cavity. The main cutaneous manifestation is the tophus, which represents the accumulation of uric acid crystals in the skin and superficial tissues. The course of gout is quite variable, with some patients experiencing only a few attacks in a lifetime and never progressing to the point of joint destruction or to the formation of tophi. Other patients experience recurrent episodes of severe and acute arthritis. At first, episodes are spaced months or years apart but, with time, attacks become more frequent and severe. The first metatarsal–phalangeal joint of the large toe is characteristically involved (Fig. 1-89), affecting 75% of people with gout. Polyarticular involvement occurs in 5–10%.

During an acute flare of gouty arthritis, the skin over the affected joints becomes red, hot, and tender. Inflammation may be so severe that the entire hand or foot may be swollen, suggesting a cellulitis, but points of extreme tenderness over the responsible joint can be identified by palpation. If untreated, an episode can last from days to weeks.

Tophi are rarely present during an initial attack of gout, appearing an average of approximately 10 years after the onset of arthritis. They frequently develop over the distal interphalangeal joints of the fingers (Fig. 1-90) and in the olecranon and prepatellar bursae. Occasionally, they are found in the rims of the ears and in the tendons of the fingers,

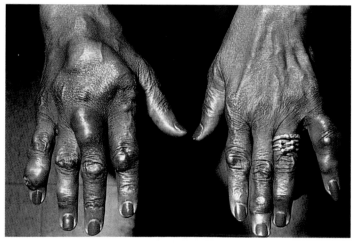

Figure 1-91

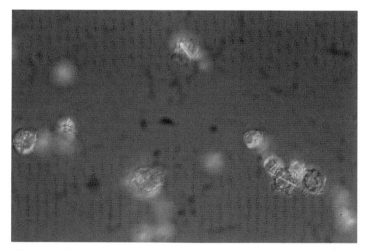

Figure 1-92

wrists, toes, and ankles. Tophi can even develop in bone, nasal cartilage, tongue, vocal cords, kidneys, myocardium, and heart valves. Tophi are white or yellow in color and range from pinhead-sized to pea-sized—even apple-sized in rare cases (Fig. 1-91). With time, tophi increase in size and number. If the overlying skin breaks down, the chalky white tophaceous material can be seen, and there can be a prolonged discharge of sodium urate crystals.

Although gout is associated with hyperuricemia, only a small percentage of hyperuricemic individuals will develop this joint disease.

Approximately 20% of gout patients will form urinary uric acid calculi. If the diagnosis of gout is in question, aspiration of an affected joint or of a tophus should be examined microscopically with polarizing lenses. Needle-shaped, **negatively birefringent uric acid crystals** are diagnostic (Fig. 1-92). It is rarely necessary to remove tophi surgically, but if histopathologic confirmation of material from a tophus is needed, the material should be fixed in absolute alcohol to prevent dissolution of the crystals.

2 Respiratory diseases

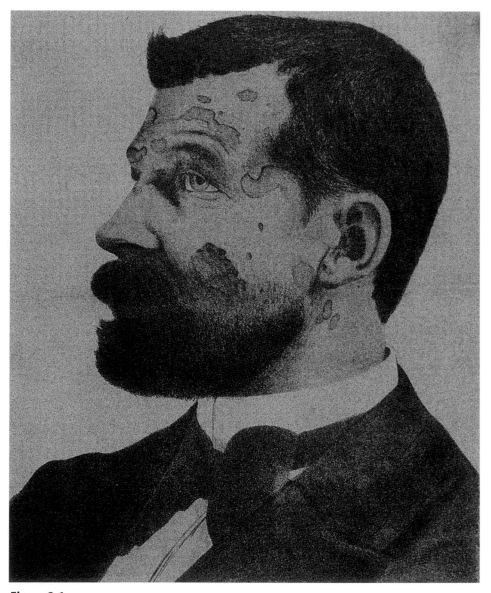

Figure 2-1

From Boeck C. Multiple benign sarkoid of the skin. Journal of Cutaneous Genito-Urinary Diseases, 1899; 17:543–550.

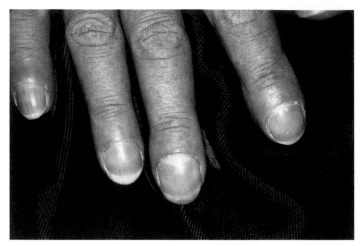

Figure 2-2

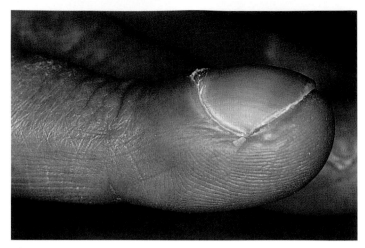

Figure 2-3

Clubbing is a nonspecific sign of pulmonary and mediastinal diseases. The distal digits are enlarged giving them a bulbous appearance. While classically associated with neoplastic lung disease, symmetric clubbing of the digits can also be found in a variety of infectious and noninfectious pulmonary diseases. The patient in Figure 2-2, for example, has sarcoidosis. Clubbing has developed in patients with nonpulmonary malignancies that have metastasized to the lungs. Identical changes in the distal digits can also occur in patients with cardiovascular disease associated with cyanosis, in cirrhosis of the

liver, and in an autosomal dominantly inherited form of clubbing that is not associated with any underlying diseases. The Lovibond angle, the angle between the proximal nail fold and the nail plate, is normally less than 180°. In patients with clubbing the angle straightens and ultimately exceeds 180° (Fig. 2-3). When clubbing is associated with subperiosteal new bone formation, the term *hypertrophic osteoarthropathy* is used. Tenderness, pain, or paresthesias of the fingertips may occur. Pain in the arms and legs is associated with concomitant new bone formation in the extremities.

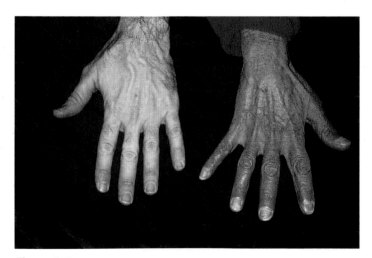

Figure 2-4

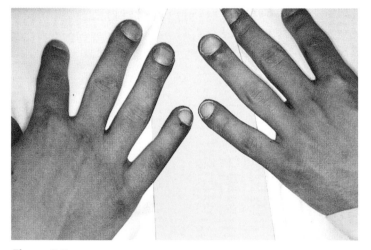

Figure 2-5

Cyanosis is a bluish skin color associated with reduced oxygen saturation of the blood in cutaneous capillaries. In fair-skinned people cyanosis may become apparent when arterial oxygen saturation is below 85%; in darker-skinned people cyanosis may not be evident until arterial oxygen saturation falls below 75%.

Cyanosis can occur in any pulmonary disease that results in reduced oxygen saturation. Figure 2-4 shows the cyanotic hand of a patient with emphysema (right) compared with a normal hand (left). Congenital

heart diseases in which venous blood is shunted into arterial blood can result in cyanosis, as can pulmonary arteriovenous fistulae. Figure 2-5 shows cyanosis of the nail beds in the fingers of a patient who was born with transposition of the great vessels. Methemoglobinemia and sulfhemoglobinemia are uncommon causes of cyanosis. Peripheral cyanosis occurs when blood flow to the extremities is reduced. It can result from localized vasoconstriction in response to cold exposure, or in states of low cardiac output such as shock or congestive heart failure.

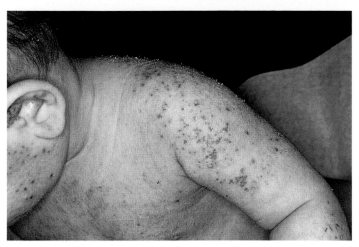

Figure 2-6

Atopic dermatitis is commonly associated with other atopic diseases, including asthma and allergic rhinitis. Patients with severe atopic dermatitis are more likely to develop either asthma or allergic rhinitis later in life. The genetic component of these atopic disorders is demonstrated by the increased incidence of asthma and allergic rhinitis in family members of patients with atopic dermatitis. Cutaneous involvement often begins at an early age. In infancy and childhood the face, scalp, and extensor surfaces of the extremities are covered with eczematous patches (Fig. 2-6).

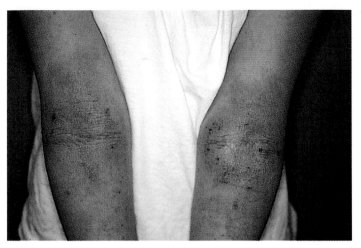

Figure 2-7

Acutely, the patches may be eroded, erythematous, oozing, or even vesicular. If the condition persists, scaling erythematous plaques studded with papules and excoriations may develop. As children get older atopic dermatitis tends to involve flexural areas such as the neck and antecubital and popliteal fossae. Chronic scratching results in thickening and lichenification of skin with increased skin markings, as shown in the antecubital fossa of the patient in Figure 2-7. In severely affected adults,

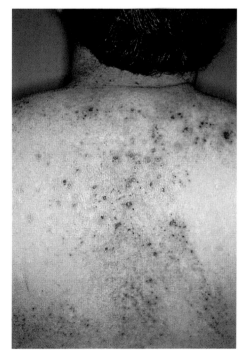

Figure 2-8

weeping, oozing, excoriated patches can become generalized (Fig. 2-8). Seasonal variation in the severity of the disease often occurs, and most patients experience periodic exacerbations and remissions. Childhood atopic dermatitis eventually resolves in most patients. However, some patients develop chronic atopic dermatitis as adults, with continuous or intermittent flares of their disease. Other patients develop hand or foot dermatitis in adulthood.

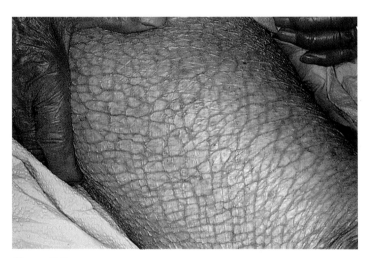

Figure 2-9

The pathogenesis of atopic dermatitis is poorly understood. Elevated levels of serum IgE have been found in many patients, and radioallergosorbent assay (RAST) often shows that the elevated IgE is directed against numerous common antigens. The severity of cutaneous symptoms, however, does not correlate with exposure to those antigens. Numerous patients benefit from treatment with systemic antibiotics, and *Staphylococcus aureus* undoubtedly plays a role in the severity of disease. External cutaneous irritants such as harsh soaps and detergents also influence the severity of this disease.

Ichthyosis vulgaris is another condition associated with atopic dermatitis. It is characterized by the presence of large fish-like scales (Fig. 2-9) that are most obvious over the shins. Flexural areas are spared, and there are increased skin markings and hyperkeratosis of palms and soles. Ichthyosis vulgaris begins in childhood and is inherited in an autosomal dominant pattern.

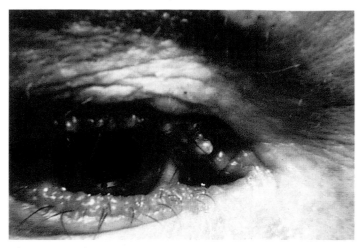

Figure 2-10

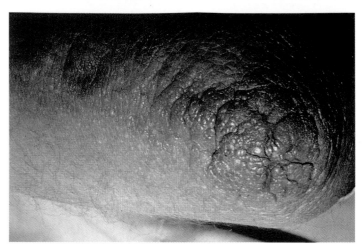

Figure 2-11

Lipoid proteinosis is an uncommon recessively inherited disorder in which hyaline material deposits in interstitial tissues. Affected patients usually have normal lifespans, but respiratory and neurological complications can be fatal. The skin is diffusely infiltrated, particularly on the face; changes may be more evident upon palpation than inspection. Translucent papules are characteristic, and scratching creates crusts and ulcerations with resulting acneiform scars on the face. Yellowish papules along the eyelid margins typically develop in most patients (Fig. 2-10). While the face is most prominently affected, papules and nodules can develop anywhere on the body, particularly at sites of

repeated injury or pressure. Involvement of the extensor surface of the elbow is shown in Figure 2-11. Diffuse infiltration of the oropharyngeal mucosa results in a pebbly appearance of the buccal mucosa and lips; the tongue is immobile, and speech is difficult. Infiltration of the vocal cords results in hoarseness. Involvement of the larynx and subglottic region can result in narrowing and eventual blockage of airways. Deposition and calcification of hyaline material in blood vessel walls of the brain can result in a seizure disorder or impaired intellect. The calcified nodules are evident on CT scan of the brain.

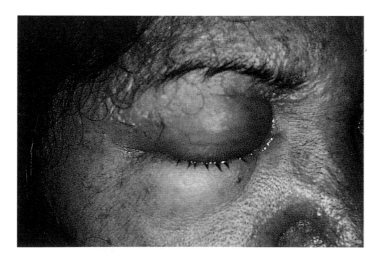

Figure 2-12

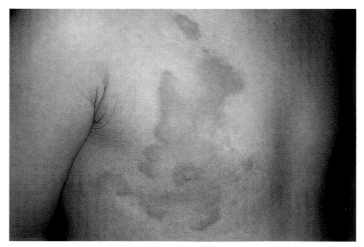

Figure 2-13

Angioedema, also called angioneurotic edema, is a localized swelling of the skin and subcutaneous tissues. Mucous membranes of the upper respiratory and gastrointestinal tracts can also be affected, resulting in airway obstruction, abdominal pain, and vomiting. Both allergic and genetic forms exist; the inherited form is autosomal dominantly transmitted and can begin at any time from infancy to adulthood. Acute episodes of facial edema (Fig. 2-12) or abdominal pain, nausea, and vomiting can last for 2–3 days. Laryngeal edema can occur and, if severe, can result in fatal airway obstruction. Hereditary angioedema is caused by an absent or dysfunctional C_1 esterase inhibitor.

Allergic angioedema is an IgE-dependent reaction that occurs upon ingestion of, or exposure to, the offending allergen. The reaction is most visible when the face, lips, or tongue are affected. Allergic angioedema is often associated with **urticaria**. Superficial dermal edema results in well-demarcated erythematous wheals with elevated serpiginous borders (Fig. 2-13). Episodes begin acutely, often within minutes of exposure to the responsible allergen. Cutaneous wheals are evanescent, lasting only hours. Fortunately, severe episodes that cause laryngeal obstruction are uncommon.

Table 2-1. Approach to the Patient: Diagnostic Steps in the Patient with Chronic Urticaria

General
- Sedimentation rate
- Complete blood count with differential
- Chemistry screen
- Thyroid function test
- Quantitative immunoglobulins

Infectious
- Stool for ova and parasites
- Indicated cultures
- Serum hepatitis antigens
- Indicated x-rays; sinus, chest, dental, others

IgE mediated
- Total IgE by PRIST
- Antigen specific IgE by RAST
- Skin tests
- Challenges

Vasculitis/immune complex mediated
- Complement levels or CH_{50}
- Antinuclear antibodies
- Immune complex assay
- Complement activation studies
- Biopsy with immunofluorescence
- Cryoglobulins

Nonimmunologically mediated
- Challenge with relevant food, additive, drug or physical stimulus (dermatographism, ice-cube test for cold urticaria, phototesting for solar urticaria, exercise for cholinergic urticaria)

Modified from Adelsberg B. Chronic urticaria. In: Lebwohl M, ed. Difficult diagnoses in dermatology. New York: Churchill Livingstone; 1988: 323.
CH_{50}: 50% hemolyzing dose of complement; IgE, immunoglobulin E; PRIST: paper radioimmunsorbent test; RAST, radioallergosorbent assay.

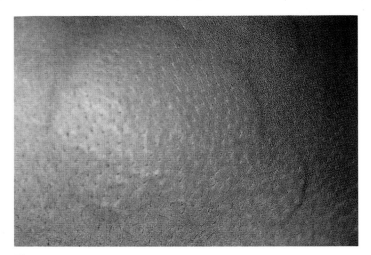

Figure 2-14

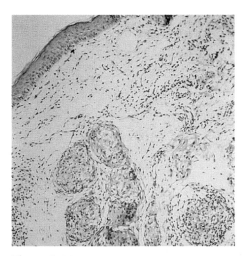

Figure 2-15

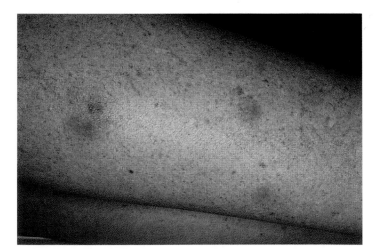

Figure 2-16

Episodes of urticaria that do not have a known cause and recur over more than 6 months are termed chronic urticaria. While extensive work-ups have been devised to find the cause of chronic urticaria (Table 2-1), diagnostic efforts are often fruitless.

Because of their transient nature, urticarial reactions are often subtle at the time of examination (Fig. 2-14). Moreover, urticarial vasculitis can mimic the clinical features of urticaria. The two conditions can be distinguished by a number of features; urticarial vasculitis burns and it can last for days or weeks, whereas allergic urticaria itches and lasts only for a few hours. Similarly, early stages of bullous pemphigoid and erythema multiforme can mimic urticaria, but these also last more than 24 hours and evolve into bullae and target lesions, respectively.

Sarcoidosis, a multiorgan system disorder of unknown etiology, can present with a wide array of skin lesions. Its diagnosis is based on clinical, radiographic, and histologic findings. **Noncaseating granulomatosis** (Fig. 2-15), the histopathologic hallmark of sarcoidosis, can be found on biopsy of many involved organs but it is nonspecific because it can occur in several other diseases. Definitive diagnosis therefore requires the addition of characteristic clinical features and exclusion of other possible causes of noncaseating granulomatosis. The Kveim–Siltzbach skin test, which involves the intradermal injection of a sarcoidal spleen extract, results in induration, erythema, and the formation of noncaseating granulomas that can be identified on biopsy 4–6 weeks later. Use of this test is limited to those with access to the antigen, but biopsy of the skin lesions usually reveals characteristic noncaseating granulomas as well.

The course of sarcoidosis can be highly variable. Approximately 20–40% of patients abruptly develop constitutional symptoms, such as fever and weight loss, over a 1–2-week period. Chest x-rays reveal bilateral hilar adenopathy, and patients with this rapidly evolving form of sarcoid may present with **erythema nodosum** (Fig. 2-16). The latter condition is characterized by bilateral deep, tender, red nodules on the

Table 2-2. Causes of Erythema Nodosum using the BEDREST Acronym

Behçet disease
Estrogens
Drugs
Recent infection
Enteropathies (e.g. Crohn's disease)
Sarcoid
Tuberculosis

Table 2-3. Approach to the Patient: Suggested Investigation of Patients with Septal Panniculitis

Chest x-ray
Gastrointestinal series with small bowel follow-through
Barium enema
Complete blood count
Erythrocyte sedimentation rate
Antistreptococcal titers
Intradermal coccidiodin or histoplasmin
Careful drug history
Microbiologic studies as indicated (e.g. *Mycoplasma, Yersinia, Trichophyton, Streptococcus*)

Reprinted from Phelps R. Panniculitis. In: Lebwohl M, ed. Difficult diagnoses in dermatology. New York: Churchill Livingstone; 1988: 401.

shins. It has been suggested that the development of erythema nodosum in association with sarcoidosis connotes a good prognosis, since these patients usually have an acute, self-limiting form of the disease.

In the absence of other signs of sarcoidosis, erythema nodosum is a nonspecific finding that occurs in association with numerous underlying etiologies (Table 2-2). The numerous causes of erythema nodosum can easily be remembered with the acronym BEDREST (*B*ehçet disease, *e*strogens, *d*rugs, *r*ecent infection, *e*nteropathies, *s*arcoid, *t*uberculosis), which can be an appropriate treatment for this condition when it is severe.

Erythema nodosum often occurs as a solitary, transient episode that resolves upon treatment with nonsteroidal antiinflammatory drugs. More severe cases may require potassium iodide, corticosteroids, or other systemic medications. Occasionally, the etiology is obvious, but

when it is not apparent work-up may be indicated. Certainly in recurrent, chronic, or severe cases of erythema nodosum, appropriate work-up should be considered (Table 2-3). Chest x-ray is a simple screening procedure, and skin testing for TB should be considered in patients who haven't received BCG (bacille Calmette–Guérin) vaccination. Gastrointestinal work-up should be undertaken in patients with abdominal pain, diarrhea, or stools containing blood. Other diagnostic steps can be taken depending on the patient history and physical examination.

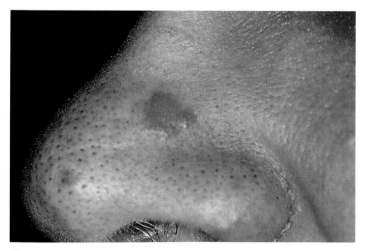

Figure 2-17

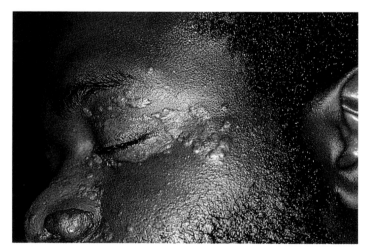

Figure 2-18

Other patients with sarcoidosis insidiously and gradually develop respiratory complaints over a period of months without constitutional symptoms or erythema nodosum. These patients develop the chronic form of sarcoid with progressive pulmonary disease.

The cutaneous manifestations of **sarcoidosis** are as varied as the systemic symptoms and can include papules, nodules, and plaques, as

well as erythema nodosum. Papular lesions can occur anywhere on the body but most commonly develop around the eyes and nose (Figs 2-17 and 2-18). The papules are usually round, red, or flesh-colored and measure 1–5 mm in diameter.

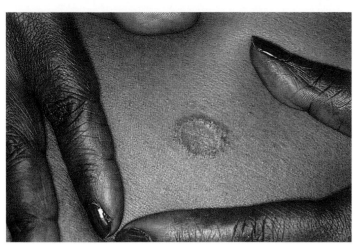

Figure 2-19

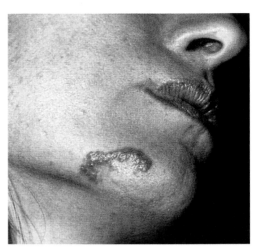

Figure 2-20

Annular lesions occur in patients with **sarcoidosis** and are particularly common in dark-skinned people (Fig. 2-19). A ring of small papules surrounding a normal or atrophic center is characteristic.

Occasionally these expand peripherally. Similar lesions can occur in light-skinned patients (Fig. 2-20) but they are less common.

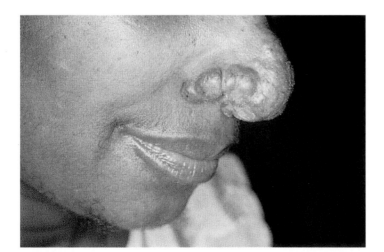

Figure 2-21

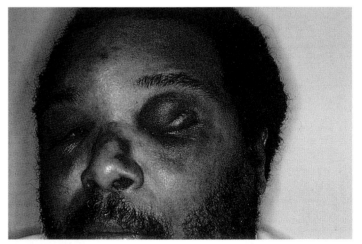

Figure 2-22

Lupus pernio refers to translucent violaceous plaques with overlying telangiectases on the ears, cheeks, nose (Fig. 2-21), and lips of patients with sarcoidosis. Involvement of the fingers and toes is associated with destructive lesions of the underlying digital bones. The nose can take on an indurated, shiny bulbous appearance as a result of lupus pernio of the nasal tip. The nasal mucosa and nasal bones are often affected.

The lung is the most commonly affected organ in sarcoidosis, and 90% of patients have abnormal chest x-rays. Respiratory symptoms, such as cough and shortness of breath, are common. Around 10–20% of patients advance to progressive fibrosis of the lung. Many other organ systems can be affected, but a number of signs and symptoms are par-

ticularly characteristic. Lymphadenopathy occurs in almost all patients and involves hilar and paratracheal nodes as well as peripheral lymph nodes. Splenomegaly and hepatomegaly may also be found. Eye involvement occurs in 25% of patients and can lead to blindness. Most patients develop anterior uveitis, but posterior uveitis occurs in some. Uveitis can be chronic, or it can have an acute onset with spontaneous remission in 6–12 months. Blockage of the lacrimal ducts can lead to keratoconjunctivitis sicca (a dry eye syndrome). Eyelid involvement can lead to marked swelling, as shown in the patient in Figure 2-22. The conjunctivae often develop small yellow nodules.

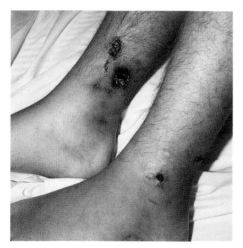

Figure 2-23

While multiple papules are the most common skin finding in **sarcoidosis**, a number of unusual forms of the disease are occasionally seen. Although ulcerations are uncommon, patients with lupus pernio can develop ulcers of the ears or nose. Ulceration may follow treatment with intralesional steroids and result from the cutaneous atrophy associated with corticosteroid therapy. The patient in Figure 2-23 presented with leg ulcers that revealed noncaseating granulomas on biopsy. Inflammation of fat can result in leg ulcers, but there was not an underlying panniculitis in this patient.

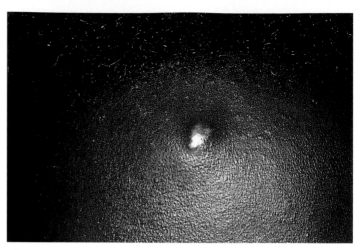

Figure 2-24

Occasional patients present with keloid-like nodules. The patient in Figure 2-24 was aware of a lesion on her forehead for several years. On biopsy it revealed characteristic, noncaseating granulomas. Physical examination revealed generalized lymphadenopathy and splenomegaly, and chest x-ray showed bilateral hilar adenopathy. Biopsy of a paratracheal node also revealed noncaseating granulomatosis.

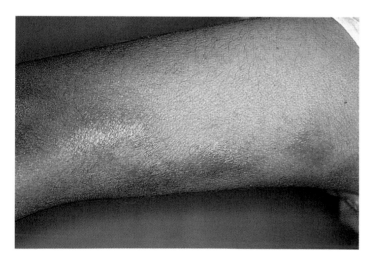

Figure 2-25

A patient with cutaneous induration simulating morphea is shown in Figure 2-25. Biopsy of an indurated plaque again revealed noncaseating granulomas. Other rare manifestations of sarcoidosis include ichthyosiform eruptions, hypopigmentation, lymphedema, and wart-like skin lesions. A psoriasiform rash of the trunk has been described in some patients. Sarcoidosis can have a predilection for scars, and biopsy of scars occasionally establishes the diagnosis. Since skin lesions are more accessible than pulmonary lesions, it is always preferable to biopsy even questionable cutaneous lesions first if the diagnosis is in doubt.

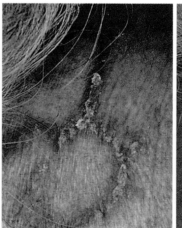 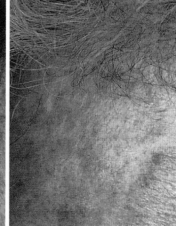

Figure 2-26A   **Figure 2-26B**

Intralesional injections of steroids improve many of the cutaneous lesions of sarcoidosis. In severe cases, antimalarials or systemic steroids are often beneficial. The patient in Figure 2-26A had annular sarcoid of the forehead. She was treated with monthly intralesional injections of triamcinolone acetonide for several months, causing resolution of her skin lesions. Unfortunately, she was left with mild atrophy, hypopigmentation, and telangiectasia of the injected areas, as shown in the post-treatment photograph (Fig. 2-26B).

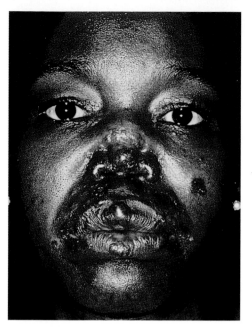

Figure 2-27

Wegener granulomatosis is a widespread granulomatous vasculitis that prominently affects the upper and lower respiratory tracts and the kidney. Upper respiratory tract symptoms include sinus pain and bloody or purulent nasal discharge. Nasal mucosal ulceration, nasal septal perforation, and saddle nose deformity occur (Fig. 2-27). Cough,

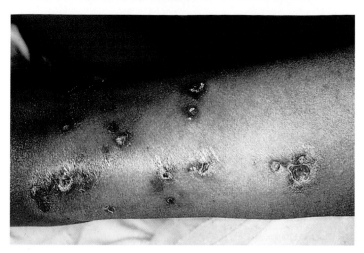

Figure 2-28

hemoptysis, rhinorrhea, pleuritic chest pain, and dyspnea are common. On chest x-ray, pulmonary nodules can be seen, which may cavitate or may resolve spontaneously. Glomerulonephritis occurs in more than 80% of patients and, if untreated, can result in the rapid development of renal failure. Approximately half of patients will develop skin lesions, including cutaneous infarcts and ulcerations (Fig. 2-28), palpable purpura, papules, nodules, and hemorrhagic bullae. On histologic examination, skin lesions may reveal a necrotizing vasculitis with thrombosis of vessels, or necrotizing granulomas.

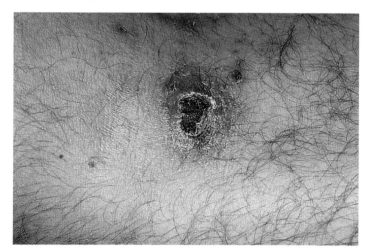

Figure 2-29

Lymphomatoid granulomatosis, a rare disorder of unknown etiology, primarily affects the lungs. A granulomatous necrotizing infiltrate concentrated in and around blood vessels is responsible for the progressive destruction of pulmonary parenchyma that occurs. The infiltrate contains atypical lymphoid cells, and in many patients, the disease evolves into a malignant lymphoma. Skin, nervous system, and kidneys can be involved, but unlike Wegener granulomatosis, lymphomatoid granulomatosis does not affect the upper respiratory tract. Erythematous macules, papules, plaques, and nodules have been described, and skin lesions often ulcerate (Fig. 2-29).

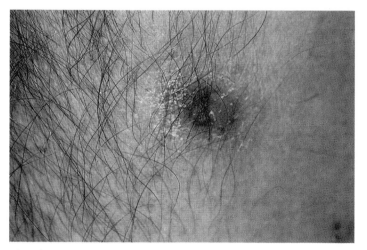

Figure 2-30

Allergic granulomatosis, also called Churg–Strauss disease, is a rare granulomatous vasculitis characterized by adult onset asthma and eosinophilia. Pulmonary findings are striking, and chest x-rays reveal recurrent pulmonary infiltrates. Involvement of other organs including heart, kidney, nervous system, or gastrointestinal tract can occur, but this is less frequent. The majority of patients have skin lesions, most commonly purpura, or cutaneous nodules. Cutaneous infarcts and ulceration can develop, as seen in the patient in Figure 2-30.

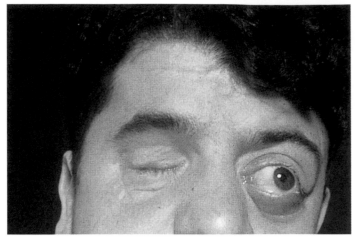

Figure 2-31

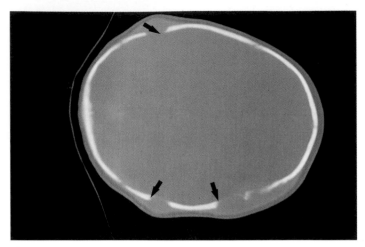

Figure 2-32

The histiocytoses are a group of conditions caused by proliferative disorders of histiocytes. Several of them involve the skin and respiratory tract. **Hand–Schuller–Christian disease** is one of three disorders that have been given the name histiocytosis X, or Langerhans cell granulomatosis, because they are derived from Langerhans cells. This disease is a chronic, slowly progressive disorder that often begins in childhood and almost always develops before the age of 30 years. The clinical triad of skull defects, diabetes insipidus, and exophthalmos is classic, but rarely occurs. Osteolytic bone lesions affect 80% of patients; diabetes insipidus is present in 50%; and exophthalmos occurs in 10%. Involvement of the orbital bones results in tumor mass in the orbital cavity, causing exophthalmos. The patient in Figure 2-31 underwent enucleation of the right eye and has exophthalmos of the left eye.

Bone defects most commonly affect the skull, ribs, pelvis, and scapulae. Multiple lesions of the skull of an infant with Hand–Schüller–Christian disease are shown on the CT scan in Figure 2-32. The cerebral hemispheres are rarely involved. Most intracranial lesions result from direct extension of skull lesions and do not penetrate the dura. Involvement of the long bones can simulate Ewing sarcoma. The histiocytic tumors in bone may grow into subcutaneous tissues where they can be felt as deep nodules. Mandibular involvement with gingival infiltration results in loss of teeth.

Histiocytic invasion of the hypothalamus has been found in most—but not all—patients with diabetes insipidus. Symptoms of polydipsia and polyuria may be present at the time of diagnosis of Hand–Schuller–Christian disease or may develop later in the course of the

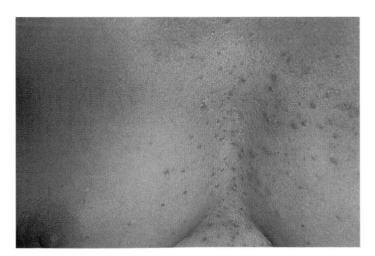

Figure 2-33

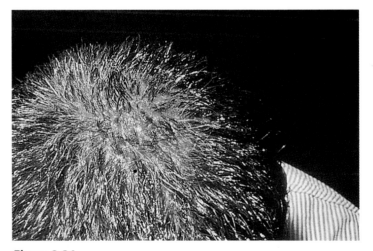

Figure 2-34

illness. Pulmonary infiltration occurs in approximately 30% of patients. Hepatomegaly, splenomegaly, and lymphadenopathy are less common. Skin lesions develop in approximately one-third of patients; they are characterized by erythematous, yellow or brown papules with a pre-

dilection for the scalp, mid-chest (Fig. 2-33), and midback. The patient shown in Fig. 2-34 has a patch of scarring alopecia after resolution of a scalp lesion.

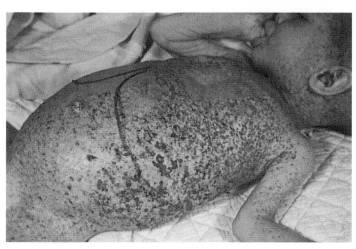

Figure 2-35

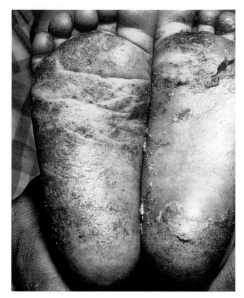

Figure 2-36

Letterer–Siwe disease, the most rare and severe form of histiocytosis X, affects children under the age of 3 years. Skin lesions are common and are often misdiagnosed as severe widespread seborrheic dermatitis. Scaling erythematous patches of the scalp, hairline, retro-auricular folds, axillae, and groin are common. Ulceration and oozing can develop, especially in intertriginous areas. Small infiltrated reddish-brown papules may distinguish this rash from severe seborrheic dermatitis, but ultimately the diagnosis is made by skin biopsy. In severe cases the rash becomes widespread (Fig. 2-35), and even the palms and soles (Fig. 2-36) may be involved. Breakdown of normal skin barriers to infection may allow a portal of entry to microorganisms, resulting in bacterial sepsis. Systemic symptoms are common, including fever, weight loss, and lymphadenopathy. Pulmonary infiltration frequently occurs with cough, tachypnea, or pneumothorax. Involvement of liver, spleen, bone, and bone marrow results in hepatomegaly, splenomegaly, osteolytic bone lesions, and severe anemia, respectively. Hypersplenism frequently leads to thrombocytopenia, causing skin lesions to become purpuric.

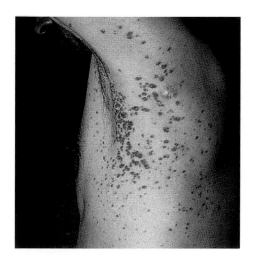

Figure 2-37

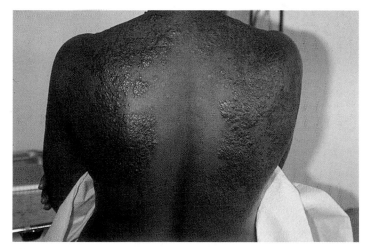

Figure 2-38

Xanthoma disseminatum is a histiocytosis that can involve the upper respiratory tract. It is not included among the histiocytosis X group of diseases, since it is not derived from Langerhans cells. This rare disorder can develop at any age, although most people develop it before the age of 25 years. Skin lesions are reddish-brown papules that coalesce to form nodules and plaques in intertriginous areas. These xanthomatous deposits are most common in the axillae (Fig. 2-37) and in the antecubital and popliteal fossae, although more generalized involvement can occur. The patient in Figure 2-38 had plaques over most of her trunk as well as nodules on her face. Xanthomatous infiltration of the oropharyngeal mucosa occurs, and infiltration of the epiglottis, larynx, trachea, and bronchi is common. Shortness of breath and airway obstruction may result, so tracheostomy has been required in several patients. Involvement of the sclera or cornea can result in obstructive blindness. Mild diabetes insipidus occurs in 40% of patients but usually resolves spontaneously. While the symptoms of xanthoma disseminatum can be severe, the condition is self-limiting, and most patients have a good outcome.

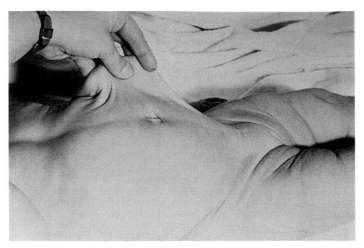

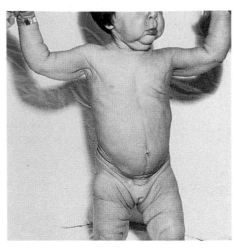

Figure 2-39

Figure 2-40

Cutis laxa, a disorder of elastic tissue, can be inherited or acquired. Both autosomal dominant and autosomal recessive forms of the disease have been described. The autosomal dominant form of cutis laxa is rare and principally affects the skin. In the autosomal recessive forms of cutis laxa, loose redundant hyperextensible folds of skin are apparent at birth (Fig. 2-39). The sagging skin of the face gives affected children a "bloodhound-like" appearance (Fig. 2-40). Pulmonary complications can be prominent with recurrent pneumonia, obstructive pulmonary disease and, in some patients, advanced emphysema and core pulmonale. Severely affected children may die of pulmonary disease before the age of 3 years. In another recessively inherited form of the disorder, hyperextensible joints and joint dislocations are common. Diverticuli of the gastrointestinal tract or the bladder can occur, as can inguinal, umbilical, and hiatal hernias. Pulmonary emphysema is also a feature of this recessive form of cutis laxa, but it is less severe.

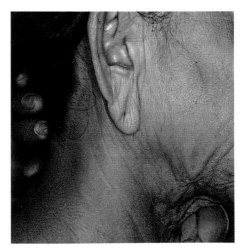

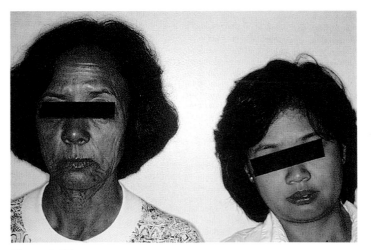

Figure 2-41

Figure 2-42

An acquired form of cutis laxa can develop in adolescents or adults. It is often accompanied by an urticarial or erythematous eruption at its onset and can develop after drug ingestion, surgery, or a febrile episode. In some patients **acquired cutis laxa** is first noted in the ear lobes, which become elongated (Fig. 2-41). The process then spreads to the face, neck, and upper trunk. The skin is hyperextensible but, unlike Ehlers–Danlos syndrome, it does not bounce back after stretching. Redundant sagging skinfolds of the face create a prematurely aged appearance. The 31-year-old woman on the left in Figure 2-42 developed acquired cutis laxa at the age of 18. Her unaffected 29-year-old relative is shown on the right for comparison. As in inherited forms of the disorder, pulmonary emphysema can develop. In all forms of cutis laxa, histologic examination of the skin reveals an absence or reduction of elastic fibers.

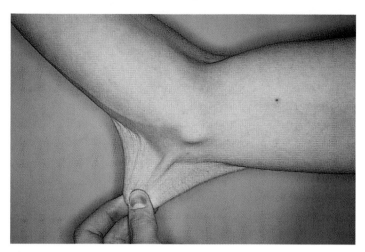

Figure 2-43

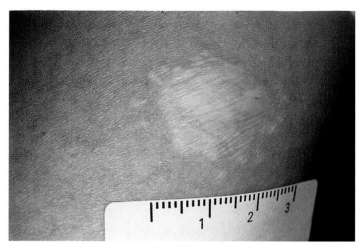

Figure 2-44

Ehlers–Danlos syndrome consists of a group of inherited disorders that have in common hyperextensibility of the skin and joints. Systemic complications are caused by fragility of blood vessels. Dissecting aneurysms of the aorta and other vessels can occur, as can gastrointestinal perforation and bleeding. Spontaneous rupture of major arteries can be catastrophic. Prolapse of the mitral valve occurs in some forms of the Ehlers–Danlos syndrome. Hyperextensibility of the skin is easily shown by pulling on skin of the arms (Fig. 2-43). Upon release, the stretched skin quickly recoils to its original position. Fragility of the skin is common and problematic. Surgical wounds often dehisce; sutures fail to hold wound edges together and tear through the skin. Scars are thin and form slowly during wound healing. They have been described as "cigarette-paper thin" (Fig. 2-44) scars or widely opened "fish-mouth scars". Hematomas result from minor trauma to the knees and heal with soft nodular scars called pseudotumors (Fig. 2-45). Pretibial scars are said to resemble necrobiosis lipoidica diabeticorum.

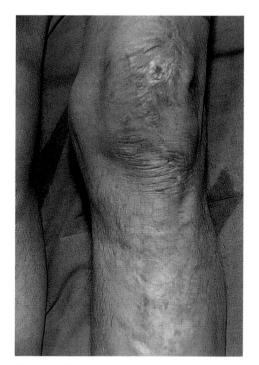

Figure 2-45

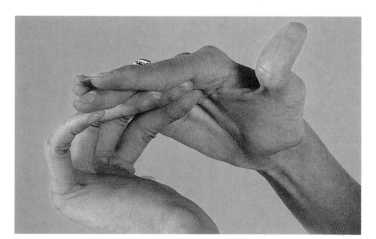

Figure 2-46

The primary defect for many of the types of Ehlers–Danlos syndrome appears to involve abnormalities of connective tissue. Type IV Ehlers–Danlos is caused by diminished synthesis of Type III collagen. Deficiencies of lysyl oxidase or lysyl hydroxylase are associated with other types of Ehlers–Danlos syndrome. The abnormal connective tissue that results is responsible for numerous complications: umbilical, hiatal, and inguinal hernias are frequent, and diverticuli of the gastrointestinal tract can develop. Pulmonary involvement may occur with spontaneous rupture of the lung. Hyperextensibility of the joints (Fig. 2-46) is another common feature of this syndrome. Repeated joint dislocations are frequent, as are hemarthroses and joint effusions. The instability of the joints gradually leads to osteoarthritis in some patients. Kyphoscoliosis is frequently observed.

The different types of Ehlers–Danlos syndrome are genetically heterogenous. Autosomal dominant, autosomal recessive, and X-linked forms of the disorder have been reported.

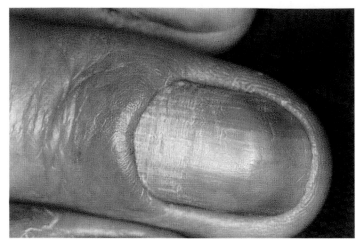

Figure 2-47

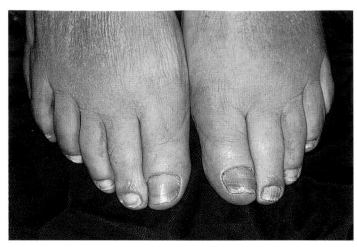

Figure 2-48

The **yellow nail syndrome** is characterized by a triad of yellow nails, lymphedema, and pleural effusion. Thickening and yellow discoloration of the nails is the initial symptom in more than a third of patients, and can affect both the fingernails (Fig. 2-47) and the toenails (Fig. 2-48). The rate of nail growth is slowed, the cuticles are absent, and paronychial infection is common. Eventually, nail abnormalities develop in 90% of those with this syndrome.

The condition has been attributed to hypoplasia or atresia of lymphatics. Peripheral lymphangiograms reveal lymphatics that are dilated and reduced in number. Lymphedema can be shown in 80% of patients and usually affects the legs, although lymphedema of face and breasts has been reported. The lymphedema can vary in severity from very mild to severe, and the resulting swelling can be pitting or nonpitting.

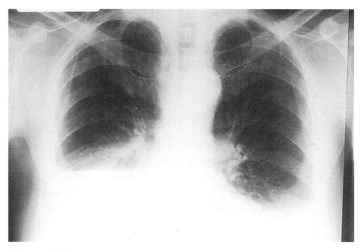

Figure 2-49

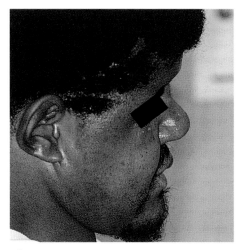

Figure 2-50

Two-thirds of patients have respiratory tract symptoms such as recurrent bronchitis. Bronchiectasis, chronic sinusitis, recurrent pneumonia, and pleuritis have been associated with the yellow nail syndrome. There have also been isolated reports of tuberculosis and pleural empyema in patients with this syndrome. On chest x-ray, pleural effusion can be seen in more than a third of cases (Fig. 2-49).

Yellow nail syndrome has been reported in several patients with thyroid abnormalities including Hashimoto thyroiditis, hypothyroidism, and thyrotoxicosis. It is also reported in patients with hypogammaglobulinemia, nephrotic syndrome, and protein-losing enteropathy. A number of malignancies have been found in patients with this syndrome including, melanoma, carcinoma of the lung, sarcoma of the liver, and adenocarcinoma of the endometrium. Some of these associations are undoubtedly coincidental.

Various topical and mechanical treatments have been attempted for the nail changes in the yellow nail syndrome, but therapy is usually unsatisfactory.

Apert syndrome is a congenital disorder characterized by numerous musculoskeletal abnormalities, respiratory obstruction, and an acneiform eruption. Children may be born with a solid cartilaginous trachea, and may develop inflexibility of the trachea or tracheal stenosis. Combined with skeletal features that reduce the size of the nasopharynx and oropharynx, these changes lead to airway obstruction in most patients with the Apert syndrome. In some instances, early death has resulted. Musculoskeletal abnormalities prominently affect the skull and extremities. Craniosynostosis with markedly dysmorphic facial features are characteristic (Fig. 2-50). Most patients have a cleft soft palate or bifid uvula, and the mouth has a trapezoidal shape. Numerous bones

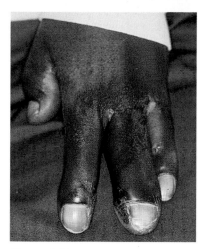

Figure 2-51

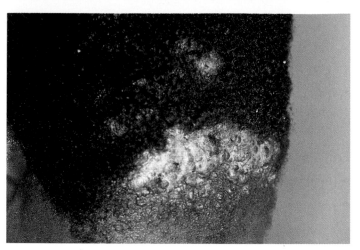

Figure 2-52

and joints are affected, and abnormalities of the hands and feet are characteristic.

Patients have short, but broad, digits. The proximal phalanx is shortened and radially deviated, and the first web space is reduced. The number of digits may be increased or decreased (Fig. 2-51). Other skeletal abnormalities include fusion of the cervical spine and limitation of elbow and shoulder motion. The craniofacial abnormalities can be so deforming that early surgical intervention has been advocated.

Oropharyngeal and upper airway changes, however, may make intubation problematic.

Patients with the **Apert syndrome** develop severe acne and related conditions. The acne can be extensive, involving not only the face, back, and chest, but also the upper arms and forearms. Figure 2-52 shows the posterior neck of a patient with Apert syndrome. The patient has acne nuchae keloidalis, a scarring condition that is associated with acneiform lesions such as follicular pustules.

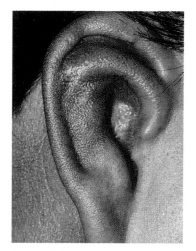

Figure 2-53

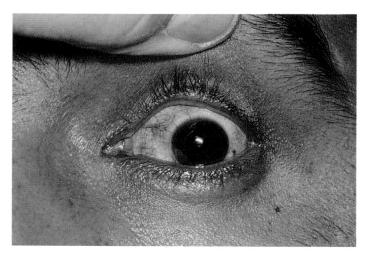

Figure 2-54

Relapsing polychondritis is an autoimmune disorder characterized by episodic inflammation and destruction of cartilaginous tissue. Antibodies to Type II collagen have been found in some, but not all, patients with relapsing polychondritis. The ears, nose, joints, and respiratory tract are commonly affected. The most common manifestation is auricular chondritis characterized by erythema, swelling, and tenderness of the external ears with sparing of the earlobe (Fig. 2-53). Progressive scarring can lead to shriveling of the cartilaginous portions of the ear, or can lead to "cauliflower" ears. Nasal chondritis can similarly result in deformities of the nose. Cutaneous manifestations of this autoimmune disorder can precede episodes of chondritis in some patients or appear concomitantly in others. Skin manifestations include aphthous stomatitis, papules, nodules, sterile pustules, purpura, ulcer-

ations, necrosis, and livedo reticularis. Superficial phlebitis can also occur. Histologic findings are variable but can include neutrophilic infiltrates or leukocytoclastic vasculitis as well as thrombosis of cutaneous vessels. Respiratory tract chondritis can lead to stenosis of airways. Symptoms include hoarseness and shortness of breath. Arthritis is frequent and can be monoarticular or migratory. Cardiovascular complications are fortunately uncommon but can include aortic insufficiency and aortic aneurysm. Ocular manifestations include conjunctivitis, episcleritis, keratitis, and iritis (Fig. 2-54). Exudative retinal detachment and bilateral vitreous hemorrhages have been reported. Relapsing polychondritis has been associated with myelodysplastic syndromes.

3 Cardiovascular diseases

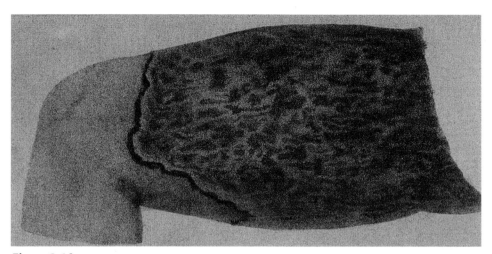

Figure 3-1A

The erythema marginatum occurs in large patches, which are bounded on one side by a hard, elevated, tortuous, red border, in some places obscurely papulated; but have no regular margin on the open side. The duration of the disease is variable, from three to six weeks.

From Bateman T. Delineations of cutaneous diseases. London: Longman; 1817.

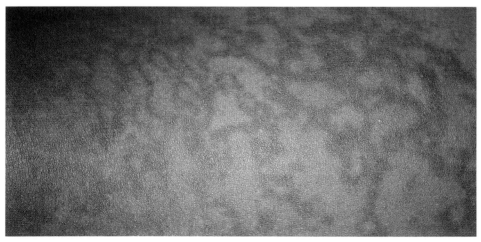

Figure 3-1B

A modern photograph of erythema marginatum, which can occur over large areas and which consists of serpiginous, erythematous patches that are often transient.

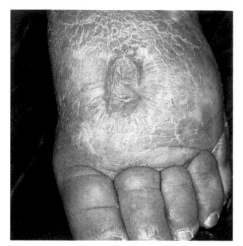

Figure 3-2

Right-sided heart failure can result from a number of conditions, including valvular heart disease, cardiomyopathies, ischemic heart disease, congenital heart disease, and pulmonary hypertension. Patients with left-sided heart failure ultimately also develop right-sided failure along with its cutaneous stigmata. Finally, salt and water retention may result in circulatory congestion even in the absence of heart disease. Regardless of the underlying condition, **peripheral edema** begins in the feet, ankles and lower legs. The accumulation of fluid results in pitting, as demonstrated on the dorsal foot in Figure 3-2. Pressure applied by a single finger results in an indentation in the fluid-congested tissues.

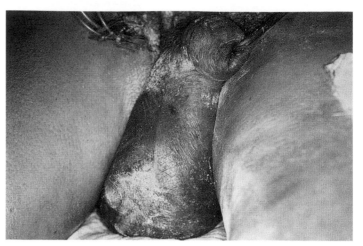

Figure 3-3

With extensive edema, the contour of the skin may take 30 seconds or longer to return to normal.

If edema is chronic, patients develop thickening of the skin with papillomatous changes, especially in flexural creases. These changes are evident on the flexural surface over the anterior aspect of the patient's ankle in Figure 3-2. Leg edema can begin on one side, but it eventually becomes symmetrical. When severe, edema extends up the legs and involves the scrotum (Fig. 3-3). The scrotal skin becomes macerated, and a serous exudate leaks from cutaneous fissures. Peripheral edema is dependent, resulting in more severe symptoms at the end of the day with complete resolution in the morning after bed rest.

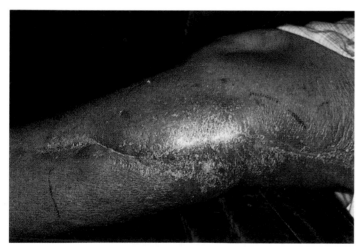

Figure 3-4

Several complications of **cardiac bypass surgery** develop in the skin. In the immediate postoperative period, local infection of the saphenous vein graft scar is frequent. Inflammation develops around the surgical wound on the medial aspect of the leg (Fig. 3-4), especially on the thigh. When mild, there may be simple erythema along the wound edge. With more advanced infection, erythema, tenderness, swelling, and heat are evident. Occasionally, purulent material drains from the wound. High fever and chills result from severe infection. Wound or blood cultures may grow *Staphylococcus aureus* or other Gram-positive or Gram-negative organisms.

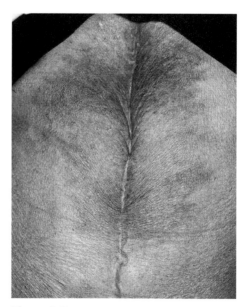

Figure 3-5

Sternal wound infection (Fig. 3-5) occurs in 0.5% of patients who undergo cardiac surgery, including coronary artery bypass surgery. S. *aureus* infection is the most common, but Gram-negative bacilli and other organisms have also been isolated. Osteomyelitis and mediastinitis can result in longer hospitalizations, bacteremia, and even death. Infection increases with diabetes, obesity, and emergency surgery. Infection is also increased in people with large wounds that do not allow primary closure but require flap reconstruction.

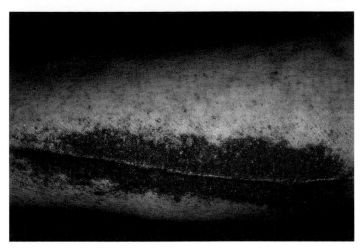

Figure 3-6

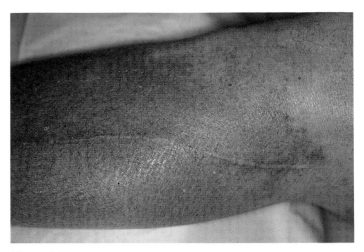

Figure 3-7

Two to six months following coronary bypass surgery, some patients develop an eczematous eruption around the vein graft scar, usually involving the distal half of the scar on the lower leg. This **vein graft dermatitis** is characterized by reddish-brown scales, erythema and fissures (Fig. 3-6) with exudation and crusting in more severe cases. Involved skin can be very pruritic, and excoriations are common. Until the dermatitis develops, skin around the saphenous vein graft scar appears normal, and there is no evidence of preceding skin disease, cellulitis or phlebitis. Vein graft dermatitis responds to treatment with topical steroids but it frequently recurs.

Recurrent cellulitis of the leg may develop many months after bypass surgery. Local inflammation characterized by fiery red erythema, tenderness, and swelling may develop along large portions of the donor graft surgical site (Fig. 3-7). Induration and tenderness can be linear, simulating thrombophlebitis. This postbypass donor site cellulitis may be caused by chronic venous disease, tinea pedis, or vein graft dermatitis that allows entry of pathogenic bacteria. β-Hemolytic streptococci have been cultured from some patients.

Thromboembolic phenomena complicate a number of cardiac conditions, including atrial fibrillation, cardiomyopathy, myocardial

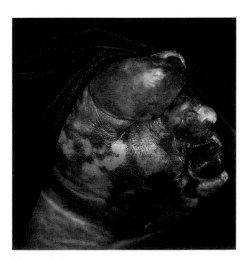

Figure 3-8

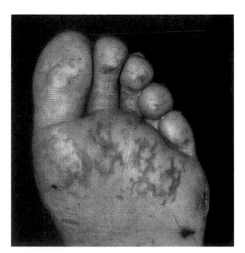

Figure 3-9A

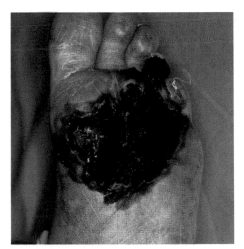

Figure 3-9B

infarction, ventricular aneurysm, and atrial myxoma. When emboli are small, splinter hemorrhages or tender purpuric lesions of the digital pads occur, simulating the cutaneous lesions of endocarditis. Larger arterial emboli result in cold, cyanotic, mottled skin that can become necrotic (Fig. 3-8). In some instances entire limbs become painful, cold, and pulseless.

Cholesterol emboli are rare complications of atherosclerosis. The typical patient has extensive atherosclerotic vascular disease, and the emboli arise from atherosclerotic plaques within arterial lumina. The cholesterol crystals are dislodged either spontaneously or during

procedures such as aortography or surgical correction of aortic aneurysms. Patients usually have normal arterial pulses because these microemboli occlude smaller arterioles. Early lesions often begin with a livedo reticularis-like pattern associated with pain. Not surprisingly, acral areas are typically affected, especially the volar surfaces of the feet. In Figure 3-9A reticulated erythematous and purpuric patches are shown on the sole of a patient after surgical correction of an abdominal aortic aneurysm. This patient went on to develop cutaneous ulceration and necrosis (Fig. 3-9B). Histologic examination of a deep skin biopsy revealed diagnostic cholesterol clefts within arteriolar lumina.

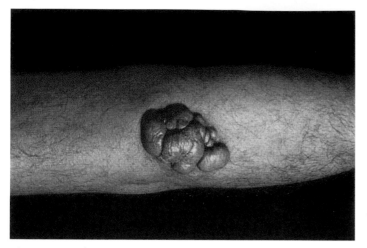

Figure 3-10

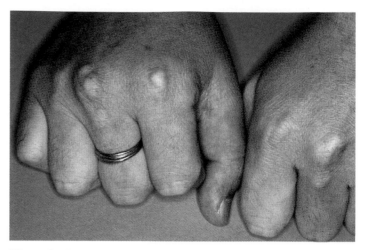

Figure 3-11

Accelerated atherosclerosis is strongly associated with several of the hyperlipoproteinemias. **Xanthomas** result from disorders of lipid metabolism that cause the deposition of lipids in skin, tendons, fascia and periosteum. **Tuberous xanthomas** are among the most dramatic and appear as yellow or red nodules ranging in diameter from a few millimeters to 5 cm or more. They often occur over the extensor surfaces of joints such as the elbow (Fig. 3-10) and on the hands. The nodules result from deposition of lipid in the dermis and subcutaneous tissues, but, unlike tendinous xanthomas, tuberous xanthomas are not attached to underlying tendons. Tuberous xanthomas can occur in other sites, including the trunk, buttocks, and heels. Mucosal surfaces are usually spared. Tuberous xanthomas are not specific; they can develop in patients with hypertriglyceridemia, hypercholesterolemia, or elevations of both lipids. They also occur in association with tendinous

and planar xanthomas and have been reported in patients with primary biliary cirrhosis.

Tendinous xanthomas are somewhat more specific in that they characteristically occur in patients with familial hypercholesterolemia. They are also seen, however, in some patients with Type III hyperlipoproteinemia who have elevations of cholesterol and triglycerides, and in patients with cerebrotendinous xanthomatosis and sitosterolemia. They rarely occur in patients with primary biliary cirrhosis. Heterozygote individuals with familial hypercholesterolemia develop tendinous xanthomas in the third or fourth decade of their lives. Lipid infiltrates the tendon itself, resulting in firm masses over the extensor surfaces of the elbows, ankles, knees, and hands. These masses range from a few millimeters to several centimeters in diameter (Figs 3-11 and 3-12). The Achilles tendons are typically involved (Fig. 3-13). Patients have elevated

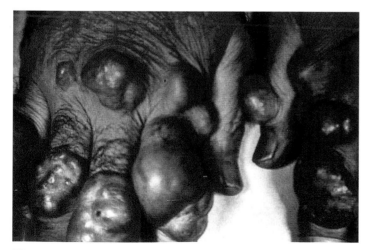

Figure 3-12

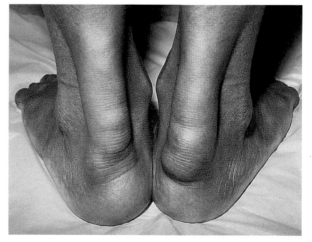

Figure 3-13

plasma cholesterol and low-density lipoprotein (LDL) levels from birth. Accelerated atherosclerosis is common, and myocardial infarctions occur at an early age. More extreme elevations of cholesterol occur in those who are homozygotic for familial hypercholesterolemia with

cholesterol levels above 700 mg/dl. In these patients, tendinous xanthomas can develop in the first decade of life, and death from myocardial infarction often occurs before the third decade.

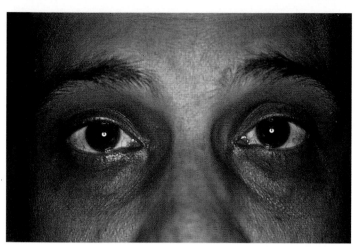

Figure 3-14

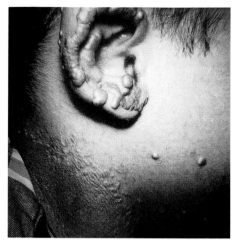

Figure 3-15

Both homozygotes and heterozygotes with familial hypercholesterolemia frequently have eyelid xanthomas that are called **xanthelasma** (Fig. 3-14). These consist of small yellow papules, a few millimeters in diameter, and they involve the upper and lower lids. Adjacent xanthelasma can become confluent to affect the entire eyelid. Xanthelasma are the least specific xanthomas, since plasma lipids are normal in at least 50% of patients with these eyelid lesions. Xanthelasma are also seen in patients with familial hypertriglyceridemia, primary biliary cirrhosis, and multiple myeloma.

Xanthelasma belong to a class of lipid-related lesions known as **planar xanthomas**. These are flat yellow plaques that involve the palms, neck, and chest, as well as the eyelids. Plane xanthomas range in size from one to several centimeters in diameter and can become confluent to cover large areas of skin. They occasionally occur in conjunction with tuberous or tendon xanthomas. When plane xanthomas are large or occur in unusual locations, underlying disorders such as primary biliary cirrhosis or multiple myeloma should be sought. The patient in Figure 3-15 has plane xanthomas of the neck associated with biliary atresia.

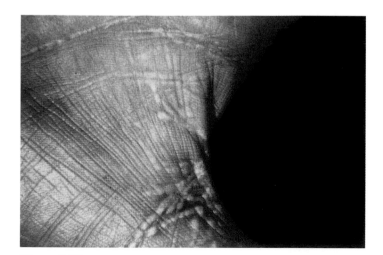

Figure 3-16

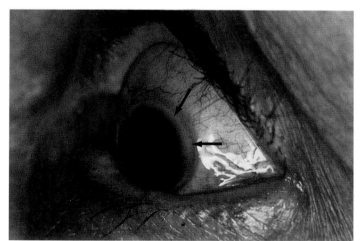

Figure 3-17

Xanthoma striatum palmare refers to plane xanthomas of the palmar creases (Fig. 3-16). Clinically, these xanthomas appear as discrete yellow macules or papules that can become confluent to form linear plaques within the palmar creases. Xanthoma striatum palmare occurs in patients with Type III hyperlipoproteinemia who have elevations of both triglycerides and cholesterol. Affected patients have an increased incidence of accelerated atherosclerotic vascular disease. Plane xanthomas of the palmar creases and the flexural surfaces of the fingers can also occur in patients with primary biliary cirrhosis.

Arcus juvenilis is commonly found in patients who are homozygous or heterozygous for familial hypercholesterolemia. It consists of a white corneal ring that is separated from the limbus by a narrow clear margin of cornea. When an arcus occurs in older patients (Fig. 3-17), it is called arcus senilis and is not necessarily associated with a hyperlipidemia. Similarly, black patients frequently exhibit an arcus in the absence of any disorder of lipid metabolism. In children, however, an arcus juvenilis usually connotes a lipid disorder.

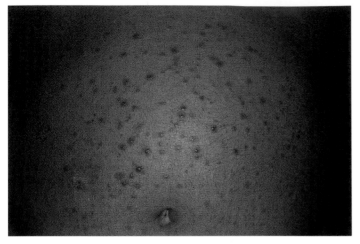

Figure 3-18A

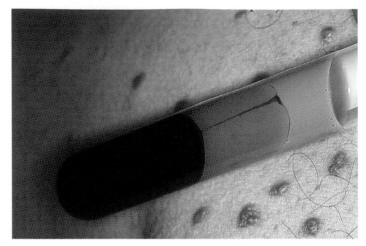

Figure 3-19

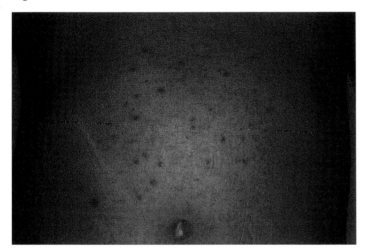

Figure 3-18B

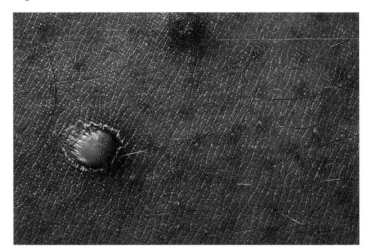

Figure 3-20

Eruptive xanthomas result from sudden increases in plasma triglycerides. They most commonly occur in patients with poorly controlled diabetes mellitus but can occur in any of the lipid disorders associated with **hypertriglyceridemia**. The patient in Figure 3-18A had uncontrolled diabetes mellitus and developed eruptive xanthomas following excessive alcohol consumption. His plasma triglycerides exceeded 2000 mg/dl. These xanthomas consist of small yellow papules on an erythematous base. The papules range in size from 1 mm to several mm in diameter and frequently form on the buttocks, elbows, back, and knees, but they can occur on any cutaneous surface including the oral mucosa. Eruptive xanthomas frequently exhibit the Koebner phenomenon, arising in sites of pressure or trauma. Lesions generally develop when plasma triglycerides exceed 1500 mg/dl, and they may recede with reduction of the triglyceride levels. Figure 3-18B shows a patient in whom many of the lesions disappeared completely with a reduction in triglycerides, although a few erythematous papules persisted. Figure 3-19 shows eruptive xanthomas on the shoulder, and thick creamy serum, in a patient with hypertriglyceridemia.

Eruptive xanthomas involving the ears and toes have been compared to gouty tophi and to pustules. A close-up of a lesion in Figure 3-20 shows their similarity to pustules; but, unlike pustules, one cannot express the white material within eruptive xanthomas. Funduscopic examination of patients with eruptive xanthomas and elevated triglyceride levels reveals

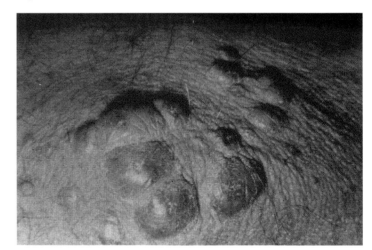

Figure 3-21

lipemia retinalis. Vision is unaffected, but circulating triglycerides give the retinal vessels a pale pink appearance. Lipid accumulation in the liver can result in hepatosplenomegaly and acute abdominal pain. Lowering of the triglycerides causes both pain and hepatosplenomegaly to improve. Acute pancreatitis is also associated with severe hypertriglyceridemia and it can be fatal. If hypertriglyceridemia persists, eruptive xanthomas can enlarge and become confluent, forming **tuboeruptive xanthomas** (Fig. 3-21) that may persist even if the hypertriglyceridemia is reversed.

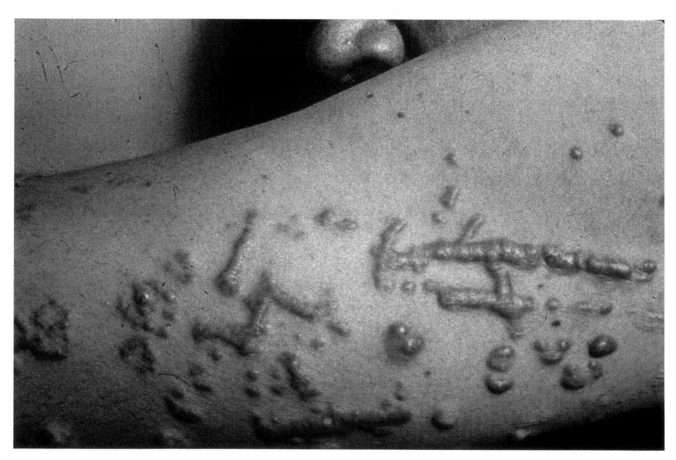

Figure 3-22

A rare, striking case of **xanthoma koebnerization** is shown in Figure 3-22; this patient developed linear xanthomas in excoriated skin.

Table 3.1. Diagnosis of Rheumatic Fever (according to modified Jones criteria) Requires Two Major Criteria, or One Major and Two Minor Criteria with Evidence of a Preceding Streptococcal Infection (throat culture, recent scarlet fever, elevated streptococcal antibodies)

Major criteria
    Carditis
    Polyarthritis
    Chorea
    Subcutaneous nodules
    Erythema marginatum
Minor criteria
    Fever
    Arthralgia
    Previous rheumatic fever or rheumatic heart disease

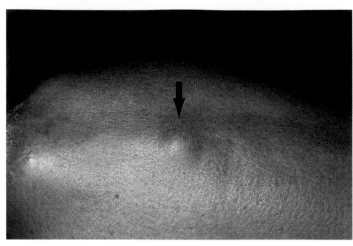

Figure 3-23

Rheumatic fever results from pharyngeal infection with group A streptococci. Depending on the virulence and "rheumatogenic" potential of the streptococcal strain, up to 3% of patients develop signs of rheumatic fever days or weeks after the acute infection. No laboratory test is specific for this disorder; thus, diagnosis depends on a combination of clinical criteria (Table 3-1). The major criteria for the diagnosis of rheumatic fever can be remembered with the acronym ACCNE (*a*rthritis, *c*arditis, *c*horea, *n*odules, *e*rythema marginatum), a useful misspelling of "acne." Acute migratory polyarthritis most commonly affects the large joints of the extremities. Joint effusions and pain are self-limited. The most severe and permanent complications of rheumatic fever involve the heart. Rheumatic carditis is manifested by new heart murmurs, congestive heart failure, or pericarditis. The acute carditis may be so severe that death from congestive heart failure results; or so mild that it is overlooked. Even in patients with mild carditis, permanent valvular damage can become apparent years later. Regurgitation or stenosis of the heart valves eventually results, most commonly affecting the mitral and aortic valves. Chorea reflects central

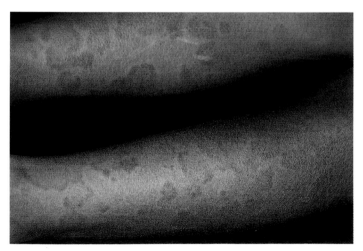

Figure 3-24

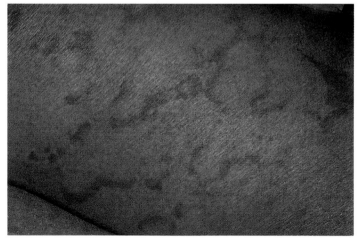

Figure 3-25

nervous system disease and is characterized by irregular, purposeless movements. It is one of the least common manifestations of rheumatic fever. Subcutaneous nodules are nontender, pea-sized, and freely moveable and usually found on the extensor surfaces of the elbows, hands, or feet or over other bones. Nodules are more palpable than they are visible, but as Figure 3-23 shows they can occasionally be seen.

Erythema marginatum, the rash of rheumatic fever, is characterized by faint erythematous macules or urticarial papules that enlarge to form annular patches with round or serpiginous borders and central clearing. When multiple lesions are present, a polycyclic pattern occurs (Fig. 3-24 and 3-25).

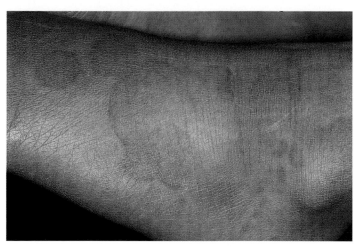

Figure 3-26

Table 3-2. Diagnostic Outlines for Kawasaki Disease
Fever of 5 days or more without other explanation and at least four of the five following criteria[a]
Polymorphic exanthema
Changes of peripheral extremities
Acute phase: erythema and/or indurative edema of the palms and soles
Convalescent phase: desquamation from finger tips
Bilateral nonexudative conjunctival injection
Changes in the oropharynx: injected or fissured lips; "strawberry tongue", injected pharynx
Acute nonsuppurative cervical lymphadenopathy (> 1.5 cm in diameter)

From the Centers for Disease Control 1985.
[a] Patients with fewer than four of these signs can be diagnosed as atypical Kawasaki disease if coronary artery abnormalities are present.

Characteristic lesions of **erythema marginatum** often develop over affected joints, as shown on a patient's ankle in Figure 3-26. The lesions can be evanescent, lasting from a few hours to days.

Kawasaki disease, also called mucocutaneous lymph node syndrome, is a recently described disorder that affects children. Almost all those affected are under the age of 5 years and most are under 3 years. The condition is rare in children above the age of 8 years. It is thought that some individuals are genetically predisposed to Kawasaki disease, and its incidence is greater in Japanese people. One group of inves-

tigators has suggested that the toxin-secreting *S. aureus* that causes toxic shock syndrome also plays a role in this disorder. In the absence of a specific laboratory test for Kawasaki disease, diagnosis depends upon a number of clinical criteria (Table 3-2). Fever is the first sign and should be present for at least 5 days before a diagnosis of Kawasaki disease is considered. High fever, typically around 40°C, starts abruptly. The temperature elevation does not respond to antibiotics and often lasts 10–14 days but can be present for several weeks. Striking erythema of the palms and soles associated with swelling of the hands and feet

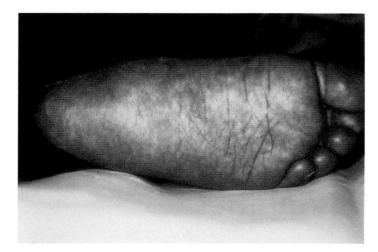

Figure 3-27

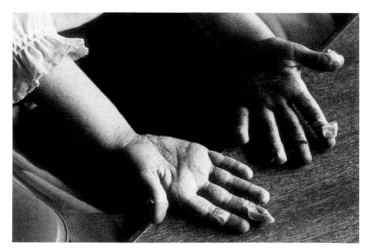

Figure 3-28

(Fig. 3-27) occurs in more than 75% of patients. Children may complain of pain on walking, and infants' shoes may suddenly not fit. Swelling and erythema gradually subside as the temperature declines. Desquamation of the hands and feet follows, beginning approximately

2–3 weeks after the first symptoms of the disorder. The skin of the palms and soles peels off in large thick pieces (Fig. 3-28), and this pattern of desquamation is one of the most characteristic features of Kawasaki disease.

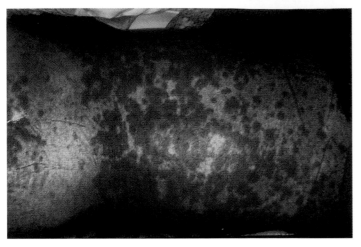

Figure 3-29

More than 90% of patients with Kawasaki disease develop a rash that can be variable in appearance. The rash often begins after 3–5 days of fever and is usually generalized and erythematous (Fig. 3-29). Papular, pustular, urticarial (Fig. 3-30) and erythema multiforme-like skin

Figure 3-30

lesions can occur. Diffuse erythema similar to that seen in scarlet fever has been described and consists of 1–2-mm papules. In flexural areas purpuric lesions resembling Pastia's lines of scarlet fever have also been reported.

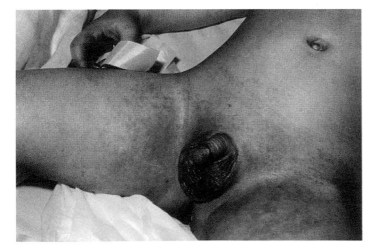

Figure 3-31

Although the exanthema of **Kawasaki disease** can be variable, peri-anal and scrotal erythema and desquamation (Fig. 3-31) are characteristic; occasionally the rash is limited to the diaper area.

More than 90% of patients with Kawasaki disease have oral mucosal abnormalities. The lips are often red, swollen, fissured, and covered with crusts (Fig. 3-32). Erythema of the oropharyngeal mucosa is common,

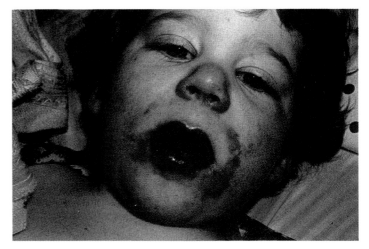

Figure 3-32

and occasionally small ulcerations form. Lingual swelling with hypertrophy of the lingual papillae occurs in many patients, and a white coating of the tongue develops. A strawberry tongue likened to that seen in scarlet fever may necessitate differentiation of the two disorders. Unlike scarlet fever, patients with Kawasaki disease have conjunctivitis, peripheral edema, and inflammation of the lips, and they do not have a group A β-hemolytic streptococcal throat infection.

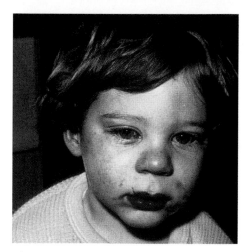

Figure 3-33

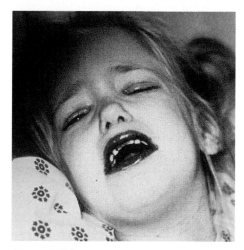

Figure 3-34

Bilateral conjunctival injection occurs in almost all patients (Fig. 3-33). Lids are not swollen, and usually there is no exudate, but the conjunctival vessels are enlarged. Uveitis can be seen on slit-lamp examination, and patients may complain of sensitivity to light. Enlargement of lymph nodes occurs in up to 75% of patients and usually involves a solitary cervical node that is nontender, firm, and at least 1.5 cm in diameter. Less commonly, nodes can be multiple, tender and can occur in the supraclavicular or axillary areas. Affected children are ill-appearing, and lethargic or irritable (Fig. 3-34).

Cardiac complications are responsible for a mortality rate of up to 2% with two-thirds of deaths occurring within 7 weeks of the onset of fever. The majority of patients show abnormalities during electrocardiography or echocardiography, although most are asymptomatic.

Coronary artery occlusion and myocardial infarction have occurred up to 14 months after the onset of Kawasaki disease. More commonly, aneurysms of the coronary arteries, as well as iliac, femoral, or hepatic arterial aneurysms have been reported. Cardiac arrhythmias and inverted T-waves are found by electrocardiography in patients with myocarditis. Pericardial effusion is common. Arrhythmias, cardiac valvular disease, and rupture of coronary aneurysms can be fatal.

Thrombocytosis, the solitary characteristic laboratory abnormality of Kawasaki disease, is not apparent at first; but over 2 weeks the platelet count usually increases to more than 1 000 000 per microliter. Other abnormalities have been described, including aseptic meningitis, cranial nerve palsy, hepatitis, pancreatitis, and hydrops of the gallbladder. Treatment with intravenous gamma globulin together with aspirin may be beneficial.

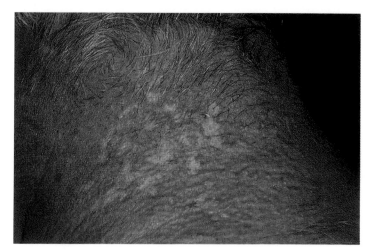

Figure 3-35

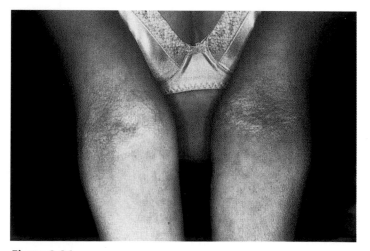

Figure 3-36

Pseudoxanthoma elasticum, an inherited disease of elastic tissue, is associated with numerous systemic manifestations, including significant cardiovascular complications. While autosomal dominant and autosomal recessive inheritance patterns have been described, mutations in an ABCC transporter protein have been identified, demonstrating autosomal recessive inheritance. Mildly affected individuals

may be asymptomatic, and the diagnosis can easily be missed; ophthalmologic and dermatological examination of family members is therefore crucial. Skin lesions primarily involve flexural areas, the most frequent sites being the neck, axillae, antecubital and popliteal fossae, and periumbilical area. Lesions begin as yellow papules (Fig. 3-35) that gradually enlarge and become confluent to form plaques (Fig. 3-36) or,

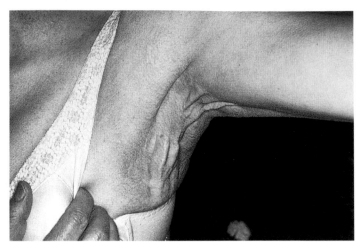

Figure 3-37

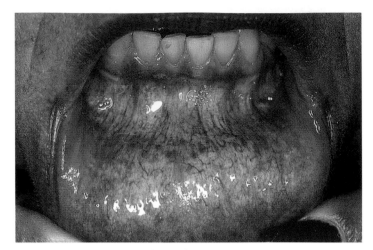

Figure 3-38

in severe cases, redundant folds of skin (Figs 3-37). The yellow color of the skin lesions resembles that of xanthomas, and the lesions have been likened to plucked chicken skin.

The complications of pseudoxanthoma elasticum are related to calcification of elastic tissue in various organs. Calcification of the internal elastic lamina of the coronary arteries results in a clinical picture simulating accelerated atherosclerosis. Typical exertional angina can occur at an early age, and myocardial infarctions have been reported in adolescents. A diagnosis of pseudoxanthoma elasticum should be considered in any patient who presents with signs of accelerated arteriosclerosis without any other risk factors for early heart disease.

Calcification of arteries can be seen on radiographs in pseudoxanthoma elasticum, and patients may have diminished peripheral pulses. Intermittent claudication is a common complaint. Calcification

and degeneration of elastic fibers in the heart valves can result in a number of cardiac valve abnormalities, including mitral valve prolapse. Because endocarditis has occurred in pseudoxanthoma elasticum, antibiotic prophylaxis before dental procedures has been recommended for patients with evidence of abnormal heart valves. A restrictive cardiomyopathy has been reported, and renal artery calcification in this disorder has been associated with hypertension.

Mucous membrane involvement is common in pseudoxanthoma elasticum, and yellow papules are frequently seen on the mucosal aspect of the lips and under the tongue (Fig. 3-38).

A characteristic horizontal crease associated with deep lines often develops on the chin in patients with pseudoxanthoma elasticum (Fig. 3-39). Similar changes can occur in older individuals without this disorder but are seldom seen under the age of 50 years, except in

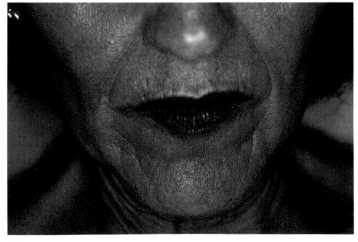

Figure 3-39

patients with pseudoxanthoma elasticum who frequently develop this sign early—in their 30s or 40s.

Biopsy of skin or mucosal lesions reveals fragmentation and clumping of elastic tissue in the middle and deep dermis in **pseudoxanthoma elasticum**. These changes are readily seen with elastic tissue Verhoeff–van Gieson stains (Fig. 3-40A), and calcification of the middle and deep dermis can be shown by the von Kossa stain (Fig. 3-40B). Using these stains, calcification and fragmentation of the internal elastic

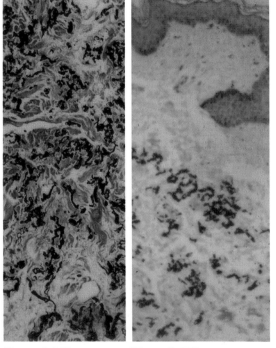

Figure 3-40A   **Figure 3-40B**

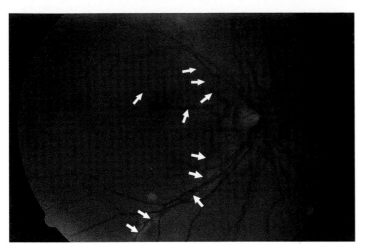

Figure 3-41

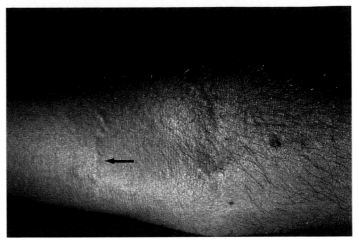

Figure 3-42

lamina of arteries can be shown in many tissues. There have been numerous reports of gastrointestinal bleeding, as well as bleeding from the uterus, bladder, and nose in patients with pseudoxanthoma elasticum. Hemarthroses have also occurred. The bleeding diathesis seen in patients with pseudoxanthoma elasticum has been attributed to calcification and subsequent cracking of arteries. Because of the bleeding diathesis, avoidance of platelet inhibitors such as aspirin has been advocated. In patients with gastrointestinal bleeding, endoscopic examination may reveal yellow xanthoma-like papules on mucosal surfaces, but sources of bleeding are often not apparent. Because of reports of uterine and gastrointestinal bleeding during pregnancy, it has been suggested that estrogens have a deleterious effect in patients with pseudoxanthoma elasticum. Most women with the disorder have uncomplicated pregnancies, however, and the role of estrogens remains unclear. Despite all of the reported complications of pseudoxanthoma elasticum, most patients have relatively normal lifespans.

One of the most common and most severe complications of pseudoxanthoma elasticum affects the eyes. On fundoscopic examination almost all adults have **angioid streaks** (Fig. 3-41), which represent breaks in Bruch's membrane, an elastic tissue-containing membrane behind the retina. Retinal bleeding and loss of vision are unfortunately common occurrences.

Patients with pseudoxanthoma elasticum can develop characteristic skin lesions in scars, the so-called Koebner phenomenon (Fig. 3-42). In patients who have angioid streaks but do not have clinically apparent skin involvement, diagnosis can occasionally be made by biopsy of normal-appearing flexural skin or scar.

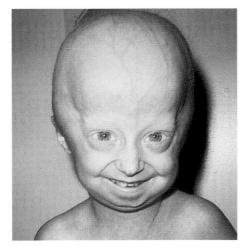

Figure 3-43

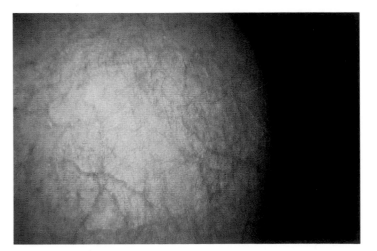

Figure 3-44

Progeria, also known as Hutchinson–Gilford syndrome, is a rare genetic disease of unclear inheritance pattern. The condition is found in many ethnic groups and is estimated to affect approximately 1 in 4 000 000 births. Abnormalities occur in the skin, bones, and cardiovascular system. Intelligence and emotions are normal. Most patients develop accelerated atherosclerosis, which leads to death between the ages of 10 and 15 years, although a few have survived into early adulthood.

Distinctive facial features allow clinical diagnosis at an early age (Fig. 3-43). The cranium is normal in size but appears large because of hypoplasia of the facial bones, short stature, and thin limbs. Patients often have micrognathia and a thin, beaked nose.

Features of accelerated aging affect both the skin and internal organs. Thinning of the skin with reduced subcutaneous fat is associated with premature wrinkling. Alopecia of the scalp begins in infancy, and prominent scalp veins are frequently visible (Fig. 3-44). Pubic and

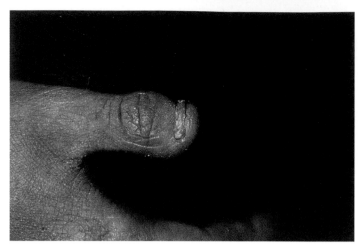

Figure 3-45

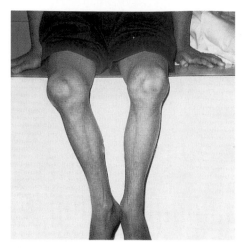

Figure 3-46

axillary hair is often sparse or absent in older patients. Facial hair, eyebrows, and eyelashes are lost as well. Thinning of the nails occurs later in life.

Bone abnormalities are prominent in this disorder, and patients can repeatedly develop fractures that do not heal. Resorption of the mandible and loss of teeth can occur in patients who live beyond adolescence. Early in life delayed cranial suture closure is characteristic. Later, osteolysis of the distal phalanges of the fingers and toes develops (Fig. 3-45). On radiographic examination, there is bone resorption of the distal ends of the clavicles. Linear lucent defects of the metaphyses, fish-mouth vertebral bodies, and general osteopenia occur as well.

Scleroderma-like skin changes are found in many children with progeria and can be present at birth. Characteristic thick, tight skin can be found on the lower abdomen, buttocks, and thighs. There is loss of muscle mass, resulting in thin limbs, but the knees and elbows are prominent (Fig. 3-46).

Other reported abnormalities include kyphosis of the thorax, a high-pitched voice due to a narrow glottic opening, hypoplastic nipples, and

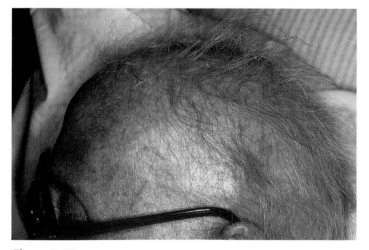

Figure 3-47

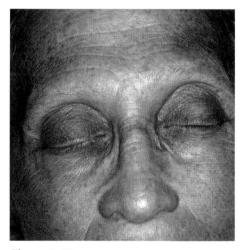

Figure 3-48

delayed sexual development. The only reported laboratory abnormality is increased urinary hyaluronic acid.

Werner syndrome resembles progeria in that it is associated with accelerated aging and scleroderma-like skin changes. Most reported cases are autosomal recessively inherited, and the incidence has been estimated to be approximately 1 in 500 000. Hair-graying occurs before the age of 20 years and alopecia often starts before the age of 25 (Fig. 3-47). Early loss of hair is not limited to the scalp but also affects body hair, including axillary and pubic hair, and the eyebrows (Fig. 3-48). Shortness of stature, bilateral juvenile cataracts, hypogonadism, and diabetes are characteristics of this syndrome. Soft-tissue calcification occurs and often involves the heart valves as well as tendons, ligaments and other tissues.

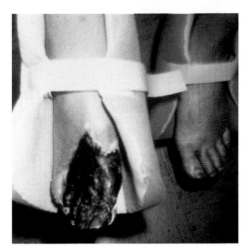

Figure 3-49

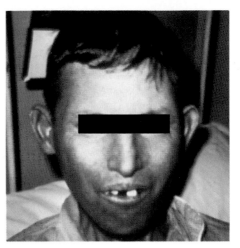

Figure 3-50

Vascular calcification in **Werner syndrome** can lead to vessel occlusion and infarction, as occurred on the foot of the patient shown in Figure 3-49. Coronary artery involvement frequently intervenes, although most patients live to adulthood. Skin atrophy and loss of subcutaneous fat is common. Leg ulcers characteristically develop over the heels, malleoli, Achilles tendons, and toes. Osteoporosis and characteristic osteosclerotic changes in the phalanges of the hands and feet are frequent, and periarticular calcification can

occur. Congenital absence of the tibiae and of the thumbs with polydactyly has been reported. There is an increased incidence of malignancy in people with Werner syndrome; cancers of the breast, liver, ovary, thyroid, and stomach have been reported, as has malignant melanoma, meningioma, and astrocytoma. The facial appearance of patients with Werner syndrome is not as characteristic as that of progeria, but a beaked nose and abnormal dentition are typical (Fig. 3-50).

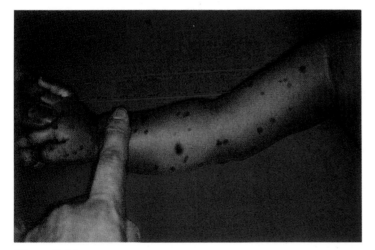

Figure 3-51

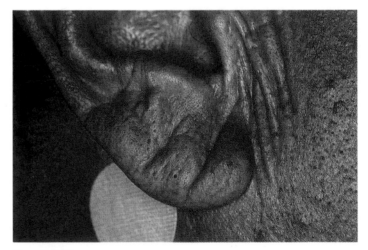

Figure 3-52

Leopard syndrome, also called lentiginosis profusa, is an autosomal dominantly inherited condition with variable expressivity. It is characterized by the presence of numerous lentigines, a few millimeters to several centimeters in diameter, on the face, neck, trunk, and extremities (Fig. 3-51). The mucous membranes are not involved. Cardiac conduction defects, subaortic stenosis, pulmonary stenosis, and electrocardiographic abnormalities that may simulate myocardial infarction can occur. The name Leopard syndrome is an acronym for the features of this disorder: *l*entigines, *e*lectrocardiograph abnormalities, *o*cular hypertelorism, *p*ulmonary stenosis, *a*bnormal genitalia, *r*etardation of growth, and *d*eafness. There have been several deaths from obstructive cardiomyopathy.

A discussion of the cutaneous manifestations of cardiovascular disease would not be complete without mention of the **ear-lobe crease**. The presence of a diagonal ear-lobe crease (Fig. 3-52) has been associated with coronary artery disease in some studies, but not in others. Some of these studies found that the association with coronary heart disease is independent of other cardiac risk factors including gender, hypercholesterolemia, smoking, and hypertension. The presence of ear-canal hair has also been associated with coronary disease. Since the prevalence of creases on the ear lobe increases with age, the specificity of this controversial sign has been questioned. Its usefulness as a predictor of coronary heart disease remains to be firmly established.

4 Gastrointestinal diseases

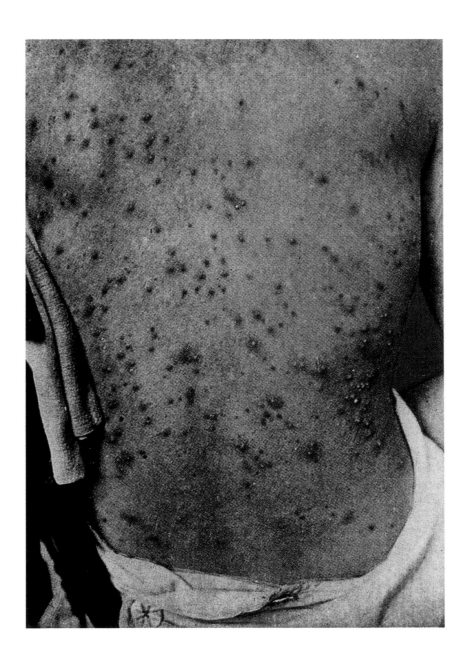

Figure 4-1

Dermatitis herpetiformis is a chronic inflammatory disease characterized by the multiformity of its lesions and the tendency of the eruption to recur and vary in form…Itching which is always severe may be present before the eruption. The lesions appear gradually or slowly over small or large areas or scattered over the greater part of the body surface. They have no predilection for any particular region but exhibit a marked tendency to appear in groups…The vesicles vary from pin head to pea size though blebs larger than cherries are exceptional.

From Rainforth SI. The stereoscopic skin clinic. New York: Medical Art Publishing; 1911.

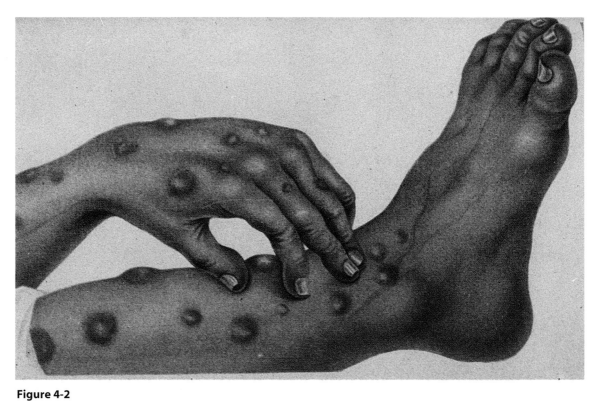

Figure 4-2

Erythema nodosum.
From Kaposi M. Handatlas der Hautkrankheiten für Studirende und Arzte. Vienna and Leipzig; 1898–1900.

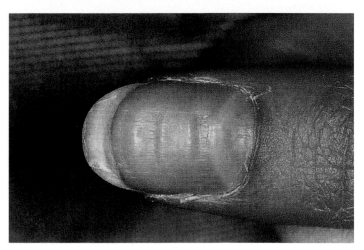

Figure 4-3

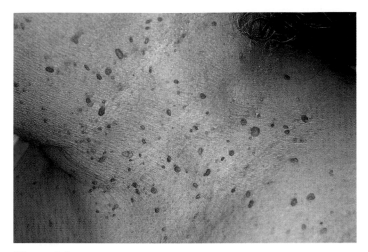

Figure 4-4

A number of nonspecific cutaneous manifestations are occasionally associated with gastrointestinal diseases. **Beau's lines** of the nails, for example, can occur weeks after episodes of acute gastrointestinal bleeding just as they can develop after any extreme physical stress. The patient in Figure 4-3 developed parallel horizontal ridges of several fingernails following two episodes of hematemesis and melena. These horizontal depressions in the nail plate grew out over several months.

Acrochordons, also called skin tags (Fig. 4-4), are common cutaneous lesions that have been associated with pregnancy and obesity. These skin-colored or pigmented papules are pedunculated and usually occur in flexural or intertriginous areas, including the neck, axillae, and medial aspects of the thighs. Several reports have correlated the presence of acrochordons with an increased incidence of adenomatous polyps of the colon, but this association is controversial.

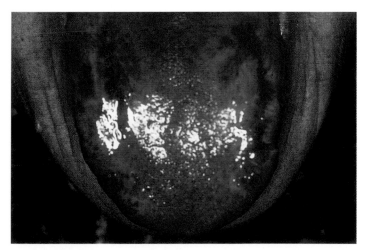

Figure 4-5A

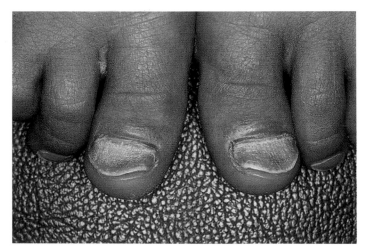

Figure 4-6

The dermatological stigmata of iron deficiency anemia (koilonychia, glossitis, and cutaneous pallor) commonly result from gastrointestinal bleeding, although dietary causes and chronic blood loss of any etiology will cause the same symptoms. **Glossitis** (Fig. 4-5A), manifested by papillary atrophy and pain and burning of the tongue, results from deficiencies of B complex vitamins and folic acid, as well as iron. Additional cutaneous signs of malabsorption occur as a result of celiac sprue or any other disorder that interferes with intestinal absorption. **Angular stomatitis** (Fig. 4-5B), characterized by fissures and crusts at the oral commissures, is a manifestation of vitamin B_2 (riboflavin) deficiency, but more commonly occurs as a result of excessive licking or monilial infection. Other nonspecific cutaneous features of malabsorption include dry skin, hair fragility, and impairment of hair and nail growth.

Koilonychia is the term for spoon-shaped nails (Fig. 4-6). It is another manifestation of iron deficiency that can also occur as a normal variant.

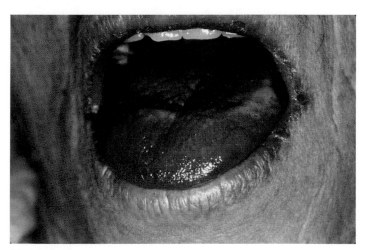

Figure 4-5B

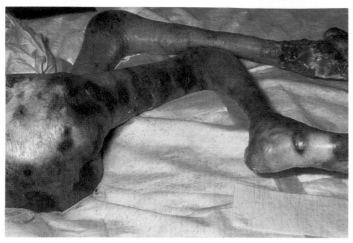

Figure 4-7

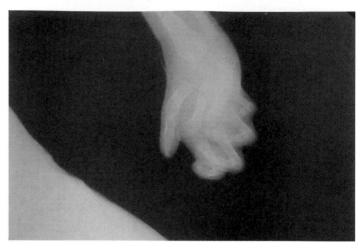

Figure 4-8

The term **epidermolysis bullosa** (**EB**) includes a group of diseases characterized by bulla formation. At least 16 types of EB have been described, including autosomal dominant and autosomal recessive forms of the disease, and an acquired form that does not have a genetic basis. The types are further subdivided into scarring (dystrophic) and nonscarring (simplex) forms.

One of the most severe forms of the disease is **recessive dystrophic epidermolysis bullosa**. Blisters are noted at birth, or shortly thereafter, and continue to occur throughout life. Sites of pressure, friction, or trauma are most commonly involved, and rupture of bullae may leave painful erosions and large areas of denuded skin (Fig. 4-7). Recurrent blistering and scarring typically occurs on the hands and feet, resulting in flexion contractures, shown in the x-ray of a hand in Figure 4-8.

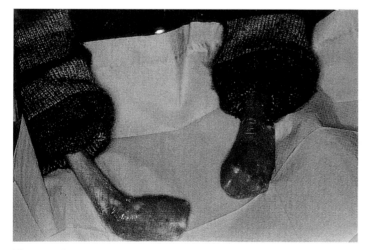

Figure 4-9

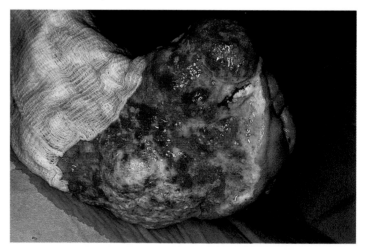

Figure 4-10

Patients develop characteristic mitten-like hands (Fig. 4-9) caused by pseudofusion of the digits (**pseudosyndactyly**). Nail-bed involvement frequently occurs. Fingernails are often severely dystrophic or absent. Scarring can be severe, and metastasizing squamous cell carcinomas can arise in the scars. Figure 4-10 shows a huge squamous cell carcinoma of the foot in a patient with recessive dystrophic EB.

Involvement of the gastrointestinal tract also occurs primarily in patients with the recessive dystrophic form of EB. Gastrointestinal symptoms often begin with complaints of **dysphagia** or odynophagia in childhood. Mucosal bullae of the esophagus can be caused by ingestion

of coarse food or can arise spontaneously. Dysphagia can improve with healing of bullae, but scarring and stricture formation often follow. Strictures generally involve the upper third of the esophagus and range in length from 2–70 mm. Esophageal dilatation can result in further progression of the strictures. Malignant degeneration can occur and metastatic **squamous cell carcinoma of the esophagus** is a leading cause of death. Perianal lesions cause pain on defecation, and constipation is another common complaint. Liquid or puréed diets are often prescribed to minimize esophageal trauma, but these may exacerbate the constipation.

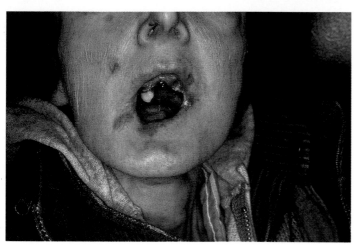

Figure 4-11

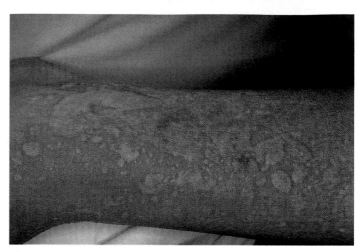

Figure 4-12

Oral involvement in recessive dystrophic EB includes dental caries and malformation of the teeth. Tooth-brushing unfortunately leads to intraoral bulla formation, and repeated intraoral scarring can prevent patients from opening the mouth widely (Fig. 4-11) and can cause difficulty with mastication.

Dominant dystrophic epidermolysis bullosa has far milder clinical manifestations than the recessive dystrophic type, and several forms exist. One of these is a form which heals with hypertrophic scars (Cockayne–Touraine variant) and one is characterized by the development of white papules (Pasini "albopapuloid" variant) (Fig. 4-12). Bullae are occasionally present at birth, but may develop

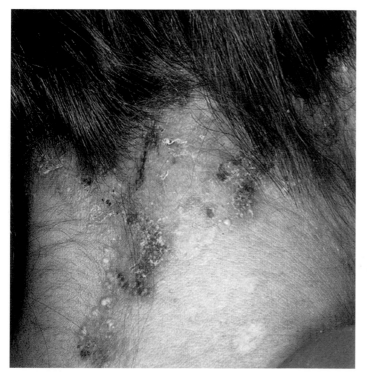

Figure 4-13

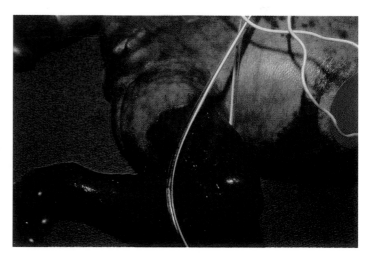

Figure 4-14

later in life. Bullae sometimes develop on the elbows and knees when an infant begins to crawl. There can be scarring and milium formation (white pinpoint epidermoid cysts) (Fig. 4-13).

Junctional epidermolysis bullosa (also called Herlitz disease or epidermolysis bullosa letalis) is a frequently fatal form of EB that is inherited in an autosomal recessive pattern. Skin lesions are almost always present at birth and large areas of sloughing and denuded skin are characteristic. Almost any area of skin can be affected but leg and scalp involvement is common. Perioral lesions with sparing of the lips

are said to be pathognomonic of junctional EB. Large areas of denuded skin can lead to fluid loss, electrolyte abnormalities, and sepsis, and approximately 50% of infants with junctional EB die by the age of 2 years. Above that age the condition can improve, resulting in a milder, chronic blistering, nonscarring eruption. Figure 4-14 shows extensive denudation of the leg in an infant with junctional EB. Pyloric and duodenal stenosis and atresia, presumably due to mucosal bulla formation and scarring, have been described in junctional EB and recessive dystrophic EB.

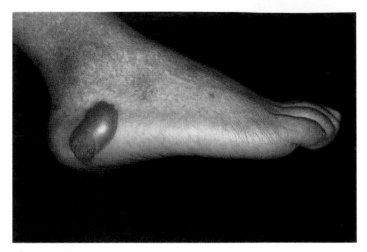

Figure 4-15

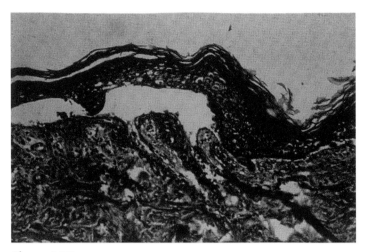

Figure 4-16

Epidermolysis bullosa simplex is an autosomal dominant condition that has much milder clinical manifestations than recessive dystrophic EB. Bullae and erosions develop at sites of trauma or rubbing and the extremities are prominently involved (Fig. 4-15). Mucous membranes are rarely affected, and nail involvement occurs in only 20% of patients. The condition gradually improves with age, and lesions are usually limited to the hands and feet in children of 3 years or more. Clinically significant gastrointestinal involvement does not occur with this form of EB.

Differentiation between the various types of EB depends upon identification of the level of cleavage that results in bulla formation (Fig. 4-16). Electron microscopy or immunofluorescent mapping may be helpful in delineating the site of cleavage. Separation of the dermis from the epidermis below the basal lamina is typically seen in dystrophic forms of EB.

Junctional EB, as the name implies, results from separation at the dermal–epidermal junction. Electron microscopy shows separation between the plasma membrane of basal cells and the basal lamina. Hemidesmosomes are abnormal and reduced in number in junctional EB. In EB simplex, cleavage occurs in the epidermis within or above the level of the basal keratinocytes.

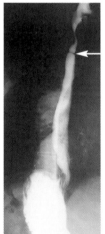

Figure 4-17

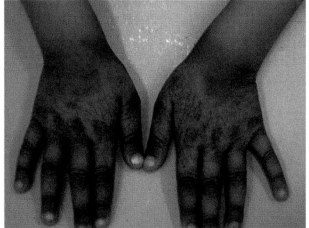

Figure 4-18A

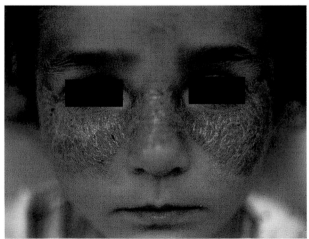

Figure 4-18B

The **Plummer–Vinson syndrome** is a condition characterized by dysphagia associated with iron deficiency anemia. Koilonychia, glossitis, and angular stomatitis occur. The cutaneous lesions are reversible with iron supplementation, which corrects the dysphagia as well. Dysphagia has been attributed to esophageal spasm, which can lead to irreversible anatomic changes. On esophagram, a postcricoid web appears with swallowing (Fig. 4-17). The web begins as a fold of normal mucosa that extends into the esophageal lumen. Strictures are occasionally seen near the web, and squamous cell carcinoma can develop in the postcricoid area after some years. Iron replacement can result in disappearance of the web and relief of dysphagia.

Hartnup disease is a rare autosomal recessive disorder that results from defective transport of tryptophan and other neutral amino acids by jejunal mucosa and renal tubules. It is associated with mental retardation, seizures, and intermittent cerebellar ataxia due to neuronal degeneration and cerebral demyelination. Some patients present with a normal IQ, with normal growth, and few neurologic symptoms. Skin lesions consistent of a photosensitivity reaction similar to pellagra. Sharply demarcated, hyperpigmented patches are characteristic (Fig. 4-18A and Fig. 4-18B).

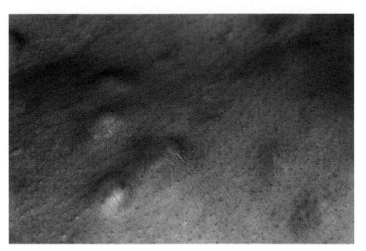

Figure 4-19

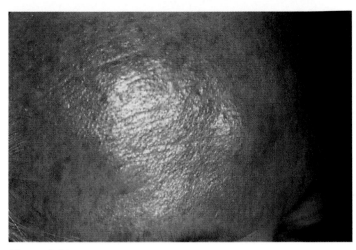

Figure 4-20

Gardner syndrome is an autosomal dominantly inherited disorder characterized by the development of premalignant polyps of the colon and rectum. Malignant degeneration of colonic polyps occurs in approximately 50% of patients. Colectomy is advised for affected patients, but gastric and small intestinal polyps can develop that also carry a small risk of malignancy.

Cutaneous lesions include epidermoid cysts (formerly called "sebaceous cysts") that are present at birth or develop early in life. They can be large, often occurring on the face, but they can also be found on the trunk and extremities.

The patient in Figure 4-19 had multiple epidermoid cysts on the chest. Osseous abnormalities consist primarily of osteomas (Fig. 4-20), benign bony tumors that may be visible or palpable. Irregular cortical thickening is common, as are dental lesions, including odontomas, rudimentary or supernumerary teeth, unerupted teeth, and dentigerous cysts. Desmoid tumors result from fibroblast proliferation in surgical scars. Fibromas can arise in the skin, the subcutaneous tissue, or abdominal cavity.

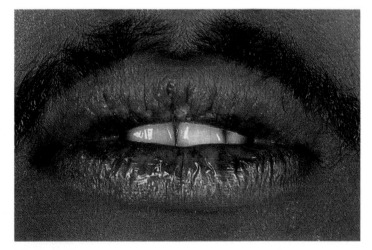

Figure 4-21

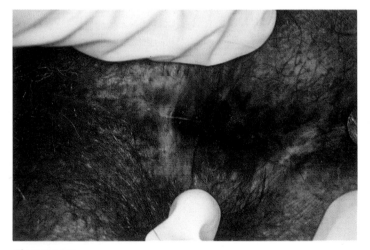

Figure 4-22

Peutz–Jeghers syndrome is another autosomal dominantly inherited condition associated with intestinal polyposis. Small intestinal polyps are characteristic, but some patients also develop large bowel and stomach polyps. Polyps of the bladder, bronchus, esophagus, mouth, maxillary sinus, and nasal mucosa have also been reported. Although the polyps are thought to be hamartomas, approximately 5% of patients with this syndrome develop gastrointestinal malignancies, most commonly in the small intestine. Ovarian tumors can occur as well.

Skin lesions are characterized by the development of pigmented macules that most commonly involve the lips and oral mucosa (Fig. 4-21). The macules range from 1–10 mm in diameter and can be associated with pigmentation of the fingers and toes, palms and soles, and the perioral, perinasal, and rectal areas. Pigmented macules of the perianal mucosa are shown in Figure 4-22.

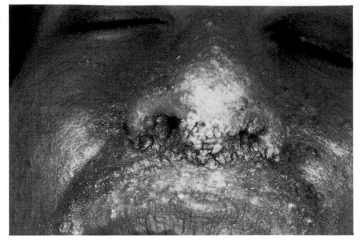

Figure 4-23

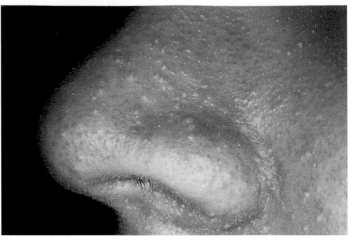

Figure 4-24

Cowden disease, also known as multiple hamartoma syndrome, is a genodermatosis associated with the development of gastrointestinal tract polyps. Fewer than 200 cases have been reported. However, the most characteristic features of the disease are cutaneous lesions that are easily overlooked. This autosomal dominant inherited disorder may therefore be more common than the small number of case reports suggests.

Cutaneous lesions are characterized by 1–3 mm skin-colored papules that most commonly occur on the face, especially on and around the nose, mouth, and ears. Lesions can be extensive (Fig. 4-23) or so mild that they are easily overlooked or mistaken for acne (Fig. 4-24). Neck lesions are also common. The patient in Figure 4-25 initially presented with a brown patch of acanthosis nigricans on the posterior neck, but further examination also revealed numerous skin-colored papules on the face and neck.

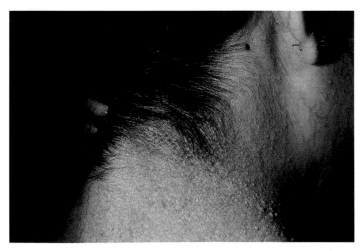

Figure 4-25

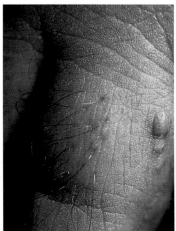

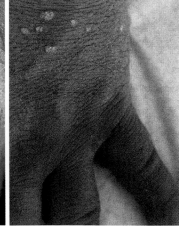

Figure 4-26A   **Figure 4-26B**

Clinically, the differential diagnosis of these lesions includes warts, syringomas, adenoma sebaceum, and trichoepitheliomas. Histologically, the papules are thought by some to be distinctive and are called **trichilemmomas**, but others have noted a similarity to verrucae vulgaris (warts). Occasionally slightly larger lesions occur on the forearms and on the dorsa of the hands and feet.

The surface of these papules may be smooth (Fig. 4-26A) or hyperkeratotic (Fig. 4-26B). Although clinically these may be indistinguishable from warts, microscopic examination reveals them to be trichilemmomas. Polymerase chain reaction (PCR) has failed to substantiate the presence of human papillomavirus in trichilemmomas.

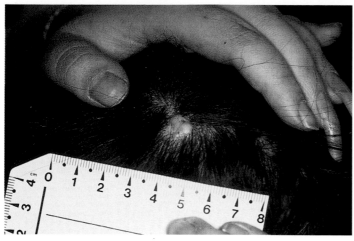

Figure 4-27

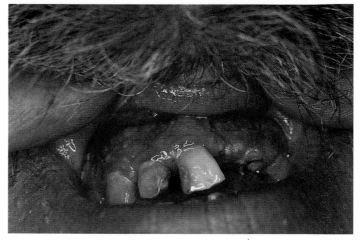

Figure 4-28

A wide array of systemic abnormalities has been reported in patients with **Cowden disease**. The vast majority of affected women have fibrocystic breast disease, and more than 50% may go on to develop breast cancer. This has led to the recommendation that affected women undergo prophylactic subcutaneous mastectomy at an early age. In one of our patients in whom mastectomy was performed prophylactically, an occult breast carcinoma was found. One man with Cowden disease was reported to have benign gynecomastia, but this is not found in most affected men. Abnormalities of the thyroid gland occur in most patients, particularly women. Goiters and adenomas are most common, but thyroid carcinoma, thyroiditis, hyperthyroidism, and hypothyroidism have all been reported. Follicular adenocarcinoma of the thyroid has been reported in several patients. Since this tumor is capable of distant metastasis, careful examination of the thyroid gland should be performed on a regular basis. Histologically distinctive fibromas have been reported in two of our patients and in several others subsequently (Fig. 4-27). **Cowden fibroma** most commonly develops on the scalp. Oral lesions are similar to those seen on the face and consist of 1–3 mm papules, which can create a "cobblestone" appearance on the gingival mucosa (Fig. 4-28).

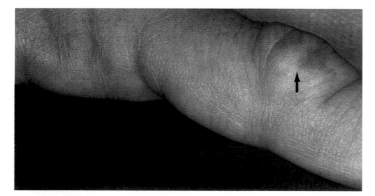

Figure 4-29A

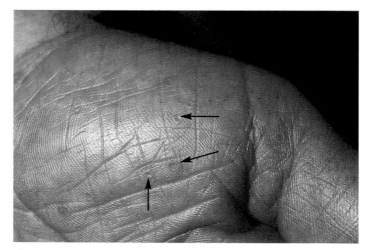

Figure 4-30

Adenocarcinoma of the uterus has been reported in women with Cowden disease, and other gynecological abnormalities can occur, including ovarian cysts, uterine fibroids, and uterine leiomyomas. Skeletal abnormalities in Cowden disease include high arched palate, pectus excavatum, scoliosis, skeletal cysts, pes cavus, and adenoid facies. Gastrointestinal polyposis has been reported in approximately a third of patients, and on biopsy these have been shown to be inflammatory or adenomatous polyps, ganglioneuromas, or fibrous polyps. Both gastric and colonic polyps have been reported, as have colonic diverticulae and an adenocarcinoma of the cecum in one patient. Hamartomatous pro-liferation of a number of tissues can occur. Figure 4-29A shows a hemangioma over the proximal interphalangeal joint of the second digit. A lipoma of the thumb is shown in Figure 4-29B. Several other cutaneous lesions are common in Cowden disease, including umbilicated papules that resemble palmar pits (Fig. 4-30).

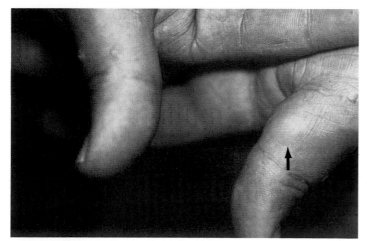

Figure 4-29B

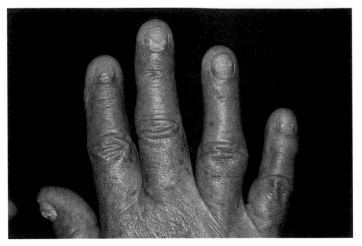

Figure 4-31

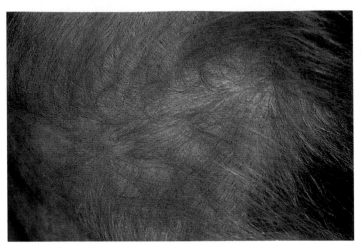

Figure 4-32

In contrast to the previously described inherited polyposis syndromes, the **Cronkhite–Canada syndrome** is an acquired disease. It is characterized by the development of polyps throughout the gastrointestinal tract, from the stomach to the rectum. Diarrhea, abdominal cramps, and weight loss are associated with a protein-losing enteropathy. Several months after the onset of gastrointestinal symptoms, brown macules develop on the arms, legs, face, palms, and soles. Other areas of the body can be affected as well, and in some patients pigmentation develops on the buccal mucosa. The pigmented macules can be faint, ranging from a few millimeters to 10 cm in diameter. On the dorsa of the hands, they can resemble solar lentigines (Fig. 4-31). Nail dystrophy, onycholysis, or complete shedding of the nails has been reported. Patchy alopecia is another feature of this syndrome. In addition to thinning of scalp hair, loss of axillary and pubic hair can occur. The patient shown in Figure 4-32 not only had alopecia of scalp hair but also lost most of her eyebrow hair (Fig. 4-33).

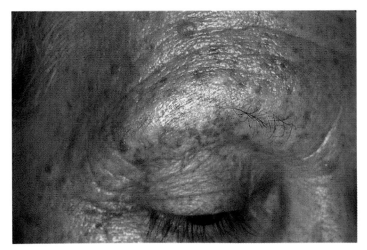

Figure 4-33

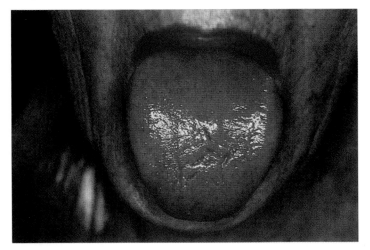

Figure 4-34

Nail and scalp changes can precede gastrointestinal symptoms and probably do not result from the protein-losing enteropathy. Other cutaneous manifestations of gastrointestinal malabsorption can occur, however. Figure 4-34 shows a patient with the Cronkhite–Canada syndrome who developed iron-deficiency anemia. Her tongue became smooth and shiny with loss of the lingual papillae. The nutritional deficiency occurring with the Cronkhite–Canada syndrome has resulted in defective immunity with cutaneous anergy, reduced serum immunoglobulin levels, and diminished lymphocyte stimulation upon exposure to mitogens.

The mortality rate of the Cronkhite–Canada syndrome is 50–75%. Malignant transformation of polyps can occur, and carcinomas of the stomach and colon have been reported. Despite the tendency to malignant degeneration, most patients die of nonmalignant complications of the bowel disease.

Occasionally, patients improve spontaneously, and remissions have been reported after gastrectomy or colectomy. In one reported case, parenteral nutrition resulted in disappearance of the gastrointestinal polyps and resolution of the cutaneous symptoms. This has led to speculation about a nutritional etiology for the syndrome. The precise cause, however, remains to be determined.

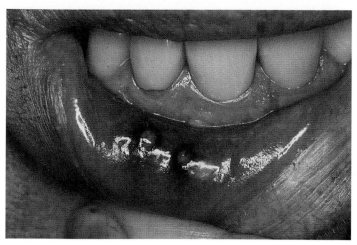

Figure 4-35

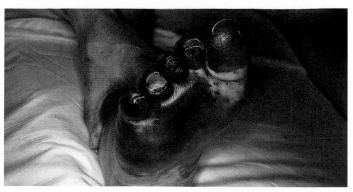

Figure 4-36

Ulcerative colitis is an inflammatory disease of the bowel associated with a number of specific and nonspecific cutaneous findings. Aphthous stomatitis that is clinically indistinguishable from ordinary canker sores is common (Fig. 4-35). A hypercoagulable state leads to clinically apparent phlebitis in up to 10% of patients. However, at autopsy, venous thromboses are found in more than 30% of people with ulcerative colitis. Arterial thromboses are fortunately rare, but they do occur. The patient shown in Figure 4-36 developed gangrene of several toes because of hypercoagulability associated with ulcerative colitis. The hypercoagulable state of these patients has been attributed to increased factor VIII activity or to thrombocytosis with reported platelet counts of 500 000/mm³ to more than 1 000 000/mm³. These abnormalities are not uniformly present, however.

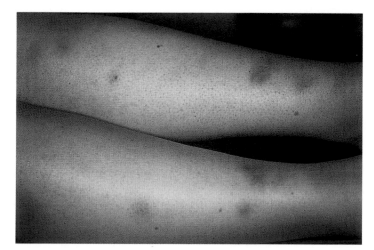

Figure 4-37

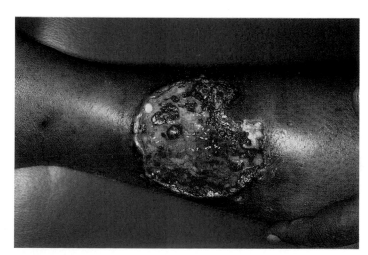

Figure 4-38

Erythema nodosum (Fig. 4-37) has been associated with numerous infectious etiologies, sarcoidosis, Behçet syndrome and Crohn's disease, as well as ulcerative colitis. It can develop along with an acute flare of gastrointestinal symptoms in patients with inflammatory bowel disease. Skin lesions are deep tender erythematous nodules most commonly distributed on the lower legs.

Pyoderma gangrenosum (Fig. 4-38) is perhaps the best known dermatosis specifically associated with inflammatory bowel disease. Of the first patients described with pyoderma gangrenosum, four out of five had ulcerative colitis. Only a minority of those with ulcerative colitis ever develop pyoderma gangrenosum, however.

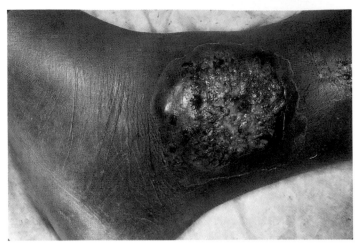

Figure 4-39

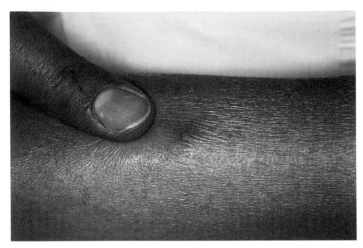

Figure 4-40

In some patients with ulcerative colitis, the skin lesions of **pyoderma gangrenosum** are closely linked to the severity of the bowel disease. In these patients exacerbation of bowel symptoms is often associated with extension of existing lesions and development of new lesions. Linkage of pyoderma gangrenosum to the severity of ulcerative colitis has been so close in some patients that severe skin disease has been used to justify surgical removal of the diseased bowel. Although this leads to improvement of pyoderma gangrenosum in some patients with severe gastrointestinal symptoms, removal of bowel is not indicated in those with limited bowel disease. The patient in Figure 4-39 had severe pyoderma gangrenosum, but only minor bowel symptoms. Colectomy was performed with the hope that his bowel symptoms would resolve, but

little improvement was noted. The independence of pyoderma gangrenosum from bowel symptoms is apparent in some patients whose skin lesions may be severe despite quiescent gastrointestinal symptoms. Moreover, in some patients pyoderma gangrenosum has preceded symptoms of ulcerative colitis, while in others the skin disease first develops years after total colectomy.

There are no laboratory findings that are diagnostic of pyoderma gangrenosum, and even the histopathology of this disorder is not specific. Clinicians must therefore rely on its distinctive clinical features, while excluding other disorders that may have a similar appearance. The initial lesion in pyoderma gangrenosum is frequently a pustule (Fig. 4-40) or occasionally a deep, painful erythematous nodule.

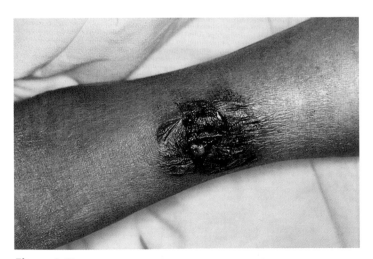

Figure 4-41

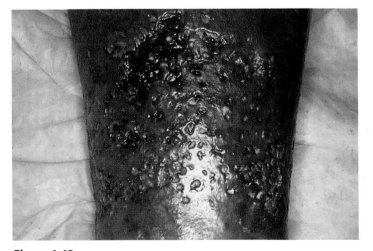

Figure 4-42

This quickly breaks down to form large ulcers containing necrotic tissue mixed with pus and blood. The lesion shown in Figure 4-40 was not treated and over the course of 1 week evolved into the ulcer in Figure 4-41. The border of the ulcer is elevated, purple, and undermined. Pustules are occasionally apparent on the ulcer base, which is studded with numerous crater-like holes (Fig. 4-42). The presence of pustules at

any stage of development of an ulcer may raise suspicion of pyoderma gangrenosum. However, other ulcers that also begin with pustules must be excluded, including necrotizing vasculitis, bacterial and fungal infections, iododerma or bromoderma, and Behçet syndrome. Cultures of the lesions of pyoderma gangrenosum are sterile, unless colonized with cutaneous flora.

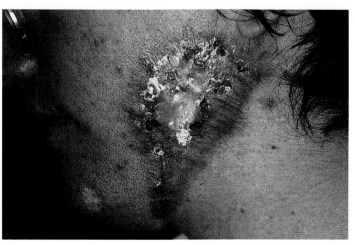

Figure 4-43

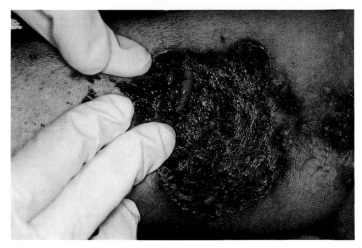

Figure 4-44

Pyoderma gangrenosum is a marker for Crohn's disease, occurring in anywhere between 0.5% and 20% of patients with this bowel disorder. Pyoderma gangrenosum occurring in patients with Crohn's disease is indistinguishable from that associated with ulcerative colitis. Pyoderma gangrenosum has also been reported in patients with chronic active hepatitis, rheumatoid arthritis, systemic lupus erythematosus, multiple myeloma, and monoclonal gammopathy without myeloma. Acute myeloblastic leukemia, myelomonocytic leukemia, and chronic myeloid leukemias have all been reported in patients with pyoderma gangrenosum, as has myeloid metaplasia and polycythemia vera. As many as 50% of patients with pyoderma gangrenosum may not have any associated internal disease.

Lesions of pyoderma gangrenosum may be solitary or multiple and most commonly affect the lower extremities. Less frequently, the buttocks and abdomen can be involved. In rare cases, patients can develop lesions on any part of the body, including the face. The patient in Figure 4-43 developed pyoderma gangrenosum of the face along with typical leg lesions. Ulcers can be superficial or may extend into the subcutaneous fat or even down to the muscle. Affected areas can be extremely painful and are occasionally associated with fever as well as gastrointestinal symptoms. The base is boggy, and when pressure is applied pus comes out through the holes (Fig. 4-44). The crater-like holes seem to form interconnected tracts under the base of the lesion. Consequently, treatment with intralesional injection of steroids on one

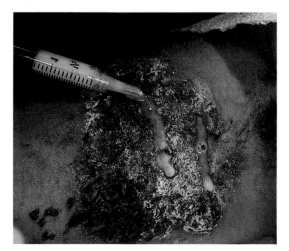

Figure 4-45

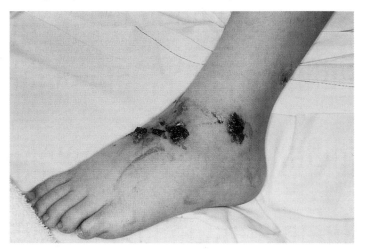

Figure 4-46

side of the lesion often results in discharge of some of the injected steroid through holes on the other side (Fig. 4-45).

The course of pyoderma gangrenosum is quite variable, with gradual, slow enlargement over weeks in some patients, and more rapid spread in others. Lesions may be limited to a few centimeters in diameter or may spread to involve entire limbs. Individual lesions may spontaneously heal in a few weeks, or they may take months or years. Healing—either spontaneously or because of therapy—usually begins with reepithelialization from the margins of the ulcer, which eventually covers the center. The resulting scar has been described as cribriform due to reepithelialization of the crater-like holes.

A phenomenon known as **pathergy** occurs in some patients with pyoderma gangrenosum. This is characterized by the tendency of

minor trauma to result in new lesions that can become extensive. The patient shown in Figure 4-46 developed several sites of early pyoderma gangrenosum because of repeated venipuncture of the foot. The occurrence of pathergy is not entirely specific for pyoderma gangrenosum, since it is also found in Behçet syndrome. Because patients with Behçet syndrome can also develop arthritis, aphthous stomatitis, uveitis, intestinal ulcerations, and ulcers that begin with sterile pustules, care must be taken to exclude this diagnosis in patients thought to have pyoderma gangrenosum associated with ulcerative colitis. Behçet syndrome can be differentiated from ulcerative colitis because of the more common development of genital ulcers or neurologic involvement in the former.

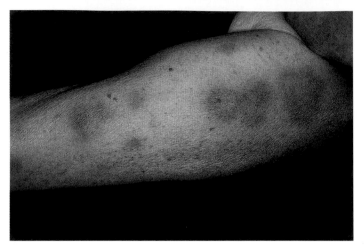

Figure 4-47

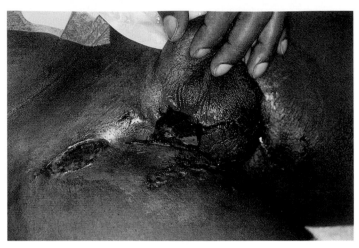

Figure 4-48

Crohn's disease has a wide array of cutaneous manifestations, most characteristic being pyoderma gangrenosum and erythema nodosum. The latter condition presents as deep tender erythematous nodules that are often more palpable than they are visible. Erythema nodosum typically affects the legs, but occasionally lesions occur on the trunk or arms (Fig. 4-47). Patients with large bowel involvement are more likely to develop erythema nodosum.

In Crohn's disease, perianal and ischiorectal abscesses and sinuses, and anal **fistulae** are common. Up to 60% of patients may have painless anal fissures. Even before symptomatic bowel disease, fistulae from the bowel to the skin can develop. Involvement of the perianal area is common, but fistulae to the inguinal area (Fig. 4-48), thighs, vagina, and other sites occur as well. Postoperative anterior abdominal wall

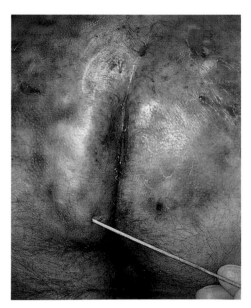

Figure 4-49

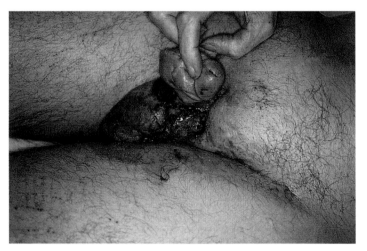

Figure 4-50

fistulae can occur in surgical scars, and these develop in up to 20% of patients with Crohn's disease.

Extensive fistulae and abscesses of Crohn's disease in the groin and perianal area can resemble severe hidradenitis suppurativa. The formation of sinus tracts with local purulent inflammation and destruction of tissue characterize the latter condition. The patient in Figure 4-49 had severe Crohn's disease with fistula formation on the buttocks and perianal area; the depth of the fistulous tract can be seen by inserting the wooden stick of a cotton-tipped applicator.

The patient in Figure 4-50 had such severe involvement of the groin that portions of the scrotum and proximal penis have been destroyed. A diagnosis of hidradenitis suppurativa was entertained, despite gastrointestinal symptoms, but work-up confirmed Crohn's disease. Fortunately, fistula formation and the associated destruction of skin responded to infusions of the new tumor necrosis factor (TNF)-α blocker, infliximab.

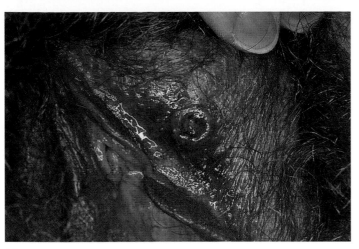

Figure 4-51

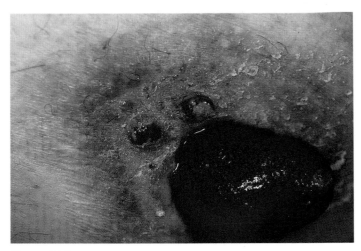

Figure 4-52

Noncaseating, granulomatous lesions of the skin have been found in patients with Crohn's disease. Perianal and peristomal inflammation frequently develops, and biopsy, especially of inflamed perianal skin, will often reveal **noncaseating granulomas**. Biopsy of fistulae to the skin can also show noncaseating granuloma formation. Aphthous ulcers of the mouth, that may be clinically indistinguishable from canker sores, may also reveal noncaseating granulomas on biopsy. Figure 4-51 shows a granulomatous ulceration of the labium majorum

in a patient with Crohn's disease. Peristomal ulcers can also develop when adjacent bowel is affected, and biopsy again shows noncaseating granulomas. The peristomal ulcers in Figure 4-52 developed granulation tissue, which often complicates healing under ostomy devices. After unsuccessful attempts to treat the ulcers with topical application of silver nitrate, biopsy revealed noncaseating granulomas typical of those seen in Crohn's disease.

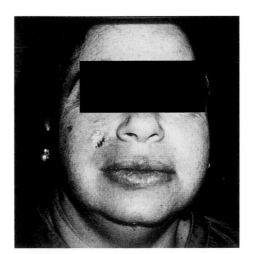

Figure 4-53

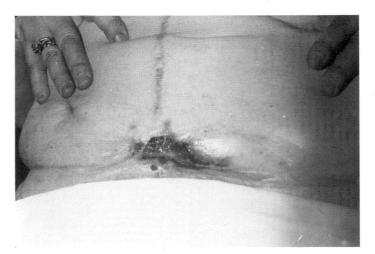

Figure 4-54

Cutaneous granuloma formation remote from the gastrointestinal tract in patients with Crohn's disease of the bowel has been called **metastatic Crohn's disease**. Fewer than 100 patients with this entity have been reported in the world literature, although the condition is undoubtedly more common than this low number suggests because there are frequent misdiagnoses of the cutaneous lesions. Figure 4-53 shows a patient with an erythematous facial plaque initially thought to be erysipelas. Biopsy revealed noncaseating granulomatous inflammation throughout the dermis. Figure 4-54 shows another patient with anterior abdominal ulcerations not contiguous with any abdominal

fistulae. Once more, histologic examination revealed the presence of noncaseating granulomas. Numerous topical and systemic therapies have been reported for metastatic Crohn's disease, but none are consistently effective. Treatment of the underlying bowel disease occasionally results in improvement of associated skin lesions.

Cases of metastatic Crohn's disease have been incorrectly diagnosed as factitial dermatitis, intertrigo, severe acne, hidradenitis suppurativa, chronic cellulitis, erythema nodosum, and severe seborrheic dermatitis. Most reported cases of metastatic Crohn's disease are associated with involvement of the colon or rectum, rather than terminal ileum alone.

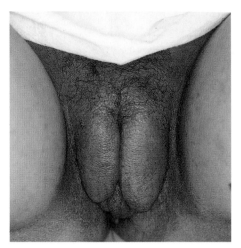

Figure 4-55

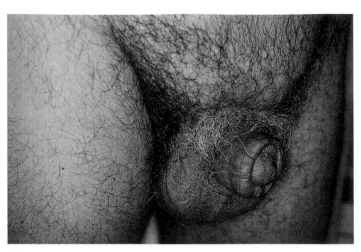

Figure 4-56

Edema of the genitalia has been reported in several patients with Crohn's disease. The patient in Figure 4-55 presented with massive enlargement of the vulva. The swelling is asymptomatic, but can be cosmetically troublesome. Topical and systemic steroids, sulfasalazine, 6 mercaptopurine, and antibiotics are of little help, but spontaneous improvement can occur after some years. Repeated biopsies may be needed to demonstrate noncaseating granulomas characteristic of Crohn's disease. Edema of the penis and suprapubic area are shown in a man with Crohn's disease in Figure 4-56.

Crohn's disease, like ulcerative colitis, is associated with an increased incidence of thromboembolic phenomena, including deep venous thromboses and pulmonary emboli. The hypercoagulation associated

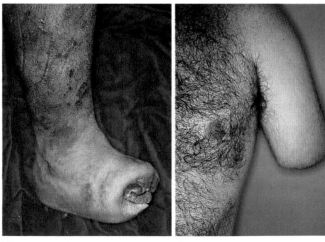

Figure 4-57A   **Figure 4-57B**

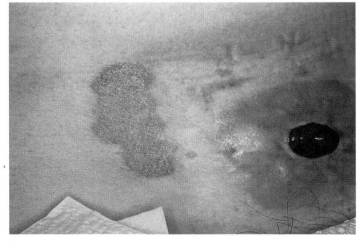

Figure 4-58

with Crohn's disease has led to ischemia and infarction of limbs and digits. The forearm, hand, distal foot, and toes of the patient shown in Figs 4-57A and 4-57B were lost through gangrene from a hypercoagulable state associated with Crohn's disease.

A number of less specific findings have been associated with Crohn's disease, including polyarteritis nodosa, and acquired zinc deficiency that produces skin lesions similar to those seen in acrodermatitis entero- pathica. A significant association between Crohn's disease and psoriasis has been reported. Several patients have developed the first signs of psoriasis in abdominal surgical scars following surgery for Crohn's disease. The patient in Figure 4-58 developed sharply demarcated erythematous scaling plaques under the tape used to secure her ostomy device. She subsequently went on to develop psoriatic lesions in more typical locations including the scalp, elbows, and knees.

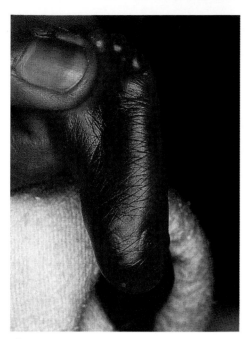

Figure 4-59

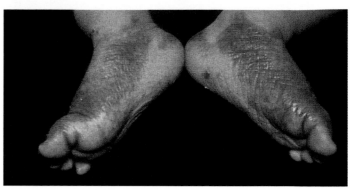

Figure 4-60

Acrodermatitis enteropathica is an autosomal recessively inherited condition caused by intestinal malabsorption of zinc. It can begin shortly after birth, or occasionally develops after the first year of life; rarely it begins later in childhood, and a few patients have been first diagnosed in adulthood. It has been suggested that impaired absorption of zinc in this syndrome is caused by reduction of a zinc binding factor or reduction of a pancreatic secretion that enhances zinc absorption.

This as yet undetermined factor appears to be present in human milk and, consequently, the symptoms of acrodermatitis enteropathica first appear after weaning from breast-milk. The primary lesion in acrodermatitis enteropathica is a bulla, as shown on the heel of an infant in Figure 4-59. The bullous nature of the skin lesions in this entity and their distribution on the hands and feet led early investigators to classify this disorder as a form of epidermolysis bullosa. When the bullae form, they are superficial and they collapse quickly, leaving an erythematous base. Many patients do not develop frank bullae, but instead form erythematous patches that are scaly, macerated, or crusted. Sharply demarcated erythematous patches of the feet are characteristic (Fig. 4-60).

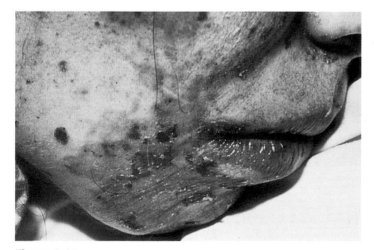

Figure 4-61

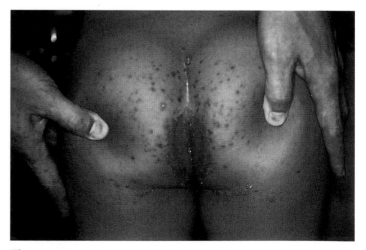

Figure 4-62

Periorificial areas are prominently involved, including the mouth (Fig. 4-61), nose, eyes, groin, and perianal areas (Fig. 4-62). Blepharitis and conjunctivitis can occur, and glossitis and cheilitis may mimic monilial infection. Secondary infection of the skin with *Candida* does occur in many patients. During periods of exacerbation, infants with acrodermatitis enteropathica are irritable and lethargic. Diarrhea is a common symptom and the stool is similar to the frothy malodorous stool of patients with sprue. As in sprue, histologic changes in the duodenal mucosa of patients with acrodermatitis enteropathica typically show flattening of villi and loss of villus architecture.

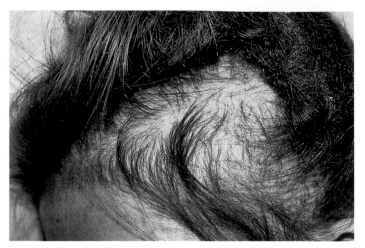

Figure 4-63

The rash of **acrodermatitis enteropathica** can also be present on extensor surfaces of the extremities and on the scalp, where alopecia results (Fig. 4-63). Loss of eyebrow hairs and eyelashes can occur as well.

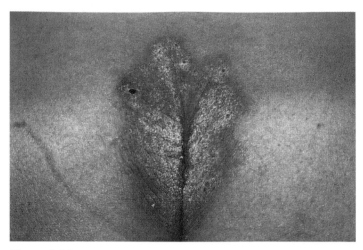

Figure 4-64

Scaling plaques of the elbows, knees, or intergluteal cleft can simulate psoriasis (Fig. 4-64). Paronychial erythema and swelling are common, and dystrophic changes of the nails develop (Fig. 4-65). When

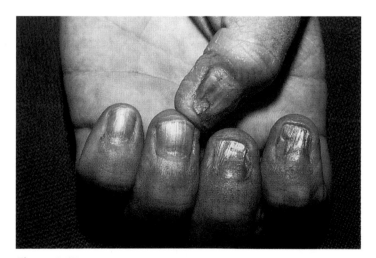

Figure 4-65

paronychial involvement is severe, nails may be lost from the hands or feet. If acrodermatitis enteropathica is not treated, failure to thrive, growth retardation, and general debilitation continue, and eventually most children die of infection. In breast-fed infants with transient zinc deficiency caused by low zinc levels in their mother's milk, skin lesions similar to those observed in acrodermatitis enteropathica have been seen. Diagnosis of acrodermatitis enteropathica is based on the demonstration of reduced serum zinc levels. Plastic syringes and tubes washed in acid must be used for drawing of blood because zinc-contaminated syringes and tubes cause false elevations. Treatment with oral zinc results in complete remission.

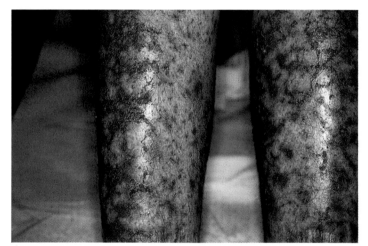

Figure 4-66

Several conditions leading to zinc deficiency have been associated with skin lesions identical to those seen in acrodermatitis enteropathica. Patients receiving parenteral hyperalimentation without supplemental zinc can develop the skin lesions of acrodermatitis enteropathica. Similar lesions have been seen in malnourished chronic alcoholics, in people with extensive Crohn's disease of the bowel who are unable to absorb adequate intestinal zinc, and those who have undergone small intestinal bypass procedures for obesity. **Eczema craquelé,** dry scaly skin with red fissures in a pattern that resembles cracked porcelain (Fig. 4-66), can also occur in adults with acquired zinc deficiency, as can angular stomatitis.

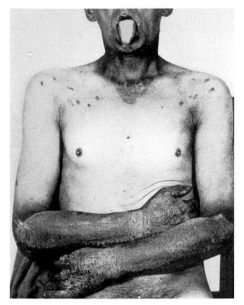

Figure 4-67

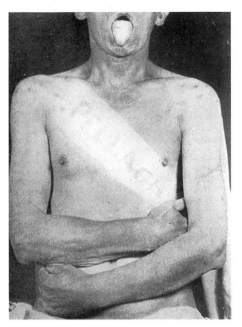

Figure 4-68

Pellagra is a condition that results from a dietary deficiency of niacin. Pellagra usually accompanies protein malnutrition, since niacin can be synthesized from tryptophan. The disorder is seen in conditions of severe malnutrition and, in Western nations, is usually seen in malnourished alcoholics. The clinical features of this disorder are summarized by "the three Ds": *d*ermatitis, *d*iarrhea, and *d*ementia. The dermatitis can be limited to areas of sun exposure, including the face, neck, and dorsa of the arms, as shown in a patient reported in 1925 (Fig. 4-67). Affected areas are sharply demarcated and can be brightly erythematous with subsequent scaling and hyperpigmentation. The

demarcation can be so striking that the collarette of dermatitis around the neck has been termed **Casal's necklace**. Mucous membranes are affected, with swelling and redness of the tongue, aphthous ulcers, and fissures at the oral commissures. Diarrhea occurs in 40–50% of patients and may be associated with steatorrhea. Mental depression and dementia follow. With institution of niacin therapy, symptoms rapidly improve. The patient shown in Figures 4-67 and 4-68 was treated with a high-protein diet, and had a dramatic improvement in cutaneous and systemic symptoms. If untreated a fourth D ensues—death.

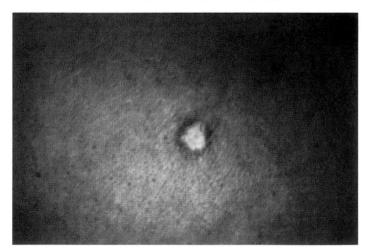

Figure 4-69

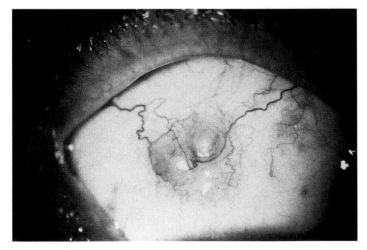

Figure 4-70

Degos disease, also called malignant atrophic papulosis, is a rare disorder that affects the skin and gastrointestinal tract. Degos disease affects males three times more frequently than females. The condition frequently begins in the second or third decades but has been reported in older patients. It is caused by an endovasculitis that results in fibrosis and, ultimately, occlusion of blood vessels. Skin lesions appear in crops of red papules that develop porcelain-white centers with surrounding telangiectases (Fig. 4-69). A similar process occurs on the gastrointestinal mucosa; these lesions create perforations resulting in peritonitis. Bowel perforation and peritonitis are the commonest causes of death.

Neurologic symptoms may include ataxia, diplopia, dysphasia, headache, and paresthesia. Several patients have died from central nervous system involvement. Lesions similar to those appearing on the skin and gastrointestinal mucosa have been found on the cerebral cortex of affected patients. Similar lesions have been found in numerous other organs, including the heart and kidneys, and on mucous membranes, including the oral, vaginal, and conjunctival linings (Fig. 4-70). This disease can be rapidly fatal, with many patients dying within a few years after onset.

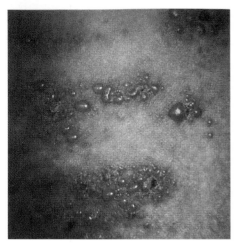

Figure 4-71

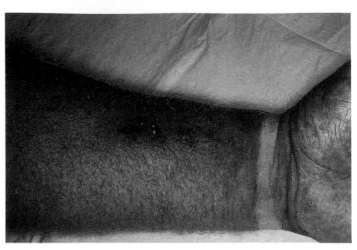

Figure 4-72

Dermatitis herpetiformis is a severely pruritic skin disorder associated with a gluten-sensitive enteropathy that does not usually produce gastrointestinal symptoms. Cutaneous lesions can develop at any age, including childhood, but the disorder most commonly begins in early adulthood. The primary lesions are vesicles, which may be grouped (herpetiform) or individual (Fig. 4-71.), and they occasionally evolve into pustules (Fig. 4-72). This disorder is usually so pruritic, however, that vesicles are quickly broken by scratching, leaving only crusts or erythematous papules (Fig. 4-73). Lesions are symmetrically distributed on the extensor surfaces of the elbows and knees, and on the buttocks, shoulders, scalp, and posterior neck. Excoriations may be the most prominent finding (Fig. 4-74). Facial lesions can occur, but

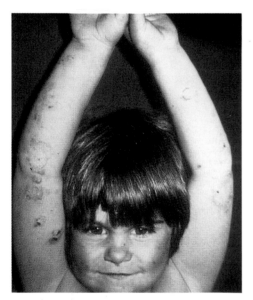

Figure 4-73

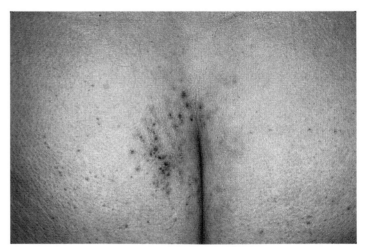

Figure 4-74

mucous membrane involvement is rare. Untreated, cutaneous symptoms follow a chronic but variable course, with occasional spontaneous remissions, or periods of milder symptomatology. Treatment with oral dapsone results in rapid improvement of symptoms.

Patients with dermatitis herpetiformis have a gastrointestinal abnormality that is histologically similar to celiac sprue. Small-bowel biopsy reveals atrophy of the villus pattern. Atrophy in celiac disease may be more severe, particularly in the distal bowel. Gastrointestinal symptoms are nevertheless rare, although some patients have asymptomatic steatorrhea, impaired absorption of D-xylose, and anemia due to malabsorption. As in celiac disease, the intestinal abnormalities found in patients with dermatitis herpetiformis resolve with a gluten-free diet. After 5 months to 1 year on the diet, cutaneous symptoms also improve. Treatment with dapsone rapidly relieves cutaneous symptoms but has no effect on the intestinal abnormality.

Diagnosis of dermatitis herpetiformis is made by direct immunofluorescence of biopsies taken from normal appearing perilesional skin and reveals granular deposition of IgA in the dermal papillae of lesional as well as normal skin. A few patients have linear deposition of IgA at the dermal–epidermal junction; there is a lower incidence of gastrointestinal abnormalities in these patients. This condition is best regarded as a distinct entity and has been called linear IgA dermatosis.

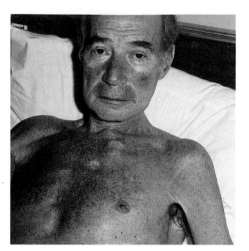

Figure 4-75

A striking syndrome with a number of cutaneous manifestations has been associated with **carcinoid** tumors, more than 90% of which originate in the gastrointestinal tract. The carcinoid syndrome most commonly occurs when intestinal carcinoid spreads to the liver, but a variant of the syndrome can occur in patients with bronchial carcinoids in the absence of hepatic metastases. Episodic flushing is the earliest symptom in many patients, although a third of patients do not experience flushing. Redness begins on the face but soon involves the upper extremities and chest (Fig. 4-75). Episodes initially last for only minutes and can occur several times the same day.

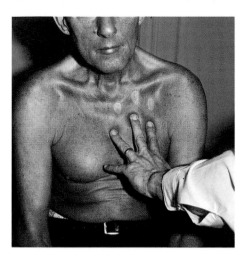

Figure 4-76

The vascular nature of flushing in the carcinoid syndrome is shown in Figure 4-76. Simple pressure by the physician's fingertips causes localized blanching on the chest of a patient with a carcinoid flush. In some patients, flushing is associated with episodic tremulousness, abdominal pain, explosive diarrhea, and paroxysmal bronchospasm characterized by shortness of breath and wheezing. Flushing can be triggered by palpation of liver metastases or abdominal tumors; by alcohol intake, exertion, anger or tension; by various foods including cheese and salty bacon; and a number of medications including epinephrine. As flushing continues, patients develop telangiectases

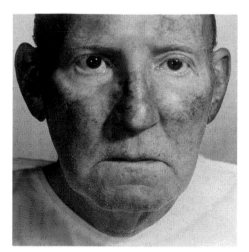

Figure 4-77

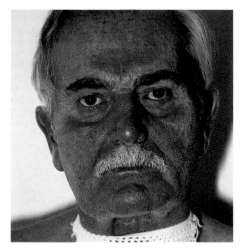

Figure 4-78

resembling those seen in longstanding rosacea (Fig. 4-77). Redness of the face and upper trunk persists between episodes of flushing and takes on a cyanotic hue (Fig. 4-78).

Right-sided endocardial fibrosis can occur as part of this syndrome and results in pulmonic stenosis and tricuspid regurgitation. The resulting right-sided heart failure leaves patients with pedal edema, hepatic congestion, and pleural effusions.

Bronchial carcinoids often produce a more severe variation of the disease with flushing that is more intense and prolonged, lasting several days. In these patients, flushing is often associated with disorientation, anxiety, tremulousness, fever, increased salivation and lacrimation, rhinorrhea, and sweating. Nausea, vomiting, diarrhea, and wheezing occur only during the flushing episodes. Headaches and hypertension are common, and left-sided cardiac valvular lesions can occur, resulting in pulmonary edema. Gastric carcinoids also differ in that flushing is sharply demarcated with serpiginous borders; diarrhea is less common, and cardiac lesions seldom occur.

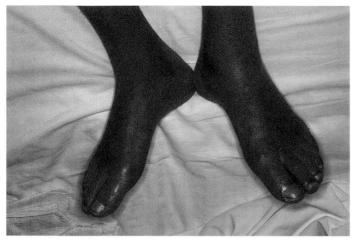

Figure 4-79

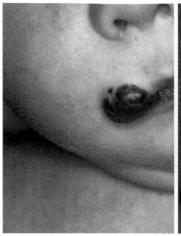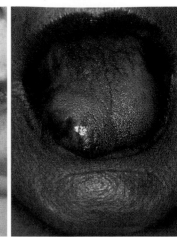

Figure 4-80A   **Figure 4-80B**

Infrequent cutaneous manifestations of the **carcinoid** syndrome include hyperpigmentation and scleroderma-like changes. The patient in Figure 4-79 developed marked induration of the skin of the feet and shins, simulating scleroderma. While cutaneous metastases are uncommon, we have observed a patient with multiple painful subcutaneous nodules as the presenting symptom of a bronchial carcinoid. Occasionally, a pellagra-like rash consisting of hyperkeratotic scaling and pigmentation of the extremities or trunk may be seen in this syndrome.

Hemangiomas of the gastrointestinal tract can be a source of bleeding. While easily recognizable on the lips (Fig. 4-80A) and tongue (Fig. 4-80B) and in the oropharynx, hemangiomas can occur anywhere in the gastrointestinal tract. Occult hemangiomas may remain asymptomatic for years before bleeding, and they may occasionally be visualized by radiography or endoscopy. Isolated hemangiomas of the gastrointestinal tract sometimes cause complications such as hemorrhages, but there have been reports of more severe syndromes — fortunately rare— involving more widespread hemangiomatosis.

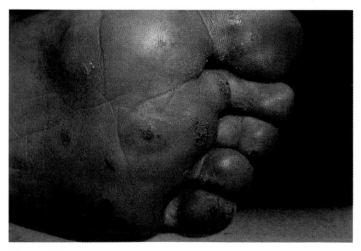

Figure 4-81

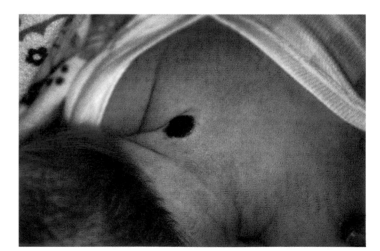

Figure 4-82

The **blue rubber bleb nevus syndrome** is characterized by the development of cutaneous and gastrointestinal cavernous hemangiomas. The hemangiomas are soft and compressible. In light-skinned people the nodules appear blue, as shown on the foot of the patient in Figure 4-81. Repeated episodes of gastrointestinal bleeding are common. In at least some patients, the condition shows an autosomal dominant pattern of inheritance. Many sporadic cases occur without any family history, however, suggesting a different mode of inheritance.

Neonatal diffuse hemangiomatosis is a rare syndrome in which multiple hemangiomas of the skin and viscera rapidly develop. Gastrointestinal bleeding, high-output cardiac failure, hydrocephalus, and a consumption coagulopathy leading to thrombocytopenia are common in affected infants. Liver involvement can result in cholestatic jaundice, and respiratory obstruction has been caused by laryngeal hemangiomas. The infant in Figure 4-82 had isolated hemangiomas on the posterior neck, face, and extremities, and CT scans revealed hemangiomas of the liver, spleen, and brain.

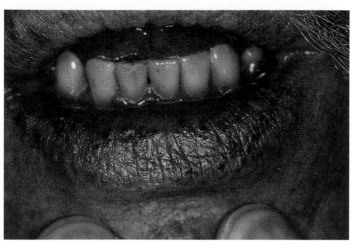

Figure 4-83

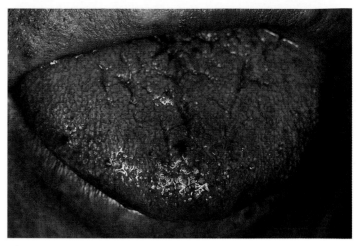

Figure 4-84

Gastrointestinal bleeding is a cardinal feature of **hereditary hemorrhagic telangiectasia**, also called Osler–Weber–Rendu disease. This autosomal dominant inherited condition often begins with repeated epistaxis during childhood. Telangiectases become apparent during the second and third decades, occurring on the nasal mucosa and lips (Fig. 4-83), the tongue (Fig. 4-84), palate, and buccal mucosa.

Telangiectases of the skin can be striking, possibly involving the palms and soles, nail beds, ears (Fig. 4-85), and nose (Fig. 4-86). Lesions appear as discrete red puncta, linear telangiectases, or spider telangiectases. After repeated episodes of bleeding, patients may be so anemic that the telangiectases become invisible. The skin and mucous membrane lesions reappear after adequate blood replacement. Gastrointestinal

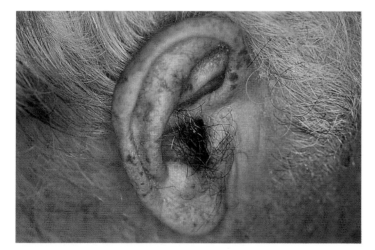

Figure 4-85

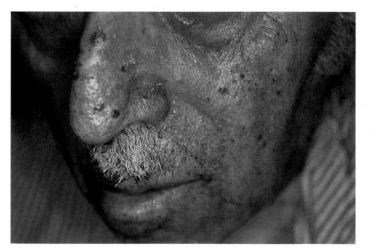

Figure 4-86

bleeding often does not occur until the fifth decade, or later, and different series report incidences of intestinal bleeding that range from 13% to 44%. Hepatic involvement is common, with passive congestion of the liver occurring in 30% of patients. Hepatic telangiectases occur in 30%, and iron overload in 50% of people with this disorder. Up to 20% of patients have evidence of pulmonary involvement on chest x-ray. Pulmonary arteriovenous fistulae can be seen as coin lesions on standard chest x-ray, and bleeding can result in massive hemoptysis. With extensive pulmonary fistula formation, clubbing and cyanosis occur, and extensive lung involvement results, paradoxically, in

secondary polycythemia. Vascular malformations develop in numerous organs and are associated with various complications depending on the organ affected.

In the absence of a diagnostic laboratory test, a history of repeated episodes of bleeding associated with cutaneous and mucous membrane telangiectases in combination with family history establishes the diagnosis of hereditary hemorrhagic telangiectasia. In patients with or without intestinal bleeding, barium studies are usually unrevealing. Telangiectases can be seen with endoscopy, but angiography may be necessary sometimes.

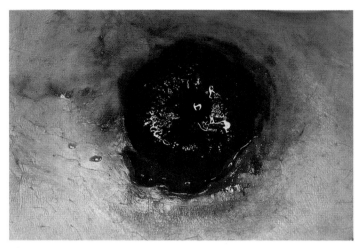

Figure 4-87

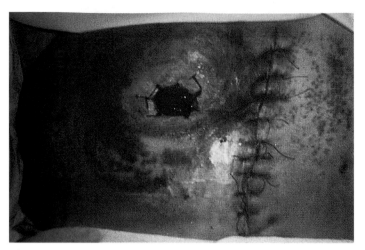

Figure 4-88

More than 100 000 patients undergo stomal surgery each year. Approximately half of these are **colostomies**, a third are **ileostomies**, and the rest are **urostomies** or combination procedures. Patients undergoing these procedures wear a device that collects intestinal or urinary contents. The device usually consists of a bag that must be attached to the skin by an adhesive. Irritation of peristomal skin is perhaps the commonest complication of ostomies, occurring in most patients if the ostomy stays in place long enough. Patients initially present with mild peristomal erythema (Fig. 4-87).

Leakage of intestinal contents has been implicated in many patients. Ileostomy patients, in particular, have stools that are watery and more frequent, resulting in an increased incidence of skin irritation. More-over, the high pH and proteolytic enzyme content of the ileostomy excretion can damage the peristomal skin. Occlusion by the ostomy device contributes to maceration, erosion, and folliculitis. Sweating adds to the creation of a warm and moist environment that permits proliferation of bacteria and fungi.

Irritating adhesives, and the solvents used to remove them, further exacerbate inflamed peristomal skin. True allergic contact dermatitis to the epoxy resin used in these devices has been shown. Figure 4-88 shows an allergic contact dermatitis around a patient's urostomy.

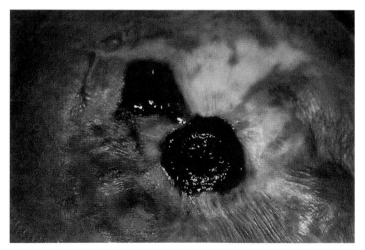

Figure 4-89

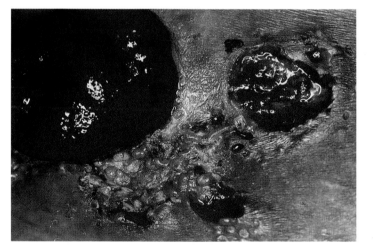

Figure 4-90

Periostomal ulcerations can occur shortly after surgery because of infected hematomas or unsuspected fistulae. Later, recurrent Crohn's disease can give rise to fistulae from the bowel to the anterior abdominal wall in the peristomal area; these may present initially as peristomal ulcerations. Pressure necrosis due to poorly fitting devices can also lead to ulceration. Although treatment with topical medications is often beneficial, it rarely becomes necessary to relocate the stoma. After a peristomal ulcer has formed, abundant granulation tissue frequently develops, preventing reepithelialization (Fig. 4-89).

Another rarely reported, but probably overlooked, complication is the development of **peristomal pyoderma gangrenosum** (Fig. 4-90). This may result from pathergy in patients with inflammatory bowel disease who are prone to develop pyoderma gangrenosum. The presence of pustules and crater-like holes helps establish the diagnosis, par-ticularly in patients with Crohn's disease or ulcerative colitis. In most cases, peristomal pyoderma gangrenosum can be successfully treated by intralesional injection of steroids.

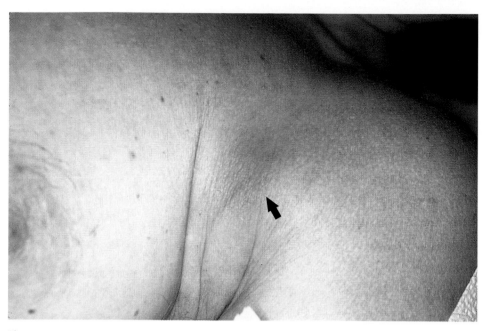

Figure 4-91

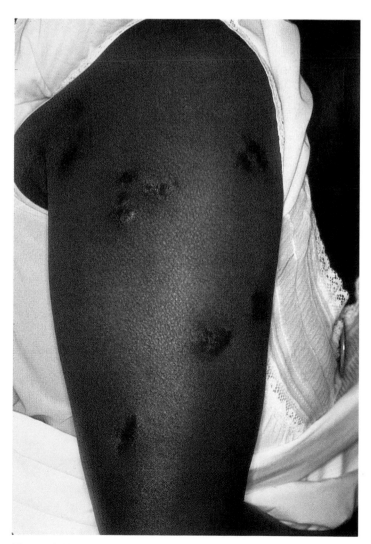

Disorders of the pancreas can have striking cutaneous manifestations. A **lobular panniculitis** has been associated with pancreatitis and pancreatic carcinoma, and is particularly increased in chronic alcoholics. Release of pancreatic enzymes leading to enzymatic destruction of fat is the mechanism that has been proposed for this disorder. Painful, deep erythematous nodules usually ranging from 2–5 cm in diameter develop, most commonly on the lower extremities, but the trunk, buttocks, or any other fat-bearing site can be affected as well (Fig. 4-91). Liquefaction and drainage of the nodules can occur, leading to formation of depressed scars (Fig. 4-92). Diagnosis of panniculitis is made by incisional biopsy that must be deep enough to obtain adequate amounts of subcutaneous fat.

Arthralgias, arthritis, pleuritis, and pericarditis can occur in association with lobular panniculitis. This constellation of symptoms has been seen in patients with acute or chronic pancreatitis and in those whose pancreatitis has been caused by trauma or associated cholelithiasis. Even though it is a rare pancreatic tumor, acinar cell carcinoma accounts for the majority of cases of lobular panniculitis associated with pancreatic cancer.

Figure 4-92

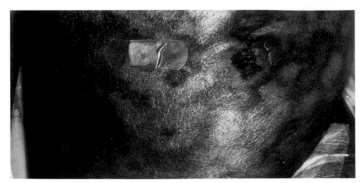

Figure 4-93A

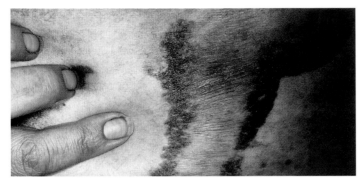

Figure 4-93B

In acute hemorrhagic pancreatitis, retroperitoneal blood can dissect along fascial planes into the skin of the flanks, the abdominal wall, and around the umbilicus. Purpura around the umbilicus has been called **Cullen's sign**. (Fig. 4-93A). Purpura in the flank (**Grey-Turner's sign**) and Cullen's sign indicate the presence of a severe necrotizing pancreatitis (Fig. 4-93B). Patients are acutely ill. Shock results from extravasation of blood into the retroperitoneal space and release of kinins and proteolytic and lipolytic enzymes.

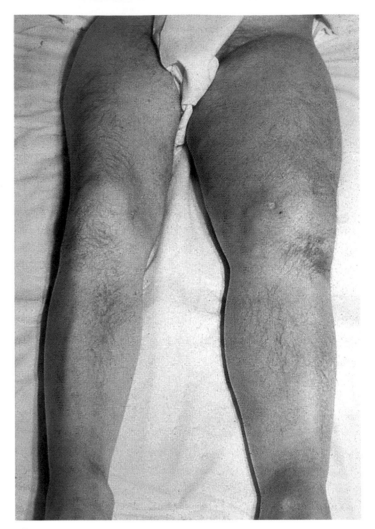

Figure 4-94

Migratory thrombophlebitis has been associated with several malignancies but most notably with pancreatic cancer. The patient shown in Figure 4-94 has obvious swelling of the left leg due to phlebitis. He developed repeated bouts of phlebitis in his arms and legs followed by the new onset of diabetes mellitus and weight loss. While thrombophlebitis and diabetes have classically been described in pancreatic carcinoma, they are actually infrequent presenting signs of this malignancy.

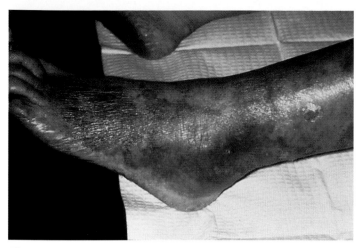

Figure 4-95

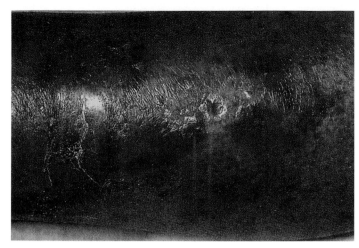

Figure 4-96

A distinctive cutaneous symptom called **necrolytic migratory erythema** has been associated with glucagon-secreting alpha cell tumors of the pancreas. The skin rash begins with irregularly demarcated erythematous patches (Figs 4-95 and 4-96) in which flaccid vesicles and bullae may transiently develop. Often a vesiculobullous component is not seen because these blisters are fragile and break quickly, leaving denuded skin surrounded by collarettes of scale or crusts.

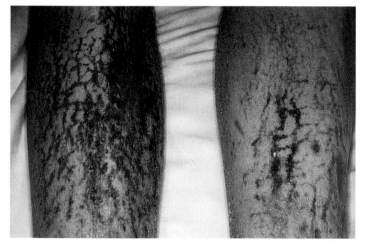

Figure 4-97

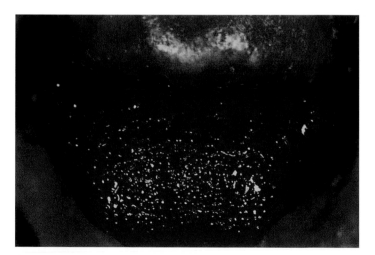

Figure 4-98

Lesions can be widespread but they characteristically affect the abdomen, thighs, and buttocks. The hands, feet, and legs can be affected too, with characteristic involvement of periorificial areas, including the perioral, perineal areas and groin. The overall severity of the rash can be variable, with unexplained periods of improvement, and even complete remissions lasting for weeks or months. Individual lesions last from a few days to a few weeks, healing with scarring and hypopigmentation. Occasional patients develop a rash that has been likened to **eczema craquelé** because of the linear fissures creating an appearance of cracked porcelain (Fig. 4-97). Other cutaneous features of the glucagonoma syndrome include alopecia, dystrophic nails, angular cheilitis manifested by crusts and fissures at the oral commissures, and **glossitis**, which presents as a beefy red tender tongue (Fig. 4-98) with atrophy of the lingual papillae. Fewer than 200 cases have been described in the world literature, and approximately 75% of these have metastasized at the time of diagnosis. The commonest sites of metastasis are the liver and bones. Nevertheless, the tumor can be slow-growing and patients occasionally survive for years, even with metastases. Resection of the tumor can result in disappearance of skin lesions. Other associated symptoms include weight loss, anemia, diabetes that is usually mild or asymptomatic, and thrombophlebitis. Diagnosis is established by finding a fasting plasma glucagon level higher than 1000 mg/l. The tumor is usually identifiable by magnetic resonance imaging or CT scan, ultrasound, or angiography.

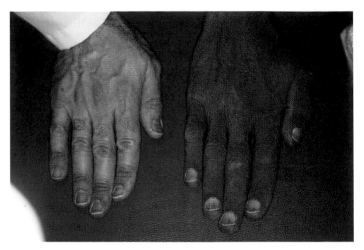

Figure 4-99

There are numerous cutaneous manifestations of liver disease, including both specific and nonspecific findings. **Jaundice** is most prominent in the various causes of obstructive liver disease, but it can also occur in acute hepatitis and other hepatic disorders and, to a much lesser extent, in the setting of hemolysis. Jaundice becomes clinically apparent when serum bilirubin levels exceed 2.5–3.0 mg/dl or 6.0 mg/dl in newborn infants. This condition is characterized by yellow discoloration of the skin and mucous membranes. A jaundiced hand is shown on the left of Figure 4-99, with a normal hand on the right.

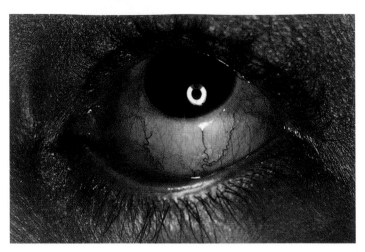

Figure 4-100

When mild, jaundice is easily overlooked, although it may be more obvious on examination of the ocular sclerae than of the skin (Fig. 4-100). It may gradually worsen over days to weeks before becoming obvious. When hyperbilirubinemia is due to excessive conjugated (direct) bilirubin, as in obstructive liver disease, urine becomes dark and tea-colored. Stools take on a tan, clay-like color. This does not occur when bilirubin is unconjugated (indirect).

Hyperbilirubinemia can result in generalized pruritus; this is a common symptom in primary biliary cirrhosis. Physical examination

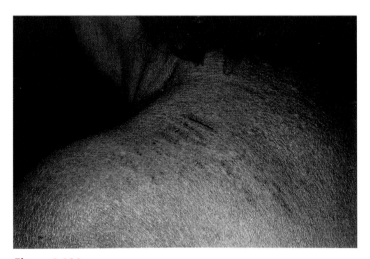

Figure 4-101

reveals only excoriations without primary skin lesions (Fig. 4-101). While deposition of bile salts in the skin has been blamed for the pruritus of hyperbilirubinemia, the precise cause of itching in this condition remains unknown. Cholestyramine and naloxone have been used to treat the pruritus associated with liver disease, but with variable success. Phototherapy with ultraviolet light is usually effective.

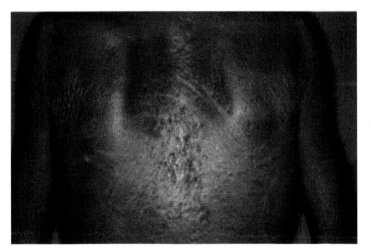

Figure 4-102

Generalized **hyperpigmentation** is another sign of cirrhosis and has been attributed to increased melanin in the basal layer of the epidermis. The pathogenesis of the increase in basal layer melanin remains unknown. While hyperpigmentation affects the entire skin surface (Fig. 4-102), it may be markedly increased in areas of freckling, or on areolar skin, and may be most noticeable in sun-exposed areas. Irregularly scattered brown macules can also develop, and a melasma-like rash can occur on the face.

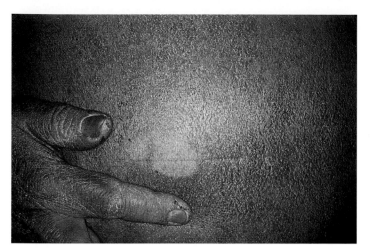

Figure 4-103

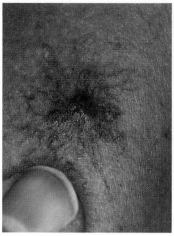 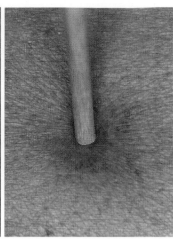

Figure 4-104A   **Figure 4-104B**

Generalized telangiectases develop in patients with chronic liver disease, and these resemble changes seen in chronically sun-damaged skin. While superficial examination gives an impression of general rubor, closer inspection reveals numerous small telangiectases that blanch on pressure. This is shown in Figure 4-103 on the abdomen of a patient with alcoholic cirrhosis and ascites.

Another vascular lesion seen in patients with cirrhosis is the **spider angioma**, also called nevus araneus. It resembles a spider in that numerous small vessels radiate from a central arteriole that may be flat or elevated (Fig. 4-104A). These range in size from 1–2 mm up to 2 cm or larger. Upon applying pressure to the central arteriole, all the radiating branches blanch (Fig. 4-104B). Spider angiomas occur

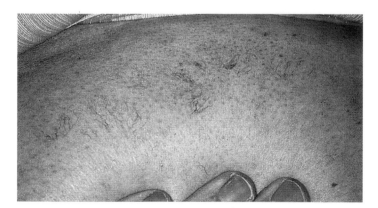

Figure 4-105

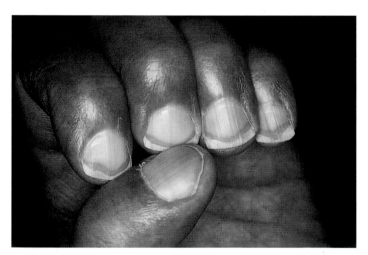

Figure 4-106

primarily on the upper chest, face, and arms. Oral estrogens and pregnancy are also associated with their development, and occasionally isolated spider angiomas develop in children.

Other stigmata of cirrhosis include palmar erythema and distension of the cutaneous veins of the abdominal wall. The telangiectatic vessels on the upper abdomen of a patient with cirrhosis in Figure 4-105 have been called "American paper-dollar markings" because of their similarity to the fibers of which American currency is made.

Hair and nails are frequently affected in patients with cirrhosis. Generalized thinning of body hair occurs and is particularly noticeable

in the pubic and axillary regions. White nails, also called **Terry's nails** (Fig. 4-106), have been described in patients with various forms of cirrhosis, including alcoholic cirrhosis. The entire nail plate becomes white, except for a narrow pink band at the distal portion of the finger. This finding has been described in numerous disease states, including congestive heart failure and diabetes mellitus. It is also seen in children and some adults without any associated diseases. **Muehrcke's nails** are parallel transverse white bands of the nail bed. These can be seen in patients with chronic hypoalbuminemia of any cause, including cirrhosis. If the hypoalbuminemia is corrected, the bands disappear.

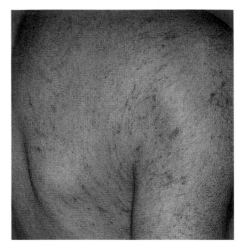

Figure 4-107

Splenomegaly, which accompanies portal hypertension, may result in thrombocytopenia and bleeding. Fibrinogen, prothrombin, and clotting factors V, VII, IX, and X are produced in the liver, as are fibrinolysis and coagulation inhibitors. Advanced liver disease can therefore result in clotting factor deficiencies. Fragility of blood vessels is also common. As a result, cutaneous purpura and petechiae are frequently seen in patients with cirrhosis (Fig. 4-107).

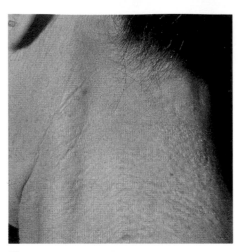

Figure 4-108

Plane xanthomas appear as yellow plaques that cover large areas of skin (Fig. 4-108). They also occur in palmar creases (xanthoma striatum palmare) and in scars. Plane xanthomas are striking in their appearance and extent; their presence should trigger a search for an underlying disorder such as primary biliary cirrhosis. Other xanthomas can also appear. Xanthelasma of the eyelids are common in primary biliary cirrhosis. Tuberous xanthomas, which appear as nodules on the extensor surfaces of the hands, elbows, and knees, rarely occur.

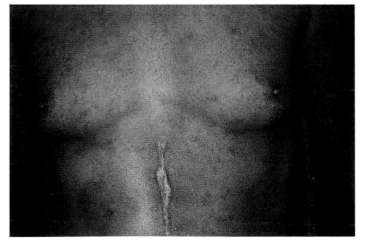

Figure 4-109

It has been thought that patients with cirrhosis develop hyper-estrogenism because of the liver's inability to metabolize estrogens. Whether or not that mechanism is correct, patients develop feminizing signs, such as loss of facial axillary and pubic hair, testicular atrophy, and **gynecomastia**. Palmar erythema and spider angiomas have also been attributed to the hyperestrogenism of chronic liver disease. The patient shown in Figure 4-109 developed progressive hepatic failure and gynecomastia as a result of severe amoebic infection.

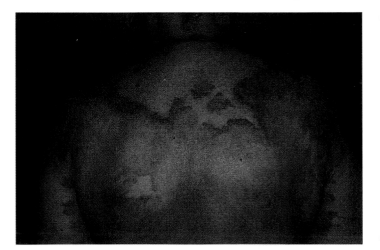

Figure 4-110

There are a number of cutaneous signs of **viral hepatitis**, and several dermatological syndromes are associated with hepatitis B, including polyarteritis nodosa, essential mixed cryoglobulinemia, and erythema nodosum. A serum sickness-like prodrome occasionally precedes other signs of hepatitis B by approximately 2 weeks. Affected patients develop an urticaria-like rash (Fig. 4-110) associated with arthralgias. Less frequently, erythematous or purpuric eruptions have been described.

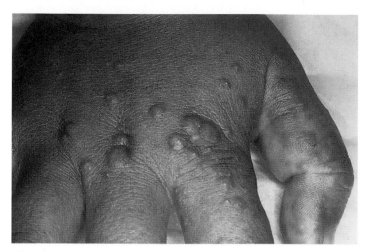

Figure 4-111

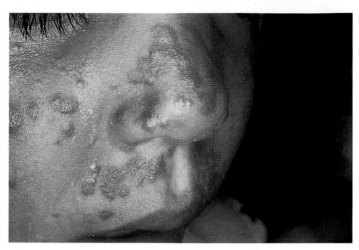

Figure 4-112

Gianotti–Crosti syndrome, also called papular acrodermatitis of childhood, was originally described in children with hepatitis B infection. This condition most commonly affects children aged 2–5 years, although it has been described in early infancy and in adolescent patients. It is characterized by discrete erythematous papules on the extremities and face (Figs 4-111 and 4-112). The papules range from 2–5 mm in diameter and do not itch. The rash resolves in 2–3 weeks and may be associated with systemic symptoms including lymphadenopathy and hepatomegaly. Cutaneous lesions with a similar distribution have been described in patients who do not have hepatitis B. Lesions can be pruritic and have a more variable appearance, being described as papulovesicular, erythematous, lichenoid, or edematous. Other viral infections including hepatitis A, Epstein–Barr virus, coxsackievirus A, parvovirus B19, and pox viruses have been found in these patients, although occasionally the rash occurs in the absence of an underlying viral infection.

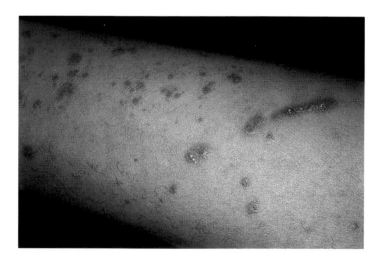

Figure 4-113

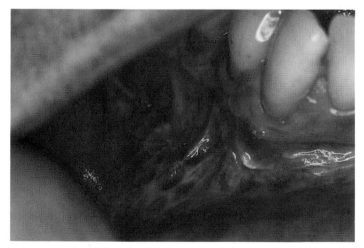

Figure 4-114

Lichen planus is an inflammatory skin disease that has been associated with hepatitis. The clinical features of lichen planus are easily remembered in that they all begin with the letter *P*: lesions are *p*urple, *p*ruritic, *p*olygonal *p*apules that are often *p*eripheral (involving hands and feet) or *p*enile. In Figure 4-113 characteristic lesions are shown on the arm of a patient with hepatitis C. Note that linear lesions have occurred at the site of scratching, an example of the Koebner phenomenon in which lesions arise at sites of trauma to the skin. Mucous membrane lesions are common in lichen planus, particularly in the mouth. The most commonly affected site is the buccal mucosa and the most characteristic lesions are known as Wickham's striae, which are characterized by white papules in a linear or reticulated pattern (Fig. 4-114). Many patients present with lesions limited to the oral mucosa. A painful variant of this disorder, oral erosive lichen planus, can be so debilitating that it interferes with eating or speaking. Old studies reported an association between lichen planus and elevated liver function tests. Subsequently, lichen planus was associated with hepatitis B, and most recently, with hepatitis C, although the association with hepatitis has not been confirmed in all studies. Treatment of hepatitis C with interferon has resulted in improvement of lichen planus in some patients, but exacerbation in others. Lichen planus has also been reported following vaccination for hepatitis B.

5 Renal diseases

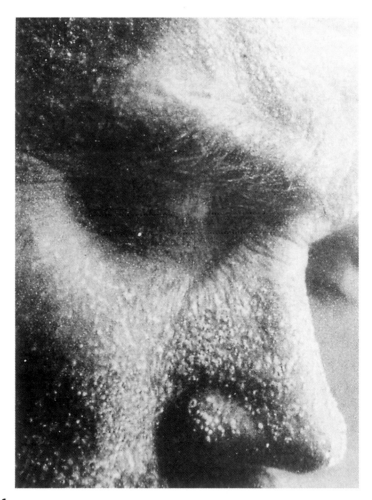

Figure 5-1

From Buttner HE, Robbers H. Schwere Uramie mit Harnstoff—und Kochsalzalbagerungen auf der Haut. Klin Wochensch 1935; 14:372.

In advanced renal failure, urea reaches high concentrations in sweat and, on evaporation, leaves a white powder that has been called **uremic frost**.

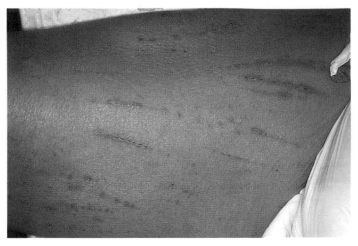

Figure 5-2

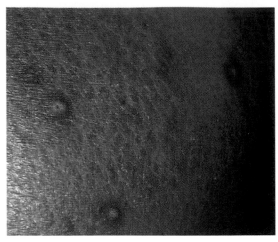

Figure 5-3

The cutaneous stigmata of **uremia** occur late in the course of renal disease and range from subtle to severe. Patients frequently develop ecchymoses as a result of a coagulation defect caused by abnormal platelet function. Hyperpigmentation is common, and the skin often has a yellow hue. Probably the most troublesome symptom of patients on dialysis is severe, unremitting pruritus. Examination of affected individuals reveals generalized excoriation without primary skin lesions (Fig. 5-2). The precise cause of **uremic pruritus** is not entirely known, but topical antipruritic agents and oral antihistamines are ineffective. However, most patients respond to phototherapy with ultraviolet B.

When discrete areas are picked, rubbed, or scratched, hyperkeratotic papules called **prurigo nodularis** develop (Fig. 5-3). These lesions, also

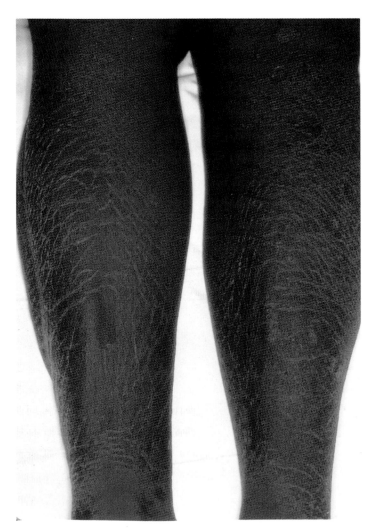

Figure 5-4

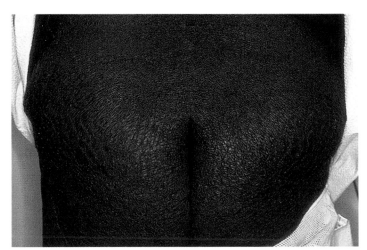

Figure 5-5

called picker's nodules, have diameters ranging from a few millimeters to 1.5 cm. They may crust, ulcerate, or bleed as a result of scratching. They most commonly occur on the extensor surfaces of the extremities, areas within easy reach of the patient's fingernails. Lesions may develop on the chest, abdomen, buttock, and scalp, but areas that are not easily scratched, such as the midback, are usually spared. Prurigo nodularis is not unique to uremic pruritus. It can occur in any patient who scratches repeatedly.

A number of different ichthyoses have been associated with elevations of parathyroid hormone. The patient shown in Figures 5-4 and 5-5 had chronic renal failure and secondary hyperparathyroidism. The large scales on her trunk and extremities correlated with elevations of her parathyroid hormone level. The skin condition cleared after parathyroidectomy only to recur when the hyperparathyroidism recurred. This presentation of **acquired ichthyosis** can be differentiated from ichthyosis vulgaris because the latter occurs in childhood. Both conditions predominantly affect the extensor surfaces of the legs.

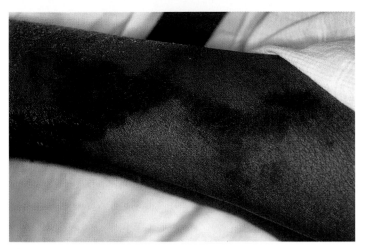

Figure 5-6

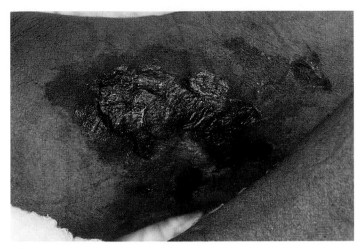

Figure 5-7

Secondary hyperparathyroidism can cause medial calcification of arteries, resulting in peripheral ischemia with necrosis of skin. This syndrome of vascular calcification and cutaneous necrosis has been called **calciphylaxis**. The condition occurs in patients with longstanding chronic renal failure and can affect those on maintenance hemodialysis, as well as people with renal transplants. Lesions begin with painful, mottled, purpuric patches resembling livedo reticularis (Fig. 5-6).

In some patients, cutaneous ischemia results in formation of bullae in affected areas (Fig. 5-7). The condition progresses to form indurated violaceous plaques that ulcerate and ultimately become gangrenous (Fig. 5-8). Ulcers are sharply demarcated, deep, painful, and are covered with necrotic eschar. The proximal extremities and fingers are typically involved, and autoamputation of the digits has occurred in people with calciphylaxis.

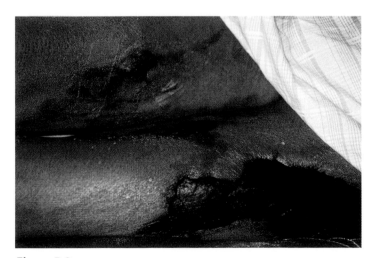

Figure 5-8

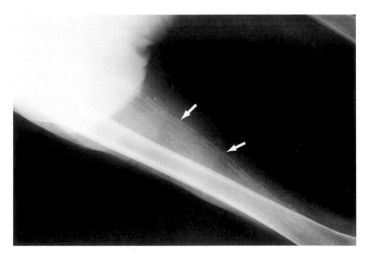

Figure 5-9

Definitive diagnosis is established radiographically. Radiographs of the affected area reveal medial calcification of small and medium arteries (Fig. 5-9). Occasionally, soft tissue calcification is apparent. In unaffected areas subperiosteal bone resorption can sometimes be seen on the radiograph.

In some patients, a painful proximal myopathy caused by muscle ischemia and necrosis precedes skin lesions. If untreated, skin lesions may fail to heal, leading to sepsis and death. Patients with calci-

phylaxis often have severe hyperphosphatemia. Reduction in serum phosphorous levels with phosphate-binding antacids may prevent the vascular calcification that causes this disorder. Withdrawal of immunosuppressive therapy in renal transplant patients improved symptoms related to calciphylaxis in at least one published report. Subtotal or total parathyroidectomy can result in rapid healing and relief of pain. Removed parathyroid tissue may be hyperplastic or adenomatous.

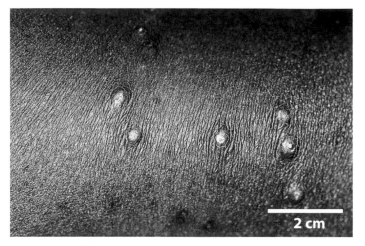

Figure 5-10

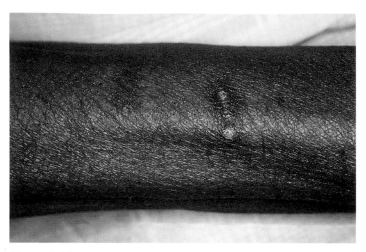

Figure 5-11

Perforating disorders of the skin are conditions in which dermal material is extruded through the epidermis. **Reactive perforating collagenosis** has been reported in patients with chronic renal failure and diabetes mellitus. Lesions are dome-shaped papules with central craters containing white keratinous debris (Fig. 5-10). Histologically, there is invagination of epidermis with perforating dermal material containing demonstrable collagen bundles. Patients with this disorder exhibit the Koebner phenomenon, in which lesions arise at the site of trauma. Figure 5-11 shows linear papules of reactive perforating collagenosis arising within a scratch mark. Some patients reporting with reactive perforating collagenosis have had diabetes without renal failure, while others have had renal failure without diabetes.

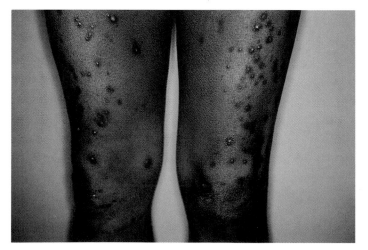

Figure 5-12

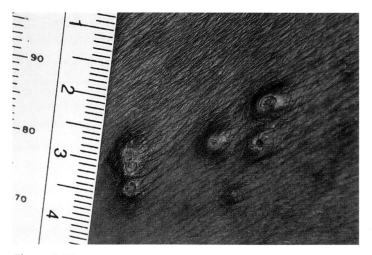

Figure 5-13

Kyrle disease, another perforating disorder, is characterized by umbilicated papules with hyperkeratotic plugs, prominently affecting the extremities (Fig. 5-12). Recently, Kyrle disease has been reported in people with diabetes and renal failure. Reexamination of histologic sections in some patients with Kyrle disease and renal failure has shown perforating collagen bundles, suggesting that when associated with renal failure Kyrle disease is identical to reactive perforating collagenosis.

Perforating folliculitis can be differentiated from other perforating dermatoses by the perifollicular location of skin lesions, by the prominent involvement of hair follicles, and the presence of hair within the dermal material penetrating through the epidermis. Not surprisingly, skin lesions most commonly occur on hair-bearing sites, especially the extremities and buttocks. Like the other perforating disorders, perforating folliculitis is characterized by skin-colored papules, with diameters of a few millimeters to a centimeter. The papules contain a central white keratinous crust and heal with pigmentary alteration (Fig. 5-13).

It has been suggested that all the perforating dermatoses associated with renal failure and diabetes represent prurigo nodularis (picker's nodules), caused by repeated scratching. Even if the perforating disorders develop simply because of repeated scratching, transepidermal penetration of dermal tissue is certainly seen more often in patients with renal failure. Reactive perforating collagenosis, Kyrle disease, and perforating folliculitis have all been seen in patients with chronic renal failure, and have been mistaken for one another. Therefore, it seems appropriate to include these conditions under a single name: **perforating disorder of renal disease**.

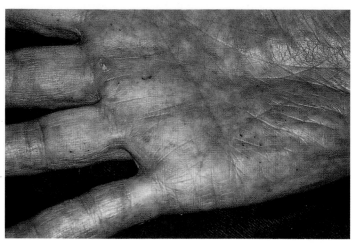

Figure 5-14

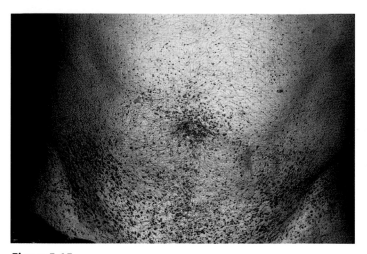

Figure 5-15

Fabry disease, an X-linked recessive disorder, is caused by defective α-galactosidase A activity. Consequently, glycosphingolipids are deposited in most viscera and in body fluids. Affected males suffer from episodes of excruciating pain that begin in childhood or adolescence. These episodic crises last from minutes to days and are characterized by extreme pain in the extremities, with severe burning of the palms and soles. Abdominal pain can occur as well. Painful crises are often misdiagnosed, and patients are frequently labeled with a psychiatric diagnosis. As patients age, the painful episodes usually decrease in severity and frequency. Apart from episodic painful crises, patients complain of constant burning and tingling paresthesias in the hands and feet (acroparesthesias).

The characteristic skin lesion in Fabry disease is the **angiokeratoma**, a pinpoint nonblanching macule or papule (Fig. 5-14). These red or purple lesions initially resemble cherry hemangiomas or pinpoint telangiectases. Other clinical features of Fabry disease include hypohidrosis, corneal and lenticular opacities, and cardiac and renal disease that frequently result in death in adulthood. Corneal opacities are the most common symptom in heterozygous women, who are usually otherwise asymptomatic. Occasionally, heterozygotes may develop isolated skin lesions and some develop cardiac involvement later in life.

Angiokeratomas develop in clusters and are usually present in the periumbilical area (Fig. 5-15). Areas most often affected include hips, buttocks, penis (Fig. 5-16), scrotum, thighs, and back. Angiokeratomas also develop on mucosal surfaces, including the oral mucosa (Fig. 5-17) and conjunctiva. Virtually all patients develop hypohidrosis or anhidrosis early in life.

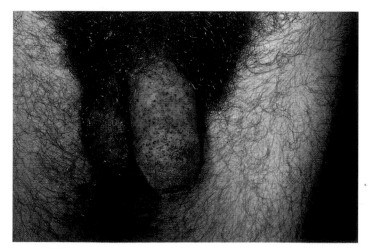

Figure 5-16

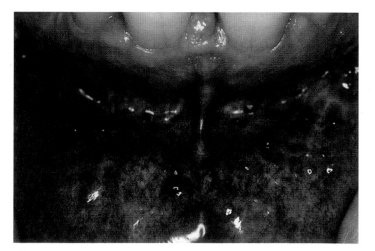

Figure 5-17

As patients reach adulthood, renal, cardiac, and cerebrovascular diseases occur. Glycosphingolipid infiltration of small vessels results in ischemia, thromboses, aneurysms, and hemorrhage. Even in the absence of a sudden cerebrovascular event, patients develop personality changes, periods of disorientation, and even psychotic behavior. Glycosphingolipid infiltration of the myocardium and coronary vessels can cause cardiac enlargement, congestive heart failure, and cardiac arrhythmias. Angina and myocardial infarction can occur. Cardiac valvular abnormalities have been described, including mitral regurgitation. Proteinuria, hematuria, and urinary casts arise from glycosphingolipid infiltration of the kidneys. There is progressive deterioration of renal function, leading to uremia in the third or fourth decade.

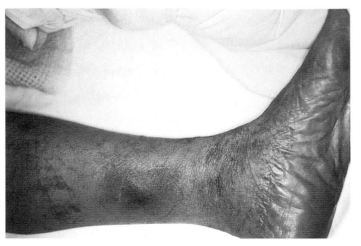

Figure 5-18

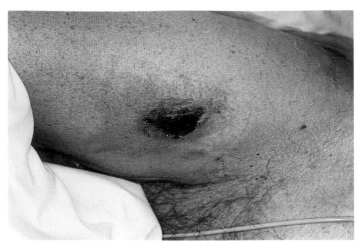

Figure 5-19

Polyarteritis nodosa results from necrotizing inflammation of muscular arteries, including small arteries in the subcutaneous tissue. Damage to the arterial wall leads to the formation of aneurysms, especially in areas where the affected artery bifurcates. Red, tender, subcutaneous nodules can develop along the course of affected arteries; these consist of thrombus-filled aneurysms. Nodules are 0.5–2.0 cm and may be solitary or multiple, occurring most commonly on the lower extremities (Fig. 5-18). They may be pulsatile if the underlying aneurysm is not filled with thrombus. Progressive vessel occlusion

results in cutaneous infarction and ulceration (Fig. 5-19), or gangrene of the digits (Fig. 5-20). Livedo reticularis can occur as well.

The diagnosis of polyarteritis nodosa may be missed on biopsy of skin lesions because the arterial involvement is not uniform; examining multiple sections will improve the diagnostic yield. If this diagnosis is suspected, renal arteriograms reveal aneurysms of the renal arteries (Fig. 5-21). Muscle or testicular biopsies may show characteristic pathologic changes even in clinically uninvolved sites.

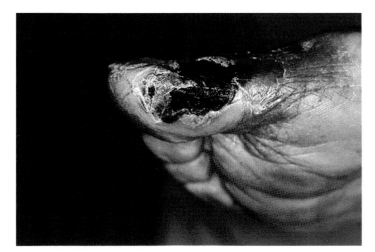

Figure 5-20

If untreated, many patients die within a few months of diagnosis. Aggressive intervention with systemic steroids may be life-saving. Renal failure resulting from glomerulosclerosis is the commonest cause of death. Involvement of the coronary arteries can cause myocardial infarction. Peripheral neuropathy results from disease of the vasa vasorum of peripheral nerves. Occlusion of mesenteric vessels with intestinal infarction gives rise to abdominal pain and gastrointestinal bleeding.

Absence of pulmonary involvement distinguishes polyarteritis nodosa from allergic granulomatosis and Wegener granulomatosis. Polyarteritis nodosa has been associated with hepatitis B infection and rheumatoid arthritis. A cutaneous form of periarteritis nodosa has been reported in patients with Crohn's disease.

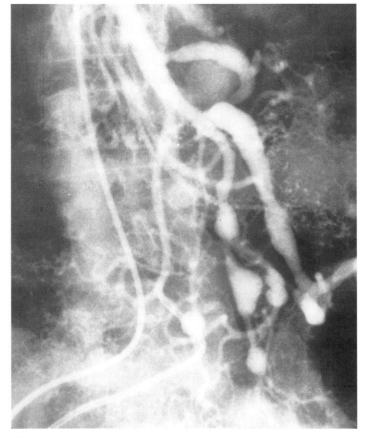

Figure 5-21

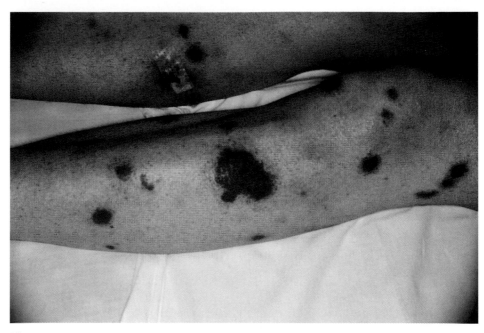

Figure 5-22

Henoch–Schönlein purpura is a leukocytoclastic vasculitis that affects the skin, kidneys, joints, and gastrointestinal tract. This syndrome can occur in adults but typically affects children. The most characteristic skin lesions are the same as those occurring in other forms of cutaneous vasculitis, namely symmetric palpable purpura of the lower extremities (Fig. 5-22). Less commonly, purpura that is macular or palpable can occur on the upper extremities or trunk. Joint involvement is variable, and patients may have arthralgias or frank arthritis with swelling and pain of the affected joints. Renal involvement is manifested by red blood cells and casts in the urinary sediment, but

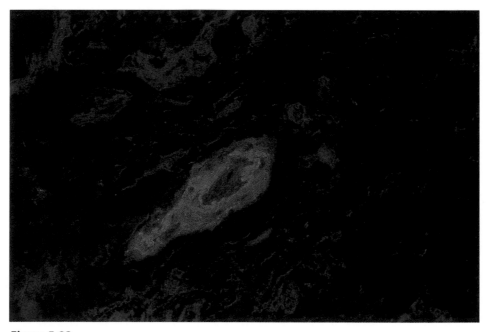

Figure 5-23

this seldom progresses to significant impairment of renal function. Gastrointestinal symptoms include hematemesis, melena, and abdominal pain. Symptoms can mimic the abdominal pain of appendicitis, leading to unnecessary surgery.

Skin biopsy shows the characteristic features of a leukocytoclastic vasculitis. The immunofluorescent examination of a biopsied skin lesion, however, is distinctive: there is deposition of IgA in and around the blood vessel walls of the superficial dermal vasculature (Fig. 5-23).

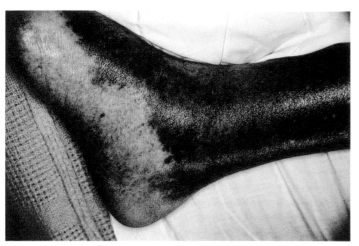

Figure 5-24

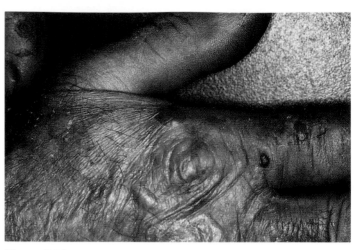

Figure 5-25

Familial Mediterranean fever is the informative name of an autosomal recessively inherited disorder that affects some patients of Mediterranean descent. Although the condition has been reported around the world, most cases occur in Sephardic Jews, Armenians, Turks and Arabs. The condition is characterized by paroxysmal attacks of fever, peritonitis, pleuritis, or arthritis. Episodes last 24–48 h and can be associated with painful, erythematous, warm, swollen plaques that have been called erysipelas-like erythema, as shown on the lower extremity of the patient in Figure 5-24. Systemic amyloidosis leads to chronic renal failure. Paroxysmal hematuria has also been reported.

Some patients with chronic renal failure on maintenance hemodialysis develop bullous lesions resembling those seen in porphyria cutanea tarda. This **pseudoporphyria** is characterized by bullae (Fig. 5-25) that are subepidermal and histologically identical to the bullae of porphyrias. Cutaneous fragility and scarring also occur but, in contrast to porphyria cutanea tarda, porphyrin levels are normal. Patients on dialysis can develop elevation of plasma porphyrins that do not cause clinical symptoms. True porphyria cutanea tarda can occur as well.

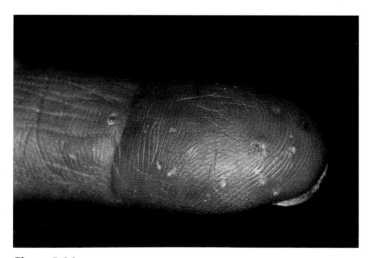

Figure 5-26

Hyperoxaluria is an autosomal recessive inherited deficiency of hepatic alanine/glyoxylate aminotransferase (type 1 hyperoxaluria) or D-glycerate dehydrogenase/glyoxylate reductase (type 2 hyperoxaluria). Patients with hyperoxaluria develop urolithiasis and progressive renal failure. Skin lesions consist of livedo reticularis, ulcers, and peripheral gangrene. Oxalate crystals can occasionally be seen in the skin (Fig. 5-26).

6　Hematologic diseases

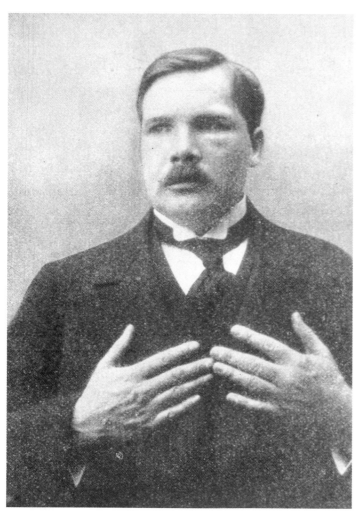

Figure 6-1

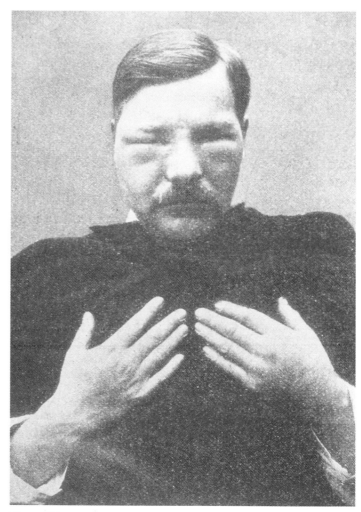

Figure 6-2

From Meyer-Betz F. Untersuchungen über die Biologische (photodynamische) Wirkung des Hämatoporphyrins und anderer Derivate des Blut- und Gallenfarbstoffs. Dtsch Arch Klin Med 1913; 112:476–503.

Meyer-Betz (Fig. 6-1) first demonstrated the photosensitizing potential of porphyrins by injecting himself with hematoporphyrin and then exposing his skin to sunlight. Marked swelling and erythema developed in the sun-exposed skin (Fig. 6-2).

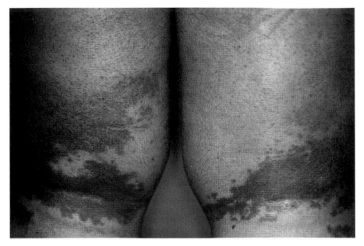

Figure 6-3

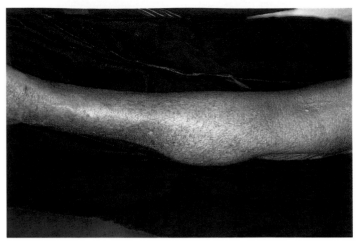

Figure 6-4A

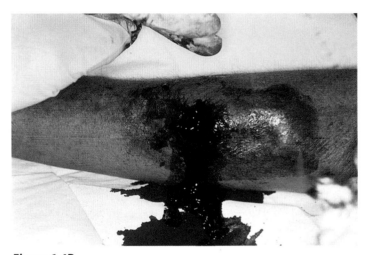

Figure 6-4B

Defects of platelets and coagulation factors result in spontaneous bleeding into the skin or easy bruising following minor trauma. Abnormalities of coagulation can be inherited or acquired but, regardless of the etiology, bleeding into the skin results in **purpura**. These purple patches are shown in Figure 6-3 in a patient with hemophilia A. This X-linked disorder affects 1 : 10 0000 men and results from a defect of factor VIII. Bleeding can occur hours or days after trauma, and symptoms are determined by the site of bleeding. Skin, muscles, and joints are commonly affected.

Advanced liver disease is responsible for acquired defects of coagulation in many instances. Patients with extensive hepatic metastases or advanced cirrhosis may bleed as a result of reduced synthesis of coagulation factors. Alternatively, the hypersplenism that accompanies cirrhosis may lead to thrombocytopenia. In patients with alcoholic cirrhosis, alcohol also suppresses bone-marrow platelet production. The patient in Figure 6-4A had alcoholic cirrhosis and spontaneously developed a large purpuric mass on the arm. The differential diagnosis included a large abscess or a neoplasm. On incision, a large hematoma was evacuated. Part of the drained clot is shown in Figure 6-4B.

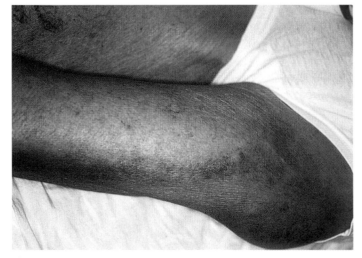

Figure 6-5

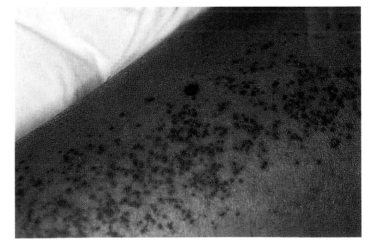

Figure 6-6

The patient in Figure 6-5 had widely disseminated colon cancer with extensive hepatic metastases. Apart from widespread bleeding into the skin, the patient ultimately succumbed to gastrointestinal hemorrhage. Purpura is also commonly seen in patients on heparin or warfarin anticoagulants.

Petechiae (Fig. 6-6) are pinpoint red or purple macules that occur at sites of bleeding capillaries in the skin. They develop in patients with abnormalities of platelet function or cutaneous vasculitis. Petechiae occur with or without purpura in several groups of patients: those on medications like aspirin that interfere with platelet function; those with

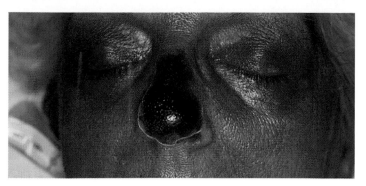

Figure 6-7

autoimmune conditions like idiopathic thrombocytopenic purpura that cause a reduction in circulating platelets; those with reduced numbers of platelets because of bone marrow destruction or hypersplenism; and those with disorders like von Willebrand disease or uremia in which platelet function is abnormal.

   Disseminated intravascular coagulation (DIC) is a life-threatening syndrome of widespread thrombus deposition in the microvasculature and concomitant bleeding. This syndrome complicates numerous conditions, including bacterial sepsis, metastatic neoplasms, obstetric disasters such as abruptio placentae, fat embolism, and extensive tissue damage from trauma or burns. The thrombotic component of

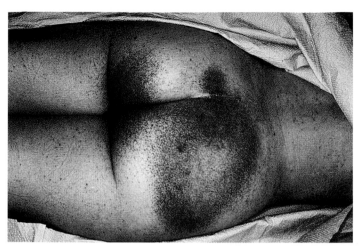

Figure 6-8

DIC results in peripheral acrocyanosis and, in some cases, gangrene of the nose (Fig. 6-7), the digits, or the genitalia. There is massive consumption of platelets, fibrinogen, and clotting factors, which eventually become depleted. This leads to paradoxical bleeding in many organs, including the skin and mucous membranes. The cutaneous surface is frequently covered with extensive patches of purpura (Fig. 6-8).

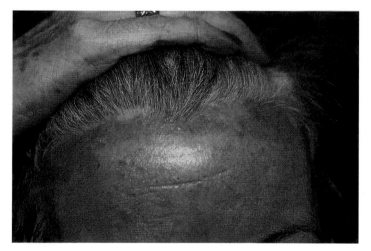

Figure 6-9

   Hermansky–Pudlak syndrome is an autosomal recessive form of oculocutaneous albinism associated with a platelet abnormality. There is a deficiency of platelet storage granules that leads to mild episodes of bleeding in various organs, including the skin and mucous membranes. Patients often complain of nose bleeds or gingival bleeding, and easy bruising of the skin is common. Most affected patients are Puerto Rican. Skin color varies from marked hypopigmentation to mild hypopigmentation in individuals whose relatives are darkly pigmented (Fig. 6-9). Pigmented nevi can occur, and freckles develop in sun-exposed areas.

   Sickle cell anemia should be considered in any young black person presenting with spontaneously appearing leg ulcers (Fig. 6-10). The ulcers affect a high proportion of people with severe anemia. Ulcers typically occur over the lateral or medial malleoli and have been attributed to vasoocclusive phenomena leading to cutaneous ischemia. Ankle ulcerations rarely occur in patients with other congenital hemolytic anemias such as thalassemia and congenital spherocytosis.

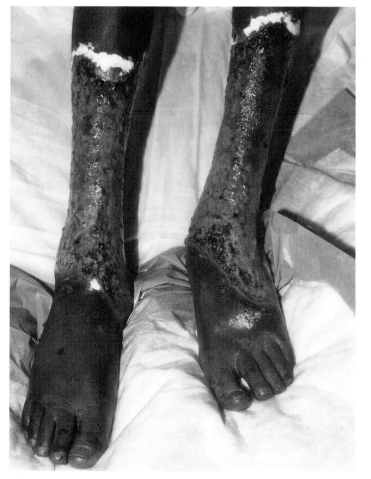

Figure 6-10

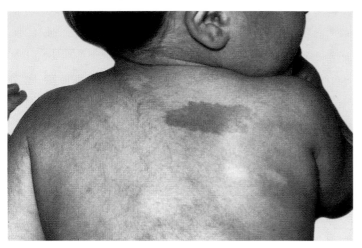

Figure 6-11

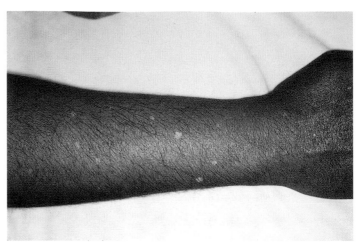

Figure 6-12

Fanconi anemia is an autosomal recessively inherited condition associated with numerous anatomic malformations and a high incidence of malignancy. Patients have increased spontaneous chromosomal abnormalities, including gaps, breaks, and translocations. Before children reach 10 years of age, they develop hypocellular bone marrow, leading to thrombocytopenia, leukopenia, and anemia. Skin lesions occur in most of those affected and consist of a number of pigmentary abnormalities. **Café-au-lait spots** are reported in many patients and are usually present at birth (Fig. 6-11). Diffuse hyperpigmentation is present early in life. Later, patients who have undergone many transfusions develop hyperpigmentation related to iron overload. **Hypopigmented macules** also occur with Fanconi anemia (Fig. 6-12). Anatomic abnormalities include renal aplasia, horseshoe kidney, patent ductus arteriosus, aortic stenosis, atrial septal defects, hypogonadism, and ear deformities leading to deafness. Mild mental retardation occurs in some patients.

The boy in Figure 6-13 has some of the features reported in patients with Fanconi anemia. He is short with microcephaly, microphthalmia,

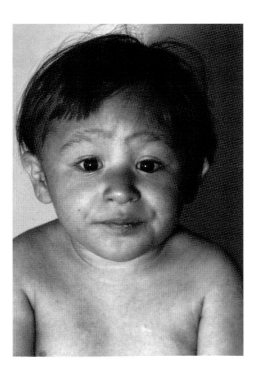

Figure 6-13

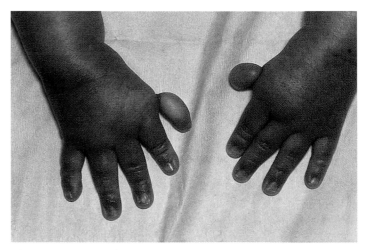

Figure 6-14

and epicanthal folds, and he has pseudostrabismus created by the epicanthal folds. Joint dislocation, scoliosis, and hypoplasia of the thumb, metacarpals, or radius also occur. The patient also has congenital hip dislocations, hypoplastic radii, and hypoplastic thumbs that are attached to the hands by thin bands of skin (Fig. 6-14).

A number of malignancies have been reported in patients with Fanconi anemia, particularly nonlymphatic leukemias. Many patients succumb to aplastic anemia. Treatment with androgens may be somewhat beneficial. Recently, bone marrow transplantation has been used successfully to treat patients with Fanconi anemia.

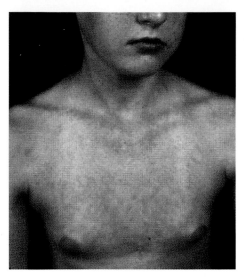

Figure 6-15

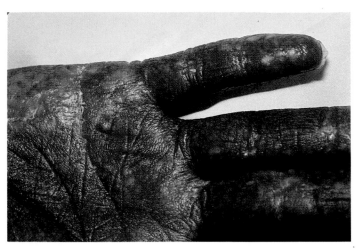

Figure 6-16

Dyskeratosis congenita in an X-linked disease associated with an increased incidence of malignancy and characteristic mucosal, cutaneous, and hematologic abnormalities. The most common clinical features include cutaneous pigmentary abnormalities, dystrophic nails, and oral leukoplakia. Subnormal intelligence is reported in approximately 50% of patients. Before the age of 10 years, patients develop reticulated erythema

with telangiectasia (Fig. 6-15) and mottled pigmentation. Dystrophic nails develop in infancy or early childhood and affect virtually all patients. Early nail changes include easy splitting and longitudinal ridging, but ultimately only small portions of the nails remain.

Hyperhidrosis and hyperkeratosis of the palms (Fig. 6-16) and soles occurs, as well as atrophic skin over the dorsa of the hands and feet. From approximately 5–10 years of age, affected children develop oral symptoms, including leukokeratosis involving the tongue (Fig. 6-17),

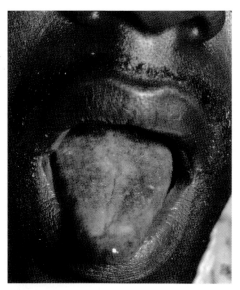

Figure 6-17

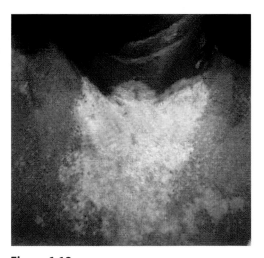

Figure 6-18

buccal mucosa, and gingiva. Lesions begin as painful ulcerations that recur. Similar lesions have been noted on other mucosal surfaces such as the anus, vagina, urethra, and conjunctiva. Involvement of the mucosae of the esophagus, lacrimal duct, and urethra may result in constriction causing dysphagia, epiphora, and dysuria. Numerous dental caries are common, as is the early loss of teeth. Squamous cell carcinomas of the mouth, esophagus, skin, vagina, cervix, and rectum are markedly increased in patients with dyskeratosis congenita. In the second or third decade of life, approximately 50% of patients develop anemia secondary to bone-marrow failure. Leukopenia and thrombocytopenia can be associated with the disorder.

Pernicious anemia is an autoimmune disorder caused by atrophy of the gastric mucosa and a reduction in the secretion of intrinsic factor. This results in cobalamin deficiency. Not surprisingly, pernicious anemia is associated with other autoimmune diseases, including vitiligo, which occurs in up to 10% of them. Sharply demarcated areas of complete loss of pigment develop around the eyes, nose, mouth, ears, and on perianal and genital skin. Hands, feet, and extensor surfaces of the extremities are also typically affected, but vitiligo can occur anywhere on the skin. The patient in Figure 6-18 was being treated for vitiligo when the macrocytic anemia and vitamin B_{12} deficiency of pernicious anemia were detected.

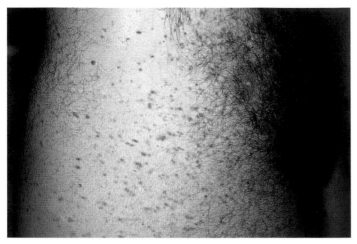

Figure 6-19

Mastocytosis refers to a number of disorders that share clinical features related to mast cell infiltration of the skin and other organs. These disorders are frequently recognized in children, but can occur at any age. The various forms of mastocytosis have been categorized. An indolent form has a good prognosis despite cutaneous lesions, ulcer disease, bone-marrow involvement, and other systemic complications. Less common forms of mastocytosis include a category associated with hematologic abnormalities; an aggressive form characterized by eosinophilia, hepato-splenomegaly, and lymphadenopathy; and mast cell leukemia.

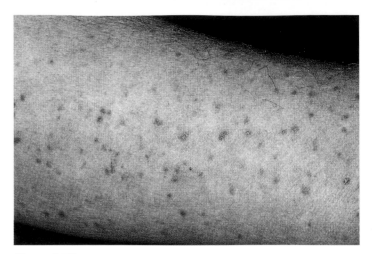

Figure 6-20

Urticaria pigmentosa is a cutaneous disorder found in patients with mastocytosis, particularly the indolent form. Skin lesions are quite variable in appearance. They consist of macules, papules, or nodules that range in size from 1 mm to several centimeters. Lesions are red, brown, or yellow and are usually truncal in distribution (Fig. 6-19). The extremities (Fig. 6-20) and scalp can be involved, but face, palms, and soles are often spared.

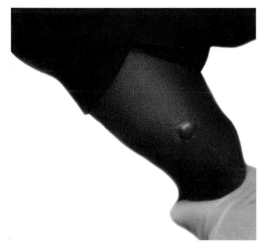

Figure 6-21

In neonates, lesions often form vesicles or bullae; the condition is then called **bullous urticaria pigmentosa** or bullous mastocytosis (Fig. 6-21).

Darier sign (Fig. 6-22) refers to the development of urticaria within minutes after firmly stroking skin lesions. This sign is pathognomonic of mastocytosis. Other cutaneous features of mastocytosis include urticaria, pruritus, and flushing. Exercise, hot baths, spicy foods, rubbing skin lesions, and a number of medications can cause symptoms. Non-

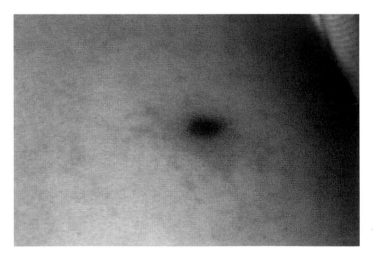

Figure 6-22

cutaneous symptoms of mastocytosis include abdominal pain, nausea, vomiting, diarrhea, and headache.

Bone marrow infiltration can be seen on radiographs and can result in bone pain and pathologic fractures. Development of anemia or thrombocytopenia is a negative prognostic factor for patients with mastocytosis. Mast cell leukemia has a poor prognosis. Most patients survive less than 6 months after diagnosis.

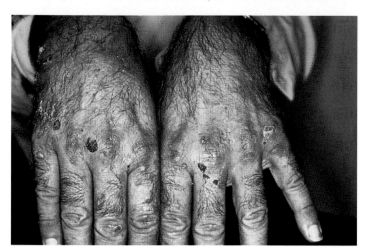

Figure 6-23

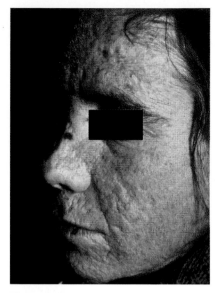

Figure 6-24

The **porphyrias** are a group of disorders caused by defects in hemoglobin synthesis, resulting in accumulation of porphyrins in body tissues and fluids. Cutaneous symptoms occur in most, but not all, of the porphyrias. Porphyria cutanea tarda is the commonest porphyria. It is caused by a decrease in activity of uroporphyrinogen decarboxylase. There are two forms of porphyria cutanea tarda: a sporadic or acquired form, and an autosomal dominantly inherited form with low penetrance. The sporadic form is precipitated by ingestion of alcohol, estrogens, iron hexachlorobenzene, or polychlorinated hydrocarbons. In recent years, human immunodeficiency virus (HIV) infection has been associated with porphyria cutanea tarda, as has hepatitis C virus infection. Clinical symptoms usually begin in the third or fourth decade. There is marked skin fragility, especially on the dorsa of the hands.

Minor trauma results in formation of vesicles and bullae, which form crusts, and eventually heal with hypopigmentation and scars (Figs 6-23 and 6-24).

Pinpoint, white, epidermal cysts—called milia—often develop in areas of scarring. Photosensitivity is not always immediately obvious, but the lesions are more common in sun-exposed areas like the face and hands, and the condition usually worsens in the summer. Hyperpigmentation, hypopigmentation, and hypertrichosis are additional cutaneous features. Hypertrichosis is particularly noticeable on the temples and cheeks. White, indurated, morphea-like plaques develop in

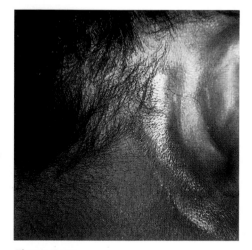

Figure 6-25

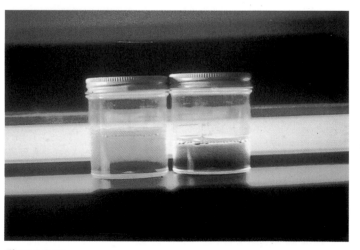

Figure 6-26

some people with porphyria cutanea tarda. The patient in Figure 6-25 had the sporadic form related to alcohol ingestion and developed a linear sclerodermoid plaque behind the ear.

For people in whom porphyria cutanea tarda is suspected, examination of the urine with a Wood's lamp provides a rapid screening test.

As shown in Figure 6-26, urine from a patient with porphyria cutanea tarda exhibits a pink–red color under fluorescence, while the normal urine (on the left) appears yellow–green. Addition of a few drops of acetic acid or 10% hydrochloric acid improves the sensitivity of this test.

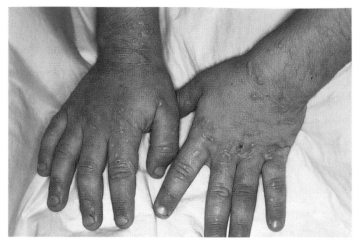

Figure 6-27A

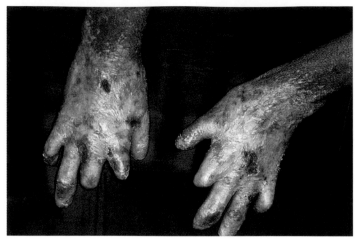

Figure 6-27B

Congenital erythropoietic porphyria, also called Gunther disease, is a rare and severe porphyria. It has autosomal recessive inheritance and is caused by deficient uroporphyrinogen III cosynthase. Symptoms begin in infancy and consist of extreme photosensitivity. With exposure to the sun, vesicles and bullae develop that ultimately heal with extensive scarring. This mutilating disorder leads to destruction of the ears and nose. Figure 6-27A shows the hands of a child with erythropoietic porphyria; the severity of the child's condition is limited by

rigorous measures to restrict sun exposure. By contrast, Figure 6-27B shows the severely mutilated hands of an adult with erythropoietic porphyria. Crusting, scarring, hypopigmentation, and loss of digits are common in this disorder.

Cutaneous lesions occurring in the scalp lead to cicatricial alopecia. Facial scarring can lead to ectropion. In sun-exposed areas, hypertrichosis is frequent and patients often have long, dark hairs on the forehead, cheeks, and sides of the face. Eyebrows and eye lashes are

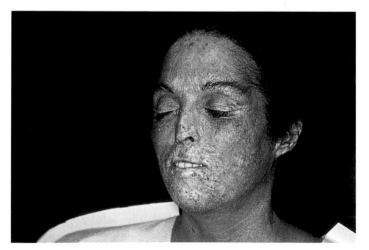

Figure 6-28

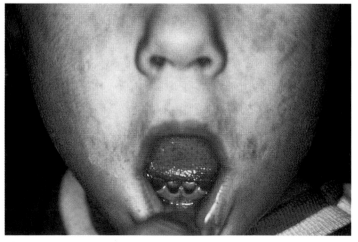

Figure 6-29

thickened. Repeated blister formation and scarring lead to irregular pigmentary alterations. The patient in Figure 6-28 exhibits numerous features of erythropoietic porphyria. There is mottled hyper- and hypopigmentation on most of the face. Hypertrichosis is apparent lateral to the eye and eyebrow.

Apart from skin lesions, erythropoietic porphyria is complicated by accumulations of porphyrins in many body tissues and fluids. Many

organs fluoresce a pink–red color. **Erythrodontia** (red teeth) is pathognomonic of this disorder and is caused by porphyrins in the teeth (Fig. 6-29). Gallstones are common and are loaded with porphyrins. Red blood cells contain porphyrins and hemolytic anemia frequently occurs. Splenomegaly is another associated finding; removal of the spleen often improves the hemolytic anemia and even the photosensitivity experienced by patients with erythropoietic porphyria.

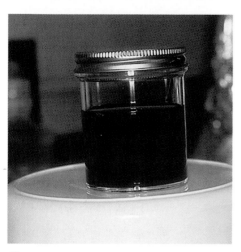

Figure 6-30

Usually the diagnosis is established on clinical grounds. Severe photo-sensitivity beginning in infancy may suggest a number of diagnoses such as xeroderma pigmentosum. In erythropoietic porphyria, however, there are other symptoms related to porphyrin deposition. Urine is pink to purple–red (Fig. 6-30); teeth are red and fluoresce with a Wood's lamp; even diapers soiled with urine and stools show characteristic purple–red fluorescence.

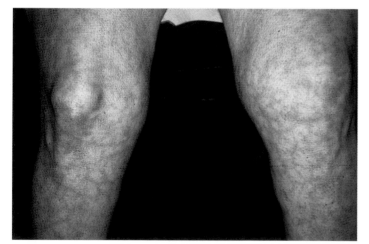

Figure 6-32

thrombus formation and infarction. It is common to see episodes of phlebitis, arterial thromboses, and repeated miscarriages in pregnant women. Some patients develop atrophie blanche—also known as livedo vasculitis—which is characterized by irregularly shaped ulcers that occur spontaneously on the feet and legs (Fig. 6-31). Occasionally patients will also have **livedo reticularis,** which appears as reticulated erythema usually involving the lower extremities (Fig. 6-32).

Cryoglobulinemia is caused by circulating proteins that precipitate at low temperatures. Cryoglobulins are occasionally found in patients with multiple myeloma, with Waldenström macroglobulinemia, and other neoplastic or inflammatory disorders.

In mixed cryoglobulinemia, activation of immune reactants and complement also occurs. The precipitated proteins mechanically block blood vessels, resulting in cutaneous infarction. Skin lesions frequently develop in acral areas that have lowest temperatures, such as the ears (Fig. 6-33), nose, and digits. Cutaneous symptoms begin with reticulated erythema or purpura resembling livedo reticularis. This

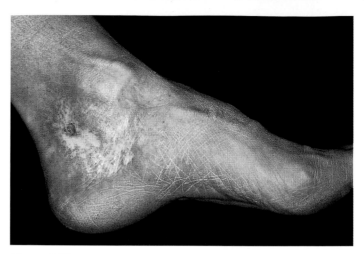

Figure 6-31

The **anticardiolipin antibody syndrome** is a recently described entity in people with circulating antiphospholipid antibodies. Patients often have false-positive serologies for syphilis, and many have positive antinuclear antibodies. The anticardiolipin antibody syndrome has been described in people with systemic lupus erythematosus who have a lupus anticoagulant. Paradoxically, the clinical features of the syndrome are caused by

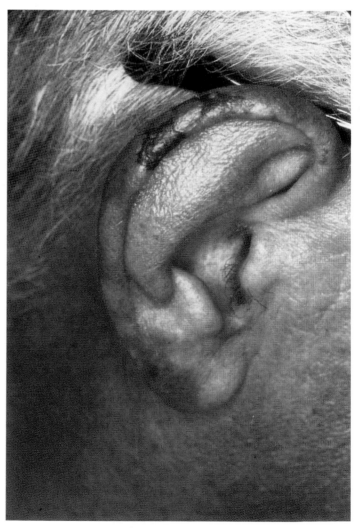

Figure 6-33

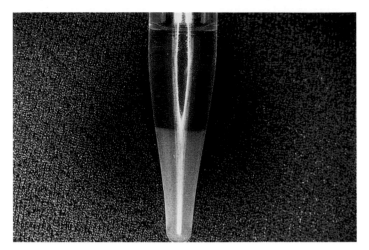

Figure 6-34

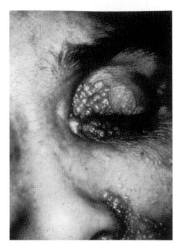

Figure 6-35

progresses to superficial, sharply demarcated ulcerations that may be covered by necrotic eschar. Gangrene of the toes or fingers may necessitate amputation. Glomerulonephritis, peripheral neuropathy, and arthritis are common systemic findings. Definitive diagnosis is aided by demonstrating the presence of circulating cryoglobulins. Blood must clot at 37° C. The serum is then allowed to stand at 4° C to allow cryoglobulins to precipitate (Fig. 6-34).

Amyloidosis consists of a group of disorders in which amyloid fibrils are deposited extracellularly in the skin or in other organs. Skin manifestations are most common in primary systemic amyloidosis or in amyloid associated with multiple myeloma. In the latter forms of amyloidosis, amyloid fibrils consist of immunoglobulin light-chain material. When this material infiltrates the dermis, the most characteristic skin lesions are waxy, shiny papules, which commonly develop on the eyelids (Fig. 6-35). Lesions are somewhat translucent and occasionally resemble

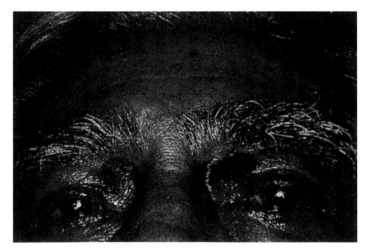

Figure 6-36

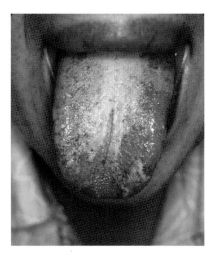

Figure 6-37

vesicles. The retroauricular folds, anogenital region, face, oral mucosa, and flexural sites, such as the neck, axillae, and periumbilical skin are typically affected.

Amyloid deposited in the blood-vessel walls results in spontaneous bleeding. Petechiae and purpura are most common on the eyelids (Fig. 6-36), face, flexural sites, and oral mucosa. "Pinch purpura" has been described after gentle pinching of the eyelids in people with amyloidosis. Periorbital purpura can develop after any maneuver that increases intrathoracic pressure— such as coughing, vomiting, or the Valsalva maneuver. An unusual but characteristic entity called "post-proctoscopic palpebral purpura" occurs in patients with amyloidosis.

Macroglossia (Fig. 6-37) affects 10% of patients with primary systemic or myeloma-associated amyloidosis. Tooth indentations may develop on the lateral borders of the tongue, and petechiae, purpura, fissures, ulcerations, or waxy papules occur on the tongue and buccal mucosa.

Half the patients with primary systemic or myeloma-associated amyloidosis develop hepatomegaly. Amyloid infiltration of the heart results in congestive heart failure, myocardial infarction, and arrhythmias. Deposition of amyloid in the gastrointestinal tract leads to malabsorption and protein-losing enteropapthy. Peripheral neuropathy, autonomic neuropathy with orthostatic hypotension,

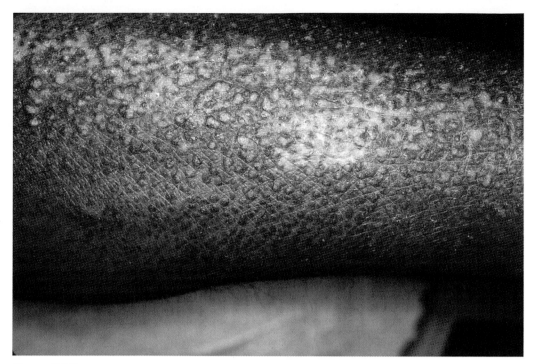

Figure 6-38

carpal tunnel syndrome, and Sjögren syndrome are complications in some cases of amyloidosis. In amyloidosis secondary to chronic disease, amyloid fibrils consist of nonimmunoglobulin proteins, and skin lesions seldom develop.

Localized cutaneous forms of amyloidosis occur without any systemic involvement. Macular amyloidosis is characterized by pruritic brown macules on the back and extremities. **Lichen amyloidosis** presents with extremely pruritic, hyperkeratotic brown papules, most commonly on the shins (Fig. 6-38). The papules often become confluent to form pruritic plaques.

7 Endocrine diseases

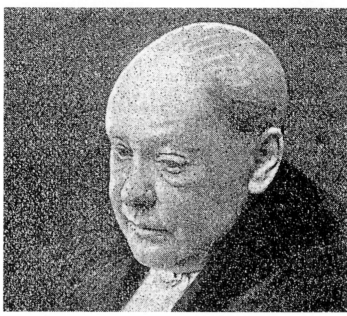

Figure 7-1

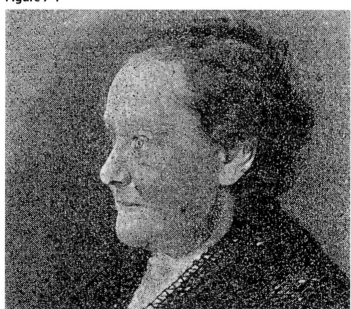

Figure 7-2

The features were thickened and swollen, the upper eyelids were swollen, and there was swelling beneath the right eye and round the neck; lips pale, but not much thickened. All the hair had disappeared from the head with the exception of two scanty tufts in each temporal region, and a few scattered hairs in the parietal region. The scalp was covered with a brown layer of dried epidermis, which was very adherent. The hands were not notably swollen; the palms were dry and cracked. She walked slowly and with difficulty, and found it required considerable effort to do anything. The memory was not good, and she was very sensitive to cold. The skin was dry (Fig. 7-1).

After seven months of thyroid extract injections: The expression of the face was brighter, and the swelling has practically disappeared. The hair had grown more than 2 inches in length. The skin had become softer, especially in the palms of the hands. By weekly injections, the temperature could be kept nearly normal. The mental and bodily activity had both improved very considerably (Fig. 7-2).

Murray G. Pathology and treatment of myxoedema. British Medical Journal 1892: August 27

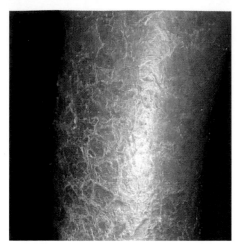

Figure 7-3

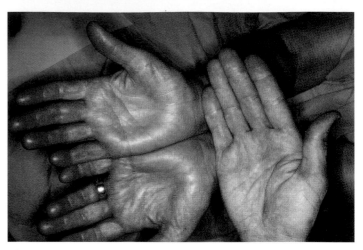

Figure 7-4

The dermatologic manifestations of **hypothyroidism** are often subtle. There is cutaneous deposition of water-binding mucopolysaccharides, which results in a puffy, water-logged feeling. The accumulation of water in the dermis results in nonpitting edema that is particularly noticeable around the eyes and in acral areas. Reduced cutaneous blood flow leaves the skin cold and pale, and reduced activity of sweat and sebaceous glands results in dry, coarse, and occasionally, pruritic skin.

Dryness and scaling can be so striking that ichthyosiform changes occur in some patients (Fig. 7-3). Reduced metabolism of β-carotene in the diet of some patients results in **carotenemia** with yellowing of the skin. The yellow discoloration is noticeable on the hands of the hypothyroid patient in Figure 7-4, and the hand of a euthyroid individual is shown for comparison.

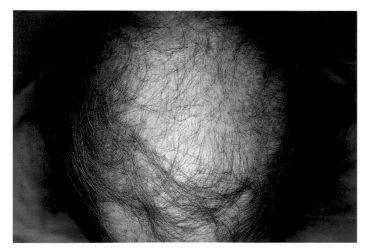

Figure 7-5

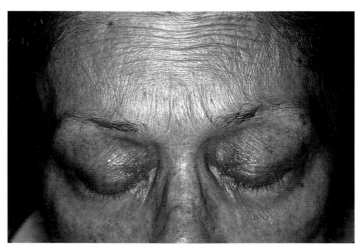

Figure 7-6

Hair loss is common and affects the entire body. Figure 7-5 shows diffuse loss of scalp hair in a woman with untreated hypothyroidism. The hair that remains is dull, coarse, and brittle, in part because of reduced sebum secretion. Loss of the outer third of the eyebrows is characteristic of hypothyroidism (Fig. 7-6). Some of the hair loss attributed to hypothyroidism can be reversed by thyroid hormone replacement therapy. Hypothyroid children occasionally develop long, fine lanugo-type hairs on their trunk, arms, and legs.

Other cutaneous features of hypothyroidism include easy bruising due to increased capillary fragility; xanthomas that arise from elevations in cholesterol and triglycerides; and rarely vitiligo. Fingernails are often abnormal, frequently described as brittle and easily broken.

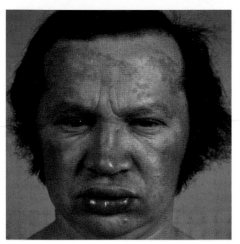

Figure 7-7A

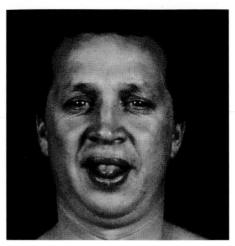

Figure 7-7B

Thyroid replacement quickly reverses many of the cutaneous features of **hypothyroidism**. Mucopolysaccharides deposited in the skin gradually disappear with administration of thyroid hormone. The patient in Figure 7-7A had a dull, listless expression with coarse features, including significant thickening of the lips and nose, as well as

nonpitting edema of the eyelids and loss of the lateral third of the eyebrows. Thyroid replacement successfully reversed many of the cutaneous features of hypothyroidism, including thickening of the lips and coarseness of facial features. Notice that the patient's tongue, which was previously enlarged, returned to its normal size (Fig. 7-7B).

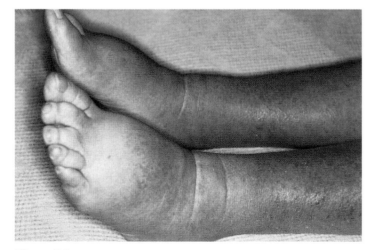

Figure 7-8

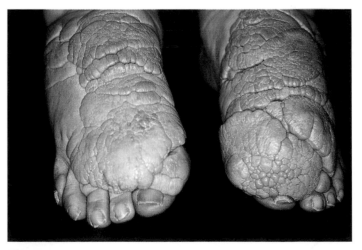

Figure 7-9

Thyroid replacement affects a number of laboratory parameters. Water bound to mucopolysaccharides is quickly mobilized, resulting in temporary reduction of hematocrit. Concomitant absorption of electrolytes from myxedematous tissue may transiently raise serum sodium. Elevated cholesterol levels return to normal after treatment with thyroid hormone.

Pretibial myxedema is one of the cardinal features of **Graves disease**. It often develops after treatment of hyperthyroidism but can develop in untreated hyperthyroid patients or in patients who are euthyroid or hypothyroid. The pretibial area develops skin-colored nodules and

plaques that can extend down to the dorsa of the feet (Fig. 7-8) and posteriorly to the calves. The plaques and nodules are usually nontender, although patients occasionally complain of pain, particularly when pretibial swelling first develops. This condition is caused by increased deposition of dermal mucopolysaccharides, especially hyaluronic acid, which can be shown histologically with Alcian blue staining. In severe cases, nonpitting thickening of the skin can be so extensive that folds extend over the ankles, and thick plaques can form on the dorsa of the feet with relative sparing of the toes (Fig. 7-9).

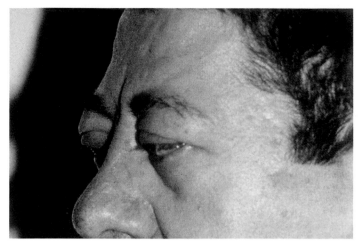

Figure 7-10

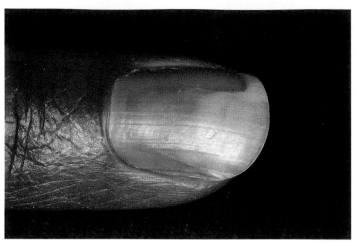

Figure 7-11

Exophthalmos is another key finding of Graves disease, and like pretibial myxedema, occurs in people who are hyperthyroid, euthyroid, or hypothyroid (Fig. 7-10). **Hyperthyroidism** is associated with peripheral vasodilatation, resulting in warm, flushed skin. Increased activity of the eccrine glands cause excessive sweating, particularly of the palms and soles. Skin is described as moist and soft or smooth.

Separation of the nail plate from the nail bed (Fig. 7-11), called **onycholysis**, occurs in more than 10% of hyperthyroid people. One or several nails can be affected and, with time, the entire nail plate may separate from the nail bed. Additional features of Graves disease include clubbing and subperiosteal new-bone formation, known as acropachy.

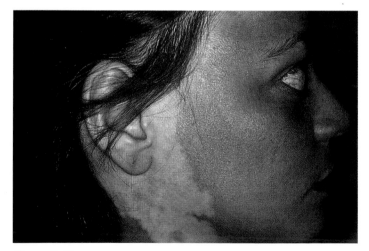

Figure 7-12

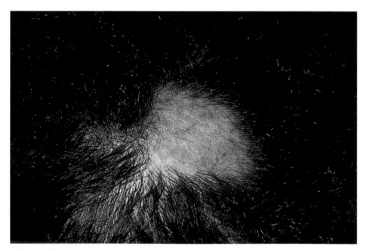

Figure 7-13

Several common dermatoses are said to be increased in patients with hyperthyroidism. These include atopic dermatitis, chronic urticaria, and generalized pruritus. An increased incidence of **vitiligo** has been noted in patients with Graves disease. Complete loss of pigmentation is found in sharply circumscribed patches as shown in a patient with exophthalmos in Figure 7-12. Other thyroid disorders such as Hashimoto thyroiditis are also found in patients with vitiligo. It is presumed that an autoimmune mechanism is responsible for the loss of pigment—as well as the thyroid disease.

Alopecia areata, another autoimmune condition, is also reported in patients with hyperthyroidism. There are sharply demarcated patches of hair loss, most commonly involving the scalp (Fig. 7-13), beard, and eyebrows. Patches can extend at their periphery, or new patches can develop. In many patients with mild alopecia areata, spontaneous regrowth of hair is common, although new patches can come and go unpredictably. The presence of "exclamation point" hairs connotes impending hair loss in a particular patch. These hairs are thick at their distal tips and thin where they originate at the scalp, resembling

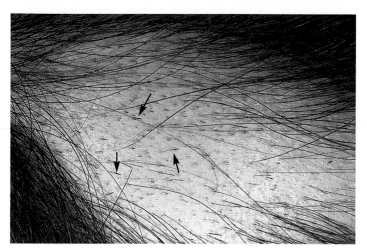

Figure 7-14

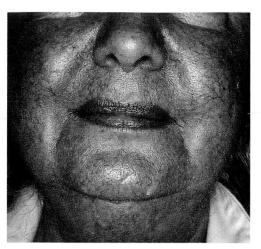

Figure 7-15

exclamation points (Fig. 7-14). In some people, alopecia areata can involve the entire scalp and is then called alopecia totalis. In other patients, all the hair is lost from the scalp, eyebrows, beard, axillary and pubic areas; this condition is called alopecia universalis. An auto-immune syndrome characterized by failure of endocrine organs has been associated with vitiligo or alopecia areata. Hypoparathyroidism, Hashimoto thyroiditis, Addison disease, pernicious anemia, diabetes mellitus, and ovarian failure have all been reported with this syndrome.

Cushing syndrome is most commonly caused by exogenous administration of systemic corticosteroids. Bilateral adrenal hyperplasia and malignant adrenal tumors, overproduction of adrenocorticotropic hormone (ACTH) by the pituitary gland (Cushing's disease) and ectopic production by nonpituitary tumors can all lead to the cutaneous stigmata of Cushing's syndrome. Patients develop central obesity with a **moon facies** (Fig. 7-15) and a "buffalo hump" caused by the deposition of fat over the clavicles and on the back of the neck.

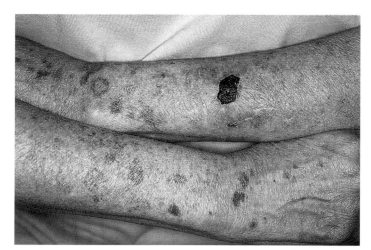

Figure 7-16

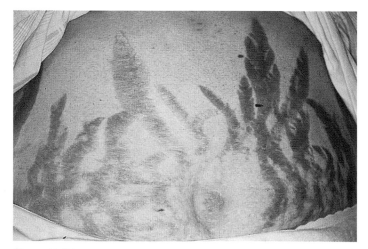

Figure 7-17

Telangiectases of the face cause a ruddy complexion. By contrast, subcutaneous fat of the extremities is reduced. The skin is atrophic, fragile, and easily damaged. Fragility of blood vessels leads to large ecchymoses even from trivial trauma (Fig. 7-16). Dermatophyte infections are common and quickly become widespread. Tinea versicolor is also common and, interestingly, can resolve with correction of the underlying hypercortisolism. Formation of large purple **striae** is characteristic, and these can affect large areas of the trunk and extremities (Fig. 7-17).

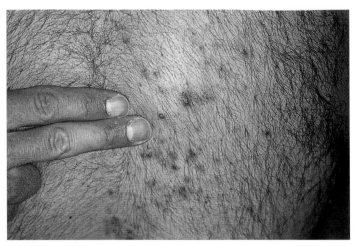

Figure 7-18

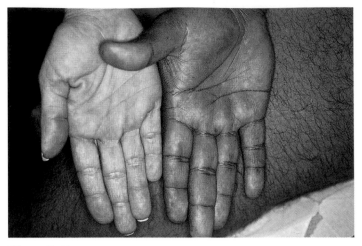

Figure 7-19

Hirsutism frequently develops, particularly of the face. Acanthosis nigricans occurs in a small proportion of patients with Cushing syndrome. An **acneiform eruption** characterized by inflamed perifollicular papules and pustules is a more common complication (Fig. 7-18), but acne cysts and comedones usually do not occur. Osteoporosis and the resulting compression fractures of the spine cause a reduction in height. When exogenous corticosteroids are responsible for Cushing syndrome, the dose and duration of treatment are related to the incidence of cushingoid side effects. The precise amount of steroid that can be administered safely varies from individual to individual. Rarely, Cushing syndrome can develop from overapplication of potent topical corticosteroids to large areas of skin. This is more likely to occur if the steroids are applied with occlusion. In addition to suppression of the adrenal-pituitary axis, local cutaneous side effects such as atrophy, fragility of skin, and formation of striae are well known to occur with overapplication of potent topical corticosteroids.

Addison disease develops with destruction of the adrenal glands by any cause. Tuberculosis used to account for the large majority of cases, but in recent years idiopathic atrophy of the glands—possibly as a result of an autoimmune mechanism—is the most frequent cause. Other causes of adrenal gland destruction, such as coccidioidomycosis, cryptococcosis, histoplasmosis, metastatic tumor, sarcoidosis, or amyloidosis, can also result in Addison disease. Diffuse hyperpigmentation of both sun-exposed and unexposed areas typically occurs. The hand and thigh of a patient with Addison disease are shown to the right of an unaffected relative's hand in Figure 7-19. The palmar creases are markedly hyperpigmented.

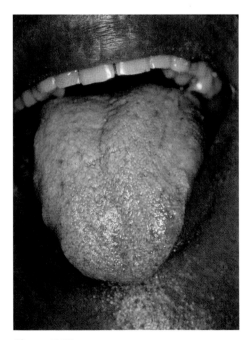

Figure 7-20

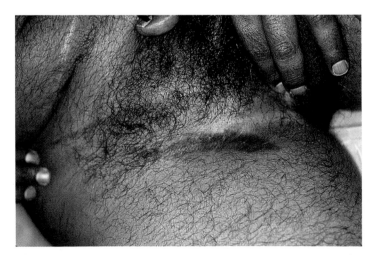

Figure 7-21

Normally pigmented areas, such as the areola of the nipple, can become even darker. Melanocytic nevi, hair, and new scars can also darken. Other characteristic sites include the elbows, knees, and knuckles. Pigmentation of oral mucosa develops in spots rather than diffusely (Fig. 7-20). The degree of hyperpigmentation is not related to the severity of other symptoms of Addison disease.

Nelson syndrome is an unusual variant of Addison disease. It develops in 10–30% of patients after bilateral adrenalectomy, even with adequate adrenocortical replacement. The syndrome can develop anywhere from 1–8 years after surgery. The patient in Figure 7-21 showed addisonian pigmentation of a new scar in the groin. By contrast, the scars resulting from his adrenalectomy healed without hyperpig-

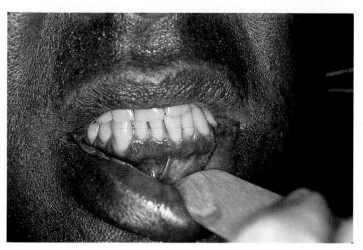

Figure 7-22

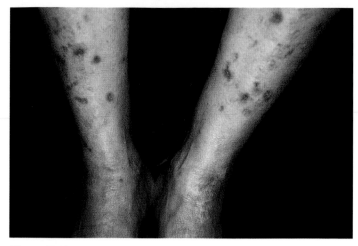

Figure 7-23

mentation. Gingival (Fig. 7-22) and lingual pigmented spots and facial hyperpigmentation developed along with a diffuse increase in pigment. Nelson syndrome occurs in the presence of an enlarging pituitary adenoma that produces large amounts of ACTH or melanocyte-stimulating hormone. These circulating hormones cause the striking hyperpigmentation seen in the syndrome. The pituitary adenomas are thought to develop as a result of the loss of feedback mechanisms from endogenous glucocorticoids after adrenalectomy.

Diabetic dermopathy, also called "shin spots," refers to depressed, atrophic, pigmented macules and patches that are commonly found on the anterior aspect of the lower legs of diabetic patients (Fig. 7-23). Lesions are asymptomatic and are occasionally preceded by erosions or erythema. They often resolve over 1–2 years, only to be replaced by new lesions elsewhere on the legs. They resemble postinflammatory changes seen after trauma to the legs, but appear much more frequently in diabetic patients—even in the absence of a history of trauma. This condition has been attributed to microangiopathic changes in the dermal blood vessels of people with diabetes. At least some of the brown discoloration is caused by hemosiderin deposition, rather than pigment.

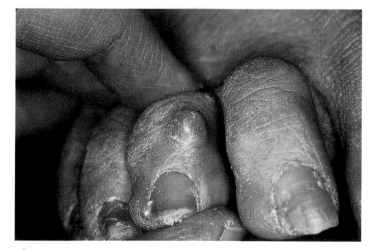

Figure 7-24

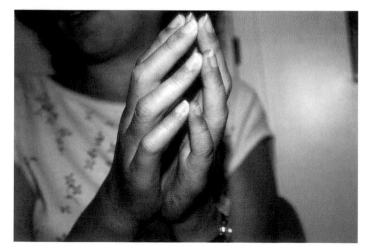

Figure 7-25

Diabetic bullae are blisters that occur in patients with severe diabetes. The blisters range from several millimeters to several centimeters in size. They are usually intraepidermal but may be subepidermal. Bullae spontaneously develop on the distal extremities, particularly the dorsa and sides of the hands and feet (Fig. 7-24). Fluid in the bulla cavity is clear. Blisters may occur individually or in crops and gradually heal without scarring. They are asymptomatic and seldom constitute a major problem for patients, although in some cases they do recur. Immunofluorescent studies are unremarkable, and the cause is unknown.

Waxy skin and stiff joints of diabetes have been described in patients with insulin-dependent diabetes mellitus and, less commonly in noninsulin-dependent diabetes mellitus. The skin over the dorsal aspects of the hands is indurated, tight, and scleroderma-like. The finger joints cannot be fully extended or flexed, particularly the proximal interphalangeal joints. Consequently, the palms cannot be approximated when the hands are held together (Fig. 7-25). This condition is associated with the complications of severe diabetes—namely retinopathy, nephropathy, and neuropathy.

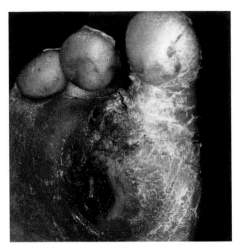

Figure 7-26

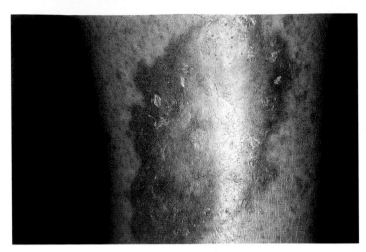

Figure 7-27

Peripheral neuropathy due to severe diabetes leads to loss of sensation. **Neuropathic ulcers**, also called mal perforans, consequently develop. The sole of the foot is usually affected, especially at sites of pressure under the metatarsal heads (Fig. 7-26). Ulcerations often occur in the middle of thick callus resulting from repeated pressure. Small vessel disease and compromised circulation result in poor healing and infection. Osteomyelitis is a common complication. Meticulous foot-care and well-fitting shoes are essential to avoid this severe complication of diabetes.

Necrobiosis lipoidica diabeticorum is characterized by chronic, indolent, asymptomatic lesions that are usually found on the anterior

and lateral surfaces of the lower legs. Lesions may be solitary or multiple and may involve one or both legs. Less commonly, they occur on the arms and trunk. They begin as erythematous nodules with sharply circumscribed borders that slowly enlarge. The center of the lesion eventually becomes atrophic, even while there is an actively enlarging red border. Epidermis overlying this center becomes shiny and atrophic, and blood vessels can be seen through the thinned skin (Fig. 7-27). The epidermis and dermis are so atrophied that subcutaneous fat is visible, giving the center of the lesions a yellow color. In some patients the condition gradually progresses to involve the entire pretibial area. With time, the lesions of necrobiosis lipoidica dia-

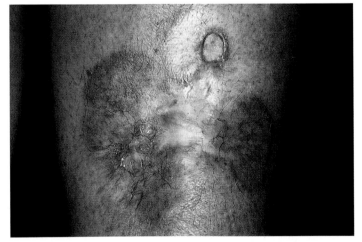

Figure 7-28

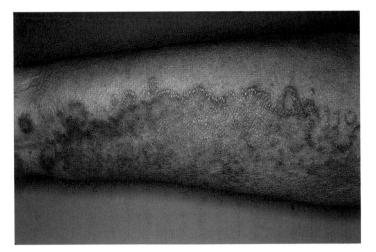

Figure 7-29

beticorum can ulcerate, becoming painful and susceptible to infection. The vast majority of patients with necrobiosis lipoidica diabeticorum have overt or latent diabetes. Even in those without evidence of diabetes, there is often a family history of the disorder, and these patients may eventually develop abnormal glucose tolerance. Only rarely does the condition develop in patients without any evidence of diabetes. Figure 7-28 shows excessive necrobiosis lipoidica diabeticorum with marked cutaneous atrophy in the center surrounded by rings of erythema at the enlarging borders and an ulcer at the superior margin of the lesion.

Granuloma annulare has been associated with diabetes by some authorities, although this association is controversial. Granuloma annulare typically involves the dorsal aspects of the hands and feet and the extensor surfaces of the elbows and knees. The classic lesion is an annular plaque with an elevated border, as shown on the tattooed arm of a concentration camp survivor with diabetes (Fig. 7-29). Skin lesions are usually asymptomatic. Diabetes is thought to be associated with a papular form of granuloma annulare that is generalized. The arms, neck, and upper trunk are involved more prominently than the legs.

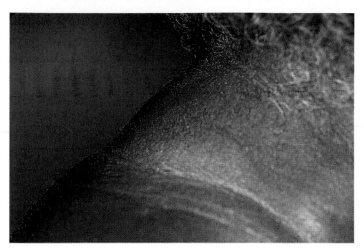

Figure 7-30

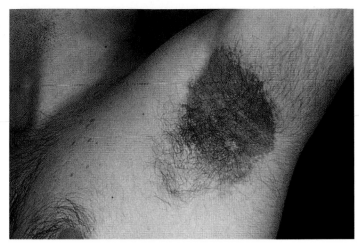

Figure 7-31

Scleredema is a condition characterized by rock-hard induration of the skin. It usually begins on the back and posterior neck (Fig. 7-30) but, in a small proportion of patients, scleredema can spread to the shoulders, arms, and chest. The face, abdomen, buttocks, and lower extremities are less commonly affected. In many patients, scleredema follows a preceding streptococcal pharyngitis or other infection. The latter form of scleredema is self-limited, resolving in 6 months to 2 years. In obese patients with noninsulin-dependent diabetes, a persistent form of scleredema commonly develops. It is associated with diabetic retinopathy and accelerated cardiovascular disease.

The prevalence of **erythrasma** is unquestionably increased in diabetic people. This corynebacterial infection is characterized by red–brown patches in the axillae (Fig. 7-31) or on the medial aspects of the thighs. The patches are often asymptomatic and can be present for years, spreading slowly at their periphery. Patients seldom complain about the discolored patches of erythrasma, which are usually incidentally noted on physical examination. Examination by Wood's lamp reveals orange–red fluorescence. This condition is often mistaken for a fungal infection, but the organism will not grow on conventional fungal media. Erythrasma is best treated with oral or topical antibiotics.

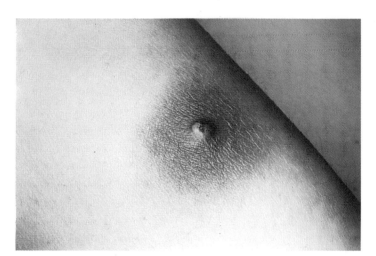

Figure 7-32

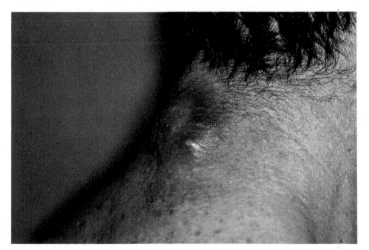

Figure 7-33

The prevalence of staphylococcal and candidal infections in diabetic patients has been controversial. For years it was thought that staphylococcal infections, such as the **furuncle** shown in Figure 7-32, occurred more in diabetic patients, but this does not appear to be true for those whose blood sugar is well controlled. Extensive cutaneous infection, however, can disrupt control of blood sugar, resulting in additional requirement for insulin. Moreover, staphylococcal infections may be more serious and more frequent in people with poorly controlled diabetes.

The patient in Figure 7-33 developed a **carbuncle** of the posterior neck. He presented with high fever and markedly elevated blood sugars. On incision and drainage of the carbuncle, his insulin requirement returned to its previous level. In contrast to furuncles, which are smaller and more superficial, carbuncles involve large areas of skin, and are red, warm, and tender. Multiple pustules develop and when treated with systemic antibiotics they ultimately form crusts. If untreated, the infection can spread to surrounding skin and soft tissues.

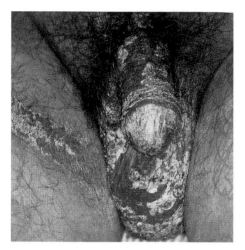

Figure 7-34

Cutaneous **candidal infections** are increased in hyperglycemic patients, but they respond well to control of blood sugar and are not increased in well-controlled diabetic patients. The patient in Figure 7-34 has a monilial infection of the groin that was refractory to topical therapy until blood sugars were brought under control by increasing his insulin dosage. The infection promptly remitted with adequate control of blood sugar. Monilial infections of the groin typically involve the genitalia and are associated with maceration, formation of pustules, and satellite lesions that are not directly contiguous with the macerated patches.

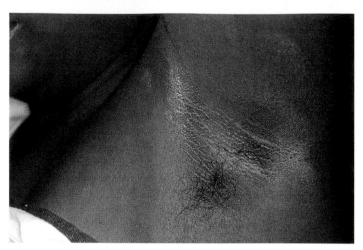

Figure 7-35

Despite a well-known association with malignancy, **acanthosis nigricans** more commonly occurs in people with a number of endocrinopathies. Cushing syndrome, acromegaly, polycystic ovary disease, hyper- and hypothyroidism, and diabetes have all been associated with acanthosis nigricans. Even in the absence of an overt endocrinopathy, obese patients frequently develop a mild form of this condition. Brown velvety patches develop on the neck and in the axillae (Fig. 7-35). Other intertriginous sites are often affected, such as the groin and inframammary creases. Papillomatous hyperplasia of the epidermis can occasionally be discerned on close inspection of the skin.

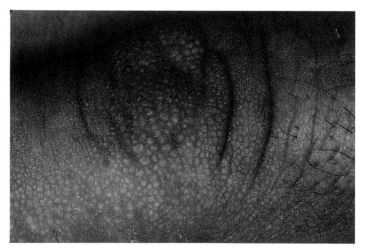

Figure 7-36

In patients with more severe acanthosis nigricans, the cutaneous lesions are more extensive and can involve sites such as the knuckles or the tongue. Although it has been suggested that severe acanthosis nigricans indicates an underlying malignancy, patients with endocrinopathies can also develop severe forms of the disease. The patient in Figure 7-36 has diabetes associated with chronic, generalized acanthosis nigricans extending to the knuckles, without any evidence of malignancy. All forms of insulin resistance have been associated with acanthosis nigricans, including insulin resistance caused by defects of the insulin receptor, anti-insulin receptor antibodies, and postreceptor abnormalities.

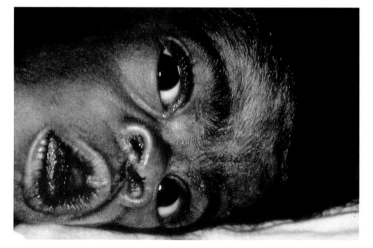

Figure 7-37

Leprechaunism is an autosomal recessively inherited syndrome caused by mutations in the insulin receptor gene. Apart from extreme insulin resistance, affected infants are born with numerous cutaneous and systemic manifestations. There is intrauterine growth retardation as well as postnatal failure to thrive. The skin is loose, subcutaneous fat is lacking, and muscle mass is reduced. Affected individuals have a characteristic "elf-like" face, with large ears and eyes, hypertelorism, a broad nose, and micrognathia (Fig. 7-37). Hands and feet are large in comparison to the body. There is hypertrophy of the male external genitalia. Additional cutaneous features include acanthosis nigricans,

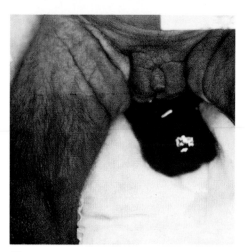

Figure 7-38

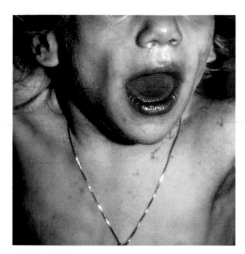

Figure 7-39

which is present at birth, and hirsutism of the face, trunk, and extremities. Hirsutism is evident in the patient shown in Figures 7-37 and 7-38. In addition to the aforementioned manifestations, the child in Figure 7-38 was born with a prolapse of the rectum. Most infants with leprechaunism survive only a few months.

Congenital lipoatrophic diabetes, a form of generalized lipodystrophy, is an autosomal recessive inherited condition of unknown cause. Patients are born lacking subcutaneous fat and extracutaneous

adipose tissue. The child shown in Figure 7-39 appears emaciated because of the complete absence of subcutaneous fat. Paradoxically, there is increased fat in the liver, resulting in hepatomegaly; the liver may be so enlarged that it causes the abdomen to protrude. In advanced cases, cirrhosis and hepatic failure develop. The kidneys are frequently enlarged, and renal failure can occur. In childhood, the muscles appear hypertrophied and the external genitalia are enlarged. Linear growth is accelerated but the epiphyses close early, so these patients ultimately attain a normal height. Cutaneous manifestations include acanthosis

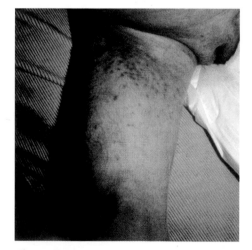

Figure 7-40

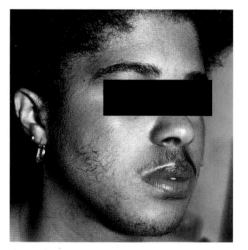

Figure 7-41

nigricans, hypertrichosis, and hyperpigmentation. Patients with lipo-atrophic diabetes may not develop clinical diabetes mellitus until the third decade of life. Affected individuals develop angiopathy, retinopathy, and nephropathy, but diabetic ketoacidosis does not usually occur. Other systemic complications include hypertriglyceridemia, polycystic ovaries, mental retardation, and bony abnormalities. Figure 7-40 shows a child with lipoatrophic diabetes. The child had severe hypertriglyceridemia, resulting in eruptive xanthomas that can be seen on the thigh.

Polycystic ovary syndrome, also called the Stein–Leventhal syndrome, consists of a constellation of clinical symptoms associated with androgen excess. Both autosomal dominant and X-linked

inheritance patterns have been described; many sporadic cases occur as well. Symptoms consist of hirsutism, obesity, enlarged cystic ovaries, and infertility due to chronic anovulation. Amenorrhea or oligomenorrhea are characteristic features of the syndrome. Menarche occurs at a normal age in most girls, although some never develop uterine bleeding.

Bleeding can occur at irregular intervals and the duration and amount of bleeding are highly variable. Not all the symptoms of polycystic ovary disease are present in every affected patient, and many symptoms are present to a variable degree. Hirsutism is evident at puberty and can be very mild in some people. The woman in Figure 7-41 has severe hirsutism of the

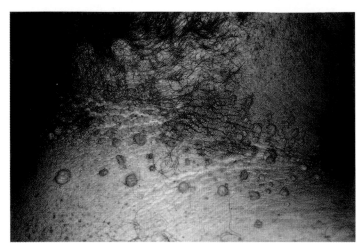

Figure 7-42

face in association with polycystic ovaries. Obesity, acanthosis nigricans, and insulin resistance have also been found. **Acrochordons** (skin tags) are reported to be increased in this syndrome and are present on the neck of the patient shown in Figure 7-42.

8 Neurologic diseases

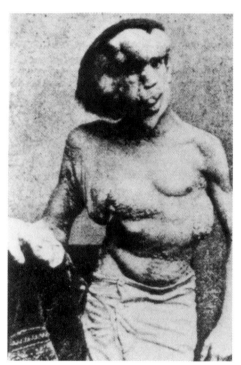

Figure 8-1

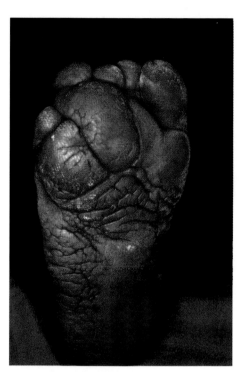

Figure 8-2

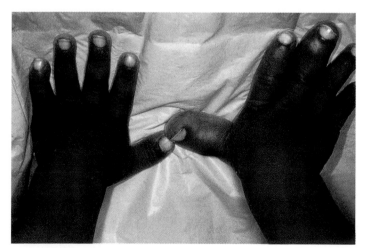

Figure 8-3

John Merrick (Fig. 8-1) was portrayed in film as "The Elephant Man" and was thought to suffer from neurofibromatosis. His condition was so severe that he was forced to become a circus-freak attraction. Recent authors have questioned Merrick's diagnosis, suggesting that he may in fact have had the Proteus syndrome. The latter condition is a recently described hamartomatous syndrome characterized by partial gigantism of the hands and feet, and skeletal hypertrophy, multiple lipomas, hemangiomas, and lymphangiomas (Figs 8-2 and 8-3).

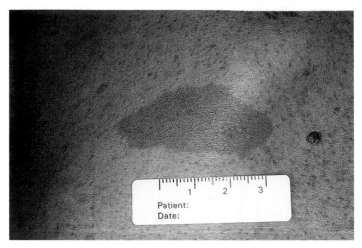

Figure 8-4

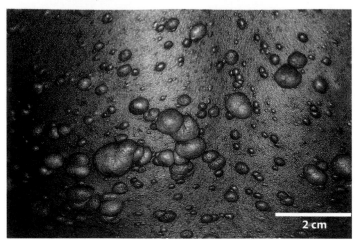

Figure 8-5

Type I neurofibromatosis, also called von Recklinghausen disease, is a fairly common inherited disorder affecting approximately 1 in 3000 births. In 50% of cases, autosomal dominant inheritance can be identified, but the rest presumably occur as a result of spontaneous mutations. The most familiar skin lesion of neurofibromatosis is the **café-au-lait spot** (Fig. 8-4). This is a completely flat, evenly pigmented brown patch that measures 1 cm to several centimeters in diameter. Café-au-lait spots can be found in 10% of the normal population, but the presence of six or more, larger than 1.5 cm in diameter, is a criterion for the diagnosis of neurofibromatosis and should trigger a search for the other stigmata of the disease. Histologically, café-au-lait spots are identified by the presence of macromelanosomes, giant pigment granules in melanocytes and keratinocytes.

Neurofibromas are soft, skin-colored nodules that can be flat or pedunculated (Fig. 8-5). Blood vessels within a neurofibroma will occasionally cause the lesion to appear violaceous. Neurofibromas have

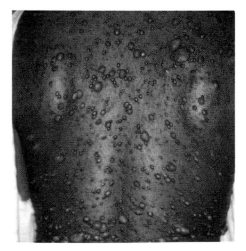

Figure 8-6

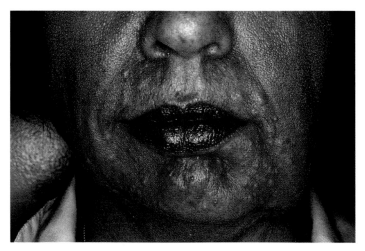

Figure 8-7

diameters of a few millimeters to several centimeters, and patients occasionally may have a few isolated neurofibromas or may be covered by hundreds (Fig. 8-6).

Neurofibromas may be present in childhood but they often increase in size and number around puberty, and in women at the time of pregnancy. Exogenous estrogens in the form of oral contraceptives will also cause an increase in cutaneous neurofibromas. The number of neurofibromas can continue to increase throughout life. The term **plexiform neuroma** refers to larger, deeper tumors that can be associated with adjacent bone and soft tissue hypertrophy, and result in marked disfigurement. In Figure 8-7, the patient's asymmetrical jaw results from an underlying plexiform neuroma.

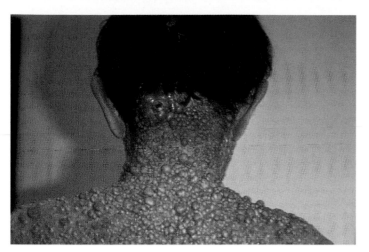

Figure 8-8

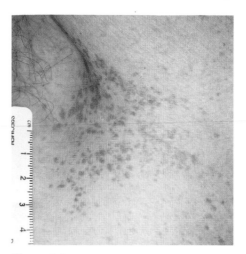

Figure 8-9

Cutaneous neurofibromas rarely undergo malignant degeneration. A small percentage of patients, however, will develop malignancies of neural origin within plexiform neuromas. Figure 8-8 shows a **neurofibrosarcoma** presenting as an ulceration on the posterior scalp. This tumor arose from a plexiform neuroma at the base of the skull. Removal of large numbers of small cutaneous neurofibromas may be warranted for cosmetic reasons, but is not likely to reduce the incidence of malignancy in these patients. Sudden enlargement or onset of pain within plexiform neuromas should be investigated, however.

Axillary and inguinal freckling refers to the presence of evenly pigmented brown macules in intertriginous areas, specifically the axillae and inguinal areas, in patients with neurofibromatosis (Fig. 8-9). Although present in only 20% of neurofibromatosis patients, this finding is also one of the criteria for establishing the diagnosis. Many neurologic complications of neurofibromatosis have been well described, including mental retardation and macrocephaly. Development of cutaneous neurofibromas or plexiform neuromas in specific locations may cause impairment of speech, hearing, or sight. Skeletal abnormalities include cystic bone changes and hypertrophy of bone adjacent to plexiform neuromas. Kyphoscoliosis is common.

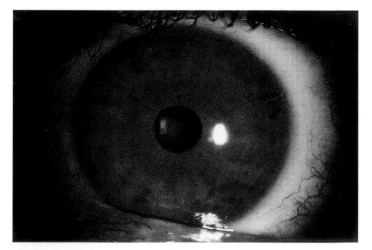

Figure 8-10

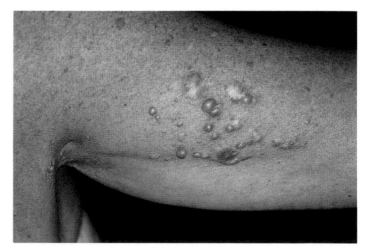

Figure 8-11

In patients who do not have a family history of neurofibromatosis and who present with multiple café-au-lait spots but have no other obvious cutaneous stigmata of the disease, the question arises as to whether they have von Recklinghausen disease. Examination for **Lisch nodules** is extremely helpful. Lisch nodules are pigmented iris hamartomas that are found in more than 90% of patients with neurofibromatosis (Fig. 8-10). They can occasionally be seen on visual examination of the eye, but may require examination by slit-lamp.

Approximately 85% of patients with neurofibromatosis have Type I disease, which refers to classic von Recklinghausen disease. Type II neu-

rofibromatosis refers to those who develop bilateral acoustic neuromas but do not have Lisch nodules and have very few skin lesions. This type has been localized to a different chromosomal abnormality, and also has autosomal dominant inheritance. Several other types of neurofibromatosis have been identified including type V, or **segmental neurofibromatosis,** in which there is a segmental distribution of café-au-lait spots and cutaneous neurofibromas. The patient in Figure 8-11 has neurofibromas that are localized to one arm. Type V neurofibromatosis is not associated with Lisch nodules and does not appear to be inherited in a dominant fashion.

Figure 8-12

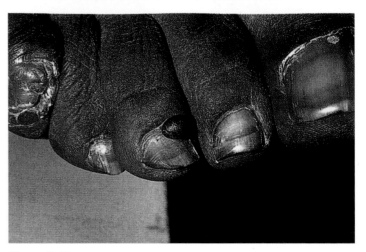

Figure 8-13

Tuberous sclerosis is an inherited syndrome with distinctive skin lesions and neurologic symptoms. The mnemonic EPILOA can be used to recall the features of tuberous sclerosis: *epi*lepsy, *lo*w IQ, and *a*denoma sebaceum. The true incidence of this disorder is not known because there is no serologic assay for its diagnosis, and the clinical features are highly variable.

Autosomal dominant inheritance can be found in approximately 25% of cases; the remaining 75% appear to result from spontaneous mutation. Hypopigmented macules are found in most patients and are present at the time of birth. Wood's lamp examination may be necessary to identify the lesions in patients who are fair-skinned. Large hypopigmented macules are 1–3 cm in diameter, occasionally larger, and have a shape that has been described as polygonal. In some cases, a macule resembles the shape of an ash leaf and is therefore called **ash leaf macule** (Fig. 8-12). The macules most frequently occur on the trunk but can develop on the head and extremities. Smaller hypopigmented macules ranging 2–3 mm in diameter are called confetti macules. **Periungual and subungual fibromas** of the fingers and toes often develop around the time of puberty (Fig. 8-13).

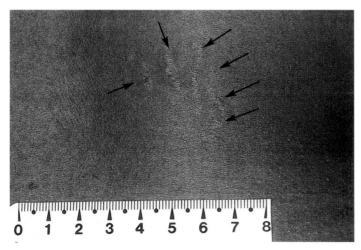

Figure 8-14

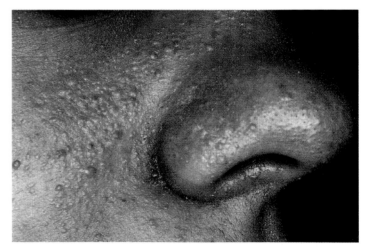

Figure 8-15

The **shagreen patch**, another distinctive feature of tuberous sclerosis, is a skin-colored plaque that consists of dermal connective tissue and develops early in childhood (Fig. 8-14). Café-au-lait spots and intraoral fibromas are among the other cutaneous features. **Adenoma sebaceum**, the characteristic skin lesion of tuberous sclerosis, consists of angio-fibromas of the cheeks and nasolabial folds. These small skin-colored papules can easily be mistaken for the lesions of acne (Fig. 8-15). Neurologic features of the syndrome include seizures, which occur in more than 80% of patients, and mental retardation, which affects almost 50%. Patients develop brain lesions called tubers, which calcify and may be visible on skull radiographs. CT scans may be helpful in establishing the diagnosis in patients who have a family history of the disorder but do not have distinctive skin lesions. A variety of other uncommon tumors and hamartomatous growths of various organs have been reported in patients with tuberous sclerosis.

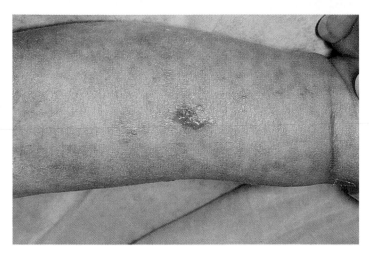

Figure 8-16

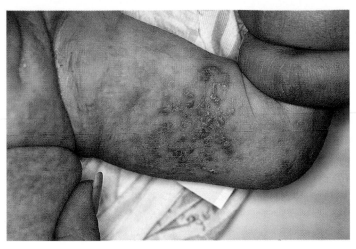

Figure 8-17

Incontinentia pigmenti is another neurocutaneous syndrome that is inherited as a sex-linked dominant trait. It is lethal in male fetuses, and almost all affected patients are female. Vesicobullous skin lesions begin either in utero or within weeks of birth (Fig. 8-16). Histologically the vesicles are intraepidermal or subepidermal and contain eosinophils.

An elevated white blood count and eosinophilia can occur during this early stage. Vesicular lesions are followed within 2–6 weeks by verrucous papules (Fig. 8-17) and, ultimately, linear pigmented macules and patches that develop in the first 6 months of life. Whorled patterns of hyperpigmentation are characteristic and can involve the trunk and

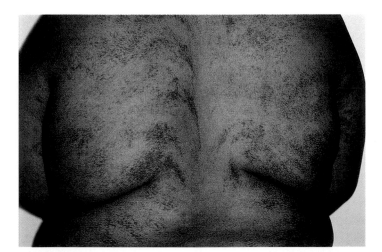

Figure 8-18

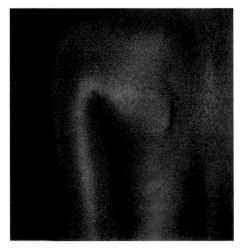

Figure 8-19

extremities (Fig. 8-18). They do not necessarily involve the same sites that had vesicular or verrucous lesions. In some infants born with pigmented macules, vesicular and verrucous stages are not seen and are presumed to have occurred in utero. With age, the pigmented areas may lighten and eventually disappear. Neurologic symptoms are common and include mental retardation, seizures, spastic paralysis, and microcephaly. Numerous ocular abnormalities have been reported, including retinal detachment, optic atrophy, cataracts, strabismus, nystagmus, uveitis, chorioretinitis, and others. Early laser coagulation of retinal vascular proliferation may preserve vision. A scarring alopecia, neural changes, ocular abnormalities, skeletal malformations, and abnormal teeth can occur as well.

Incontinentia pigmenti achromians, also called hypomelanosis of Ito, is characterized by whorls of hypopigmentation that resemble the hyperpigmented lesions of incontinentia pigmenti (Fig. 8-19). Bizarre linear hypopigmented macules and patches can be present on the trunk and extremities at birth or can develop in infancy or early childhood. Once present, these bizarre hypopigmented lesions remain for life. Neurologic symptoms, including mental retardation and seizures, affect 50% of patients. As in incontinentia pigmenti, skeletal and ocular abnormalities are common.

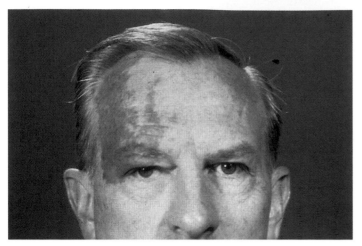

Figure 8-20

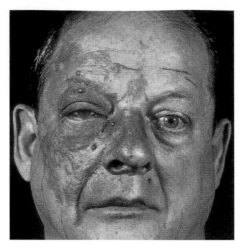

Figure 8-21

Sturge–Weber syndrome, also called encephalotrigeminal angiomatosis, is a noninherited congenital disorder characterized by a portwine stain of the face, and is associated with neurologic symptoms and ocular abnormalities. The **port-wine stain** occurs in the distribution of the first trigeminal nerve, involving the upper eyelid and forehead (Fig. 8-20). It is present at birth as a pink or red patch that remains confined to one side of the face without crossing the midline. The portwine stain can be a small patch that only covers the upper eyelid, or a much larger lesion that covers the entire side of the head and face

(Fig. 8-21); occasionally the upper trunk or an upper extremity can be involved. In children, the surface of a port-wine stain is smooth but, with age, papular or nodular components can develop. The clinical changes that occur over time correspond to the histologic changes that are seen. Telangiectasia are not apparent until age 10 years. Thereafter, dilatation of superficial capillaries increases progressively with increasing age, and even deep dermal vessels may dilate later in life. The color also darkens with time, becoming purple in older patients. Increased blood flow through a port-wine stain can result in hyper-

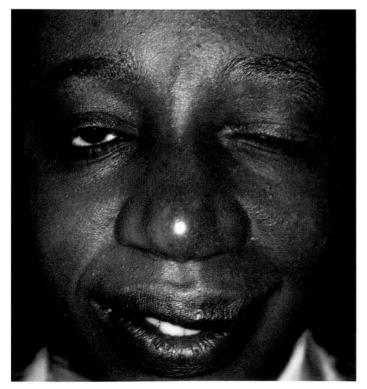

Figure 8-22

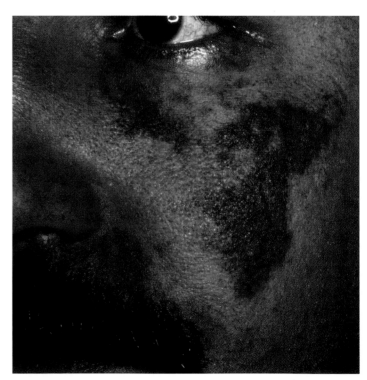

Figure 8-23

trophy of the underlying bone and soft tissue. Therefore, patients can develop marked asymmetry of the face (Fig. 8-22). In the Sturge–Weber syndrome, port-wine stains are associated with ipsilateral leptomeningeal angiomatosis that results in seizures in at least 80% of patients. These seizures, which are usually not present at birth but develop in infancy or childhood, are usually focal and contralateral to the skin lesions.

Mental retardation and hemiparesis with hemianopsia are additional neurologic abnormalities found in this syndrome. Neurologic symptoms can become more extensive over time, but rarely begin after the age of 20 years. When the **nevus flammeus** occurs only below the palpebral fissure (Fig. 8-23), central nervous system features of the syndrome do not develop, since cerebral involvement is absent.

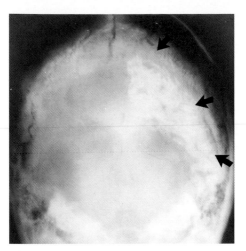

Figure 8-24

Ipsilateral cerebral calcification develops in most patients with the **Sturge–Weber syndrome**. In two-thirds of patients, skull radiographs reveal characteristic streaks that have been called "tram lines" (Fig. 8-24). These are usually absent at birth but are often visible by the age of 2 years. They represent calcification of the parietooccipital cortex and are thought to result from ischemia caused by the meningeal angioma.

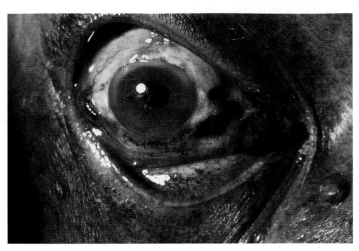

Figure 8-25

Angiomas of the conjunctiva, iris, or choroid can develop in the Sturge–Weber syndrome (Fig. 8-25). Choroidal angiomatosis may result in congenital or late onset glaucoma or retinal detachment. Nearly 50% of patients will develop glaucoma in childhood if the port-wine stain involves both the maxillary and ophthalmic divisions of the trigeminal nerve. Choroidal atrophy, exophthalmos, and megalocornea are additional ocular complications of this syndrome.

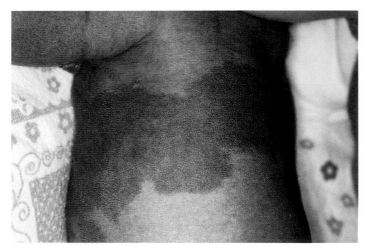

Figure 8-26

Cobb syndrome is characterized by an angioma of the spinal cord with an overlying vascular lesion such as a port-wine stain. The port-wine stain is present at birth and typically occurs in a dermatomal distribution (Fig. 8-26). Neurologic symptoms result from anoxia or compression of the spinal cord by the angioma. Motor or sensory findings can develop gradually over years or may appear suddenly. Symptoms depend on the level of involvement and can include pain, weakness, sensory loss, or loss of motor function, including paraplegia.

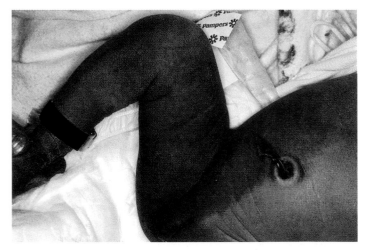

Figure 8-27

Occasionally, large areas of nevus flammeus can involve a limb. If there is associated hypertrophy of the affected extremity, patients may have features of the **Klippel–Trenaunay–Weber syndrome**. This syndrome can be associated with hemangiomas of the spinal cord in some patients. Motor and sensory symptoms are determined by the size and location of the hemangiomas. The cutaneous vascular lesions are usually unilateral and often distributed in a dermatomal pattern (Fig. 8-27). The arms, legs, or trunk are usually involved. Cerebral arteriovenous fistula and hemicranial hypertrophies have been reported in patients with this syndrome.

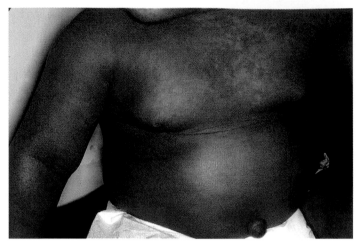

Figure 8-28

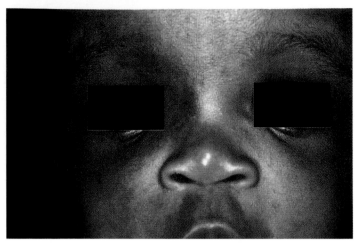

Figure 8-29

Phakomatosis pigmentovascularis is a syndrome characterized by the presence of extensive cutaneous hemangiomas and melanocytic lesions. Nevus flammeus typically involves large portions of the head, trunk, and extremities. Melanocytic lesions consist of extensive **mongolian spots**, nevus spilus, nevus anemicus, or epidermal nevi that are scattered across the face, trunk, and extremities adjacent to the hemangiomas (Fig. 8-28). Phakomatosis pigmentovascularis can be subclassified by the type of pigmented lesions that occur, and by the presence or absence of systemic symptoms. Aberrant mongolian spots, the most common pigmented lesions associated with this syndrome, are large, deep blue patches that are present at birth and persist throughout life. People with phakomatosis pigmentovascularis can develop visceral or intracranial angiomas, resulting in a variety of systemic symptoms. When the **nevus flammeus** involves the face (Fig. 8-29) and is associated with a seizure disorder, this syndrome overlaps with the Sturge–Weber syndrome. As in the Sturge–Weber syndrome, glaucoma

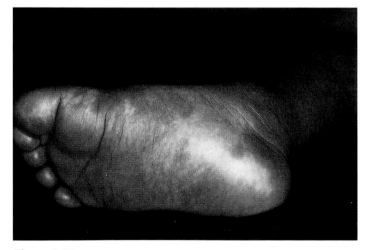

Figure 8-30

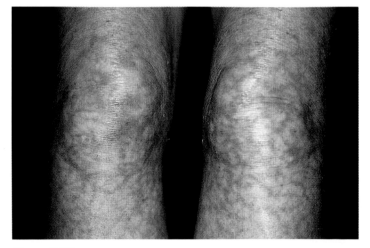

Figure 8-31

can occur. Other ocular abnormalities include melanosis oculi and iris abnormalities consisting of nodules that have been mistaken for Lisch nodules. In patients with nevus flammeus involving an extremity, there may be hypertrophy of the underlying bone or soft tissue, simulating the Klippel–Trenaunay–Weber syndrome (Fig. 8-30).

Sneddon syndrome is a rare disorder caused by blockage of small to medium-sized arteries. Skin and neurologic symptoms begin in early adulthood (ranging from adolescence to age 45 years) and often start concurrently. Cutaneous lesions are characterized by a generalized reticulated erythema that has been called **livedo racemosa** and is identical in appearance to livedo reticularis (Fig. 8-31).

After several years patients develop transient ischemic attacks or strokes. Diagnosis is established by demonstrating typical vascular changes on skin biopsy of patients with livedo racemosa and neurologic symptoms.

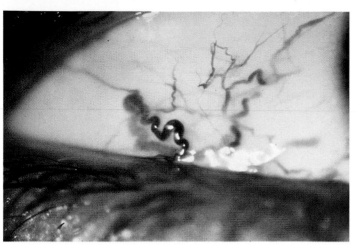

Figure 8-32

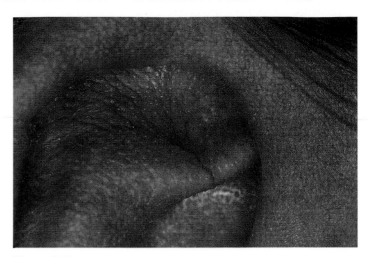

Figure 8-33

Ataxia telangiectasia is an autosomal recessive inherited syndrome characterized by the development of cerebellar ataxia and mucocutaneous telangiectasia. Cerebellar ataxia first becomes apparent as infants learn to walk. Older children develop choreoathetosis and myoclonic jerks, and most are wheelchair-bound. Telangiectases can be present at birth but are usually first seen in 3–6-year-old children, when the diagnosis is made. The telangiectases are most dramatic on the bulbar conjunctivae (Fig. 8-32). The eyelids, ears, face, buccal mucosa, antecubital and popliteal fossae, and dorsal hands and feet develop telangiectasias that may appear as linear streaks (Fig. 8-33) or as pinpoint red macules. Cutaneous atrophy with loss of subcutaneous fat and tightening of facial skin is associated with diffuse graying of the hair, giving patients a prematurely aged appearance. Some patients are affected by oculomotor dysfunction and nystagmus. Retardation of growth and mental retardation are common. Recurrent sinopulmonary infections result in bronchiectasis and are the leading cause of death in patients with ataxia telangiectasia. Lymphoreticular malignancies and cutaneous malignancies are increased in those who live to adulthood.

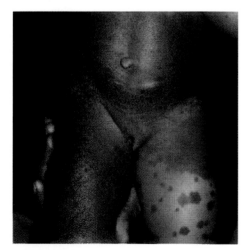

Figure 8-34

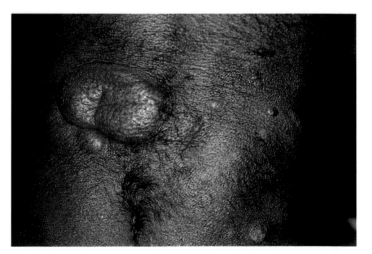

Figure 8-35

Neurocutaneous melanosis is a rare syndrome in which multiple large or giant congenital cutaneous melanocytic nevi (Fig. 8-34) are associated with leptomeningeal pigmentation. Although congenital, the condition is not hereditary. The congenital nevi may be flat or elevated at birth and often develop papules, nodules, tumors, or verrucous components with age (Fig. 8-35). They are usually hairy and can have a dermatomal distribution extending to the skin overlying the spine, without crossing the midline. Neurologic symptoms usually develop in the first 3 years of life and result from increased intracranial pressure and compression of the brain or spinal cord. Although primary leptomeningeal melanoma is rare, most patients with this syndrome are afflicted with it. CT scans should therefore be performed in children with giant congenital nevi of the scalp or posterior midline nevi; cerebrospinal fluid cytology is useful in establishing the diagnosis. Neurocutaneous melanosis has a poor prognosis even in patients who do not have leptomeningeal melanoma. Patients may present with dysarthria, weakness, or paralysis; with proptosis caused by an orbital mass; with symptoms caused by compression of the cranial nerves; or with seizures.

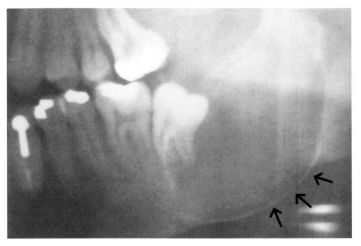

Figure 8-36

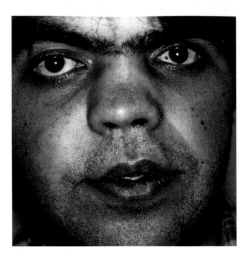

Figure 8-37

Basal cell nevus syndrome is inherited as an autosomal dominant trait and is distinguished by its combination of multiple basal cell carcinomas, cysts of the jaw, and skeletal anomalies. **Jaw cysts**, often the initial manifestation of the syndrome, appear in the first decade of life. If the syndrome is suspected, the presence of jaw cysts on x-ray may confirm the diagnosis (Figure 8-36).

These cysts, which often recur after removal, are epithelium lined. Ameloblastomas, the oral equivalent of **basal cell carcinomas**, can occur. Fibrosarcomas arising in the maxilla are also reported. Other manifestations include ocular hypertelorism, prominent supraorbital ridges, and broad nasal root, which can result in characteristic facies (Fig. 8-37). Multiple skeletal manifestations occur, including frontal and biparietal bossing, increased head circumference, kyphoscoliosis, spina bifida, bifid ribs, bridging of the sella turcica, and shortening of the fourth metacarpal. Lamellar calcification of the falx cerebri and dura are constant features of the syndrome. Tumors reported in association with the syndrome include ovarian fibromas, leiomyomas, and medulloblastoma. Several patients with medulloblastomas have been treated with radiotherapy only to develop multiple basal cell carcinomas in the irradiated area within a few years of treatment.

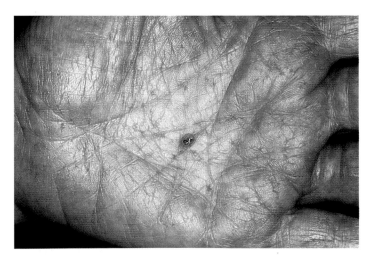

Figure 8-38

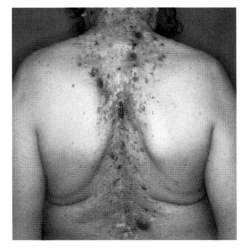

Figure 8-39

Additional neurologic findings include mental retardation in a minority of patients, agenesis of the corpus callosum, and congenital hydrocephalus. There have been several cases of meningioma in patients with the basal cell nevus syndrome. Congenital blindness due to coloboma, cataracts, or glaucoma has also been reported.

Palmar pitting is another common cutaneous feature of this syndrome, occurring in approximately 5% of patients. Pits often appear during puberty and the depressions range in size from pinpoints to a diameter of 3 mm. The pits can contain microscopic foci of basal cell carcinoma. In Figure 8-38 numerous tiny palmar pits are barely visible around the small basal cell carcinoma on the midpalm. Basal cell carcinomas can develop in infancy and continue to increase in number throughout life, until there are hundreds.

Figure 8-39 shows a patient with numerous basal cell carcinomas on the back. Sunlight and radiation may increase the numbers of basal cell carcinomas, but tumors can even arise in sites not exposed to sunlight, such as on the buttocks. All types of basal cell carcinomas can occur, and these can become erosive and invasive with large areas of local tissue destruction. Metastasis of basal cell carcinomas in this syndrome has been reported, but it is rare. Patients with the basal cell nevus syndrome can have normal lifespans, but progressive disfigurement results from the basal cell carcinomas that develop, and from their treatment.

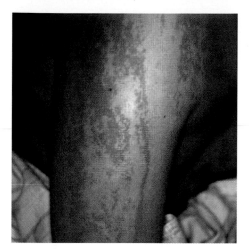

Figure 8-40

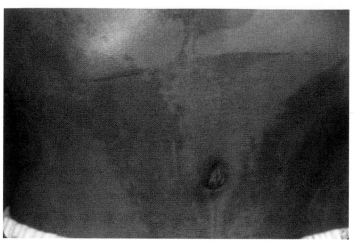

Figure 8-41

The **epidermal nevus syndrome** consists of systemic malformations occurring in association with large epidermal nevi. Epidermal nevi are present at birth or develop in early infancy and can present in a number of different forms. Long, pigmented, linear verrucous streaks involving the extremities (nevus unius lateris) (Fig. 8-40) or whorled, scaling plaques that involve large portions of the trunk (icthyosis hystrix) (Fig. 8-41) can be features of this syndrome.

Linear verrucous epidermal nevi and nevus sebaceous, which can have an orange verrucous appearance, also occur. Occasionally, skin lesions may have a dermatomal distribution or may remain localized to one side of the body without crossing the midline (Fig. 8-42). The different clinical manifestations of the epidermal nevus syndrome are undoubtedly due to different mutations leading to different clinical features.

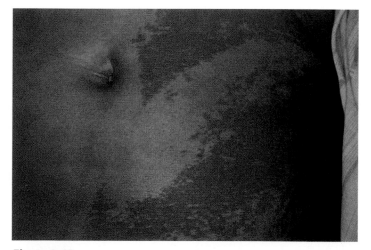

Figure 8-42

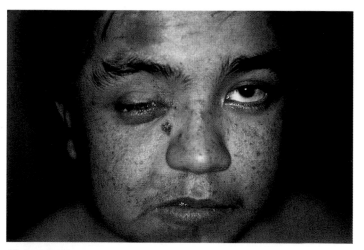

Figure 8-43

Since epidermal nevi commonly occur without associated systemic malformations, a work-up for abnormalities of the epidermal nevus syndrome should be considered in patients with epidermal nevi that are longer than 2 cm. Neurologic abnormalities are numerous and affect approximately one-third of patients with this syndrome. Seizure disorders and mental retardation are the most common. Vascular malformations of the brain, malignant astrocytomas, cortical atrophy, and hydrocephalus are less common associations. Death has resulted from intracranial bleeding or from severe seizures in a few children with the epidermal nevus syndrome.

Blindness can result from ocular involvement. Epidermal nevus of the eyelid or conjunctiva can occur, and coloboma of the eyelid, iris or retina are occasional features. Involvement of the ophthalmic nerve can result in oculomotor weakness or nystagmus. The patient in Figure 8-43 has an epidermal nevus of the right eyelids with swelling of the affected lids and a corneal opacification. Skeletal abnormalities are among the most common findings in patients with the epidermal nevus syndrome. Kyphoscoliosis, hemihypertrophy, shortening of limbs, vertebral defects, osteolytic lesions, and pathologic fractures occur. Reports of malformations of the kidney in this syndrome include horse-shoe kidney, solitary kidney, and renal tumor. Cardiovascular malformations might include patent ductus arteriosus, and coarctation and hypoplasia of the aorta.

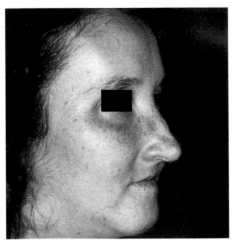

Figure 8-44

The **Hallermann–Streiff syndrome**, also called oculomandibu-lodyscephaly, is a rare condition involving skeletal, cutaneous, and neurologic abnormalities. Skeletal abnormalities include dwarfism, wing-like scapulae, syndactyly, and spinal abnormalities, including vertebral fusion, scoliosis and lordosis. Patients have a characteristic appearance of the face and head that is said to be "bird-like". The head is disproportionately short (brachycephaly) with frontal and parietal bossing and delayed suture closure. The nose is thin and beak-like (Fig. 8-44). Nasal septal deviation is common. The skin over the scalp and nose is atrophic and the underlying blood vessels may be visible.

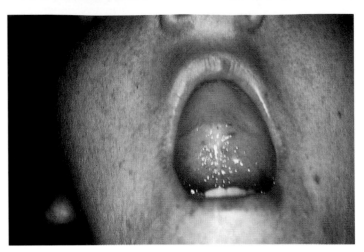

Figure 8-45

Alopecia of the scalp, eyebrows, eye lashes, and axillary and pubic hair is characteristic. Numerous dental abnormalities have been reported in patients with the Hallermann–Streiff syndrome including absence of teeth, supernumerary teeth, extensive dental caries, and mal-occlusion. Patients typically have a high-arched palate (Fig. 8-45). Neurologic abnormalities are not common but can include mental retardation. Numerous ocular abnormalities occur including, among others, nystagmus, strabismus, congenital cataracts, microphthalmia, and blue sclerae.

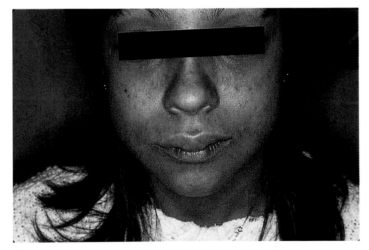

Figure 8-46

Melkersson–Rosenthal syndrome (cheilitis granulomatosa) is characterized by a triad of recurrent facial swelling, relapsing facial paralysis, and lingua plicata. Any of the three components of this triad can occur separately, and lip edema is the most common finding (Fig. 8-46). Swelling is asymptomatic, can involve one or both lips, and may be unilateral or bilateral. Individual episodes last for only a few days, but eventually the swelling can become persistent. Episodes recur at varying intervals. Neurologic symptoms are indistinguishable from Bell's palsy and are unilateral or bilateral. A plicated tongue is the least common finding.

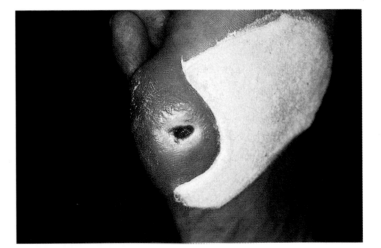

Figure 8-47

Neuropathic ulcers can occur in anyone with a sensory neuropathy affecting the feet, but they are most common in people with diabetic neuropathy. Abnormal pressure on a particular portion of the foot first results in formation of a callus, followed by breakdown of the epidermis (Fig. 8-47) and infection. Patients may unknowingly step on sharp foreign objects, perhaps needles or glass, and may remain unaware of the foreign object because of their sensory neuropathy. Therefore, radiographs of the feet should be considered if a nonhealing ulcer develops.

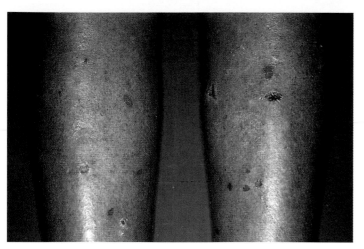

Figure 8-48

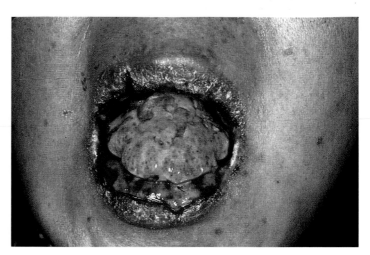

Figure 8-49

Myasthenia gravis is an acquired neuromuscular disorder in which there are circulating antiacetylcholine receptor antibodies. The severity and course of neurologic symptoms is variable, fluctuating over hours in some patients and over weeks or months in others. Ocular muscle weakness is characteristic and leads to ptosis and diplopia. Depending on the muscles affected, symptoms can be quite varied. Slurring of speech, choking on food, difficult walking, or an inability to raise the arms for even short periods of time are some of the many symptoms associated with this disorder. Anticholinesterase administration is used both therapeutically and diagnostically for myasthenia gravis and should result in improvement of muscle function. Other diagnostic criteria include the presence of antiacetylcholine receptor antibodies and electromyographic studies. Since myasthenia gravis is an auto-immune disorder, it is not surprising that other autoimmune conditions, including systemic lupus erythematosus and **pemphigus vulgaris** are associated. The patient shown in Figure 8-48 presented with generalized bullous lesions, and direct immunofluorescence of a skin biopsy revealed anti-intercellular antibodies diagnostic of pemphigus. Indirect immunofluorescence revealed circulating anti-intercellular substance antibodies. The patient with oral erosions shown in Figure 8-49 developed eyelid ptosis. A diagnosis of myasthenia gravis was made, and on CT scan the patient was subsequently found to have a thymoma (Fig. 8-50), a tumor that is found in 10–15% of people with myasthenia gravis. On further evaluation, the patient's skin lesions were found to have features of paraneoplastic pemphigus, presumably related to the thymoma. It is interesting that this patient also had another autoimmune cutaneous disease, alopecia areata.

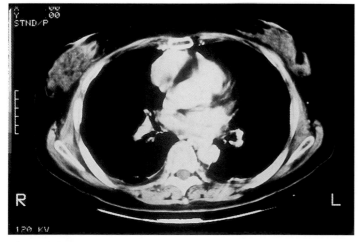

Figure 8-50

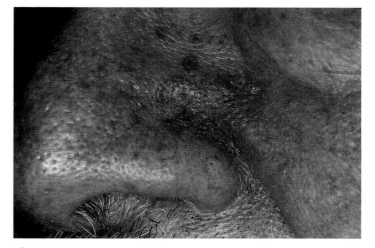

Figure 8-51

A number of nonspecific cutaneous disorders can be associated with neurologic syndromes or can cause neurologic symptoms. Seborrheic dermatitis, for example, is commonly associated with **Parkinson's disease**. The etiology of seborrheic dermatitis is not clear, but its occurrence in Parkinson's disease may be related to reduced frequency of shampooing. The rash is characterized by erythematous scaling patches on the scalp and on the face, especially involving the eyebrows, nasaolabial folds, and alar creases (Fig. 8-51). The retroauricular folds, chest, and midback can also be affected. Benign or malignant cutaneous tumors can occasionally result in neurologic symptoms by impinging upon peripheral nerves or, in some cases, on the spinal cord or brain. The child in Figure 8-50 is at risk of developing peripheral neurologic symptoms because of pressure from a midline mass overlying the spine. Symptoms depend on the level of involvement.

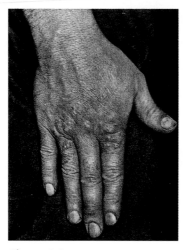

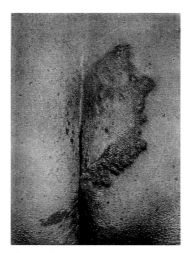

Figure 9-1   **Figure 9-2**

Tuberculosis verrucosa is shown in Figs 9-1 and 9-2.

The surface of the lesion soon shows a tendency to become knobby and furrowed, and the more prominent parts…assume at first a smooth warty and later a papillomatous appearance…The backs of the hands are the favorite sites of the malady, though it may occur on any part of the body.

From Rainforth SI. The stereoscopic skin clinic. New York: Medical Art Publishing; 1911.

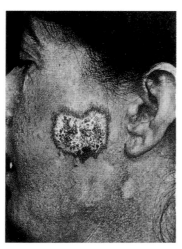

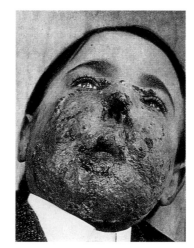

Figure 9-3   **Figure 9-4**

Lupus vulgaris is shown in Figs 9-3 and 9-4.

Lupus vulgaris is an extremely chronic tuberculous affection of the skin and mucous membranes, characterized by the presence of nodules which ulcerate or resolve with the formation of scar tissue…Looked at through a glass slide pressed firmly down upon them, the nodules have exactly the color and appearance of apple jelly…Frequently ulcers form at the sites of larger infiltrations…The disease most frequently attacks the face.

From Rainforth SI. The stereoscopic skin clinic. New York: Medical Art Publishing; 1911.

Table 9-1. An Organized Approach to the Diagnosis of Acute Fever and Rash in Immunocompetent Patients: Differential Diagnosis Based on Lesion Morphology

Erythematous eruptions	Purpuric eruptions	Vesicopustular eruptions
Infectious disorders	Infectious disorders	Infectious disorders
Viral infections	Viral infections	Viral infections
Erythema infectiosum	Atypical measles	Herpes simplex
Measles (rubeola)	Echovirus 9	Varicella and herpes zoster
Rubella	TORCHS	Kaposi's varicelliform eruption
Roseola infantum	Rickettsial infections	Variola
Enteroviruses	Rocky Mountain spotted fever	Hand-foot-and-mouth disease
Infectious mononucleosis	Epidemic typhus	Enterovirus
Hepatitis B	Bacterial infections	Rickettsial infections
Bacterial infections	Meningococcemia	Rickettsialpox
Scarlet fever	Gonococcemia	Bacterial infections
Toxic shock syndrome	Staphylococcal sepsis	Staphylococcal scalded skin syndrome
Secondary syphilis	Pseudomonas sepsis	Congenital syphilis
Lyme disease	Subacute bacterial endocarditis	Noninfectious disorders
Noninfectious disorders	Noninfectious disorders	Drug reactions
Kawasaki disease	Allergic vasculitis	
Erythema multiforme	Henloch–Schönlein purpura	
Erythema marginatum	Drug reactions	
Juvenile rheumatoid arthritis		
Systemic lupus erythematosus		
Drug reactions		

TORCHS: toxoplasmosis, other, rubella, cytomegalovirus, herpes simplex, syphilis
Modified from Fisher M, Katz S. Fever and rash. In : Lebwohl M (ed). Difficult Diagnoses in Dermatology. New York: Churchill Livingstone; 1988: 134.

The presence of fever and rash often poses a dilemma for the practicing clinician. While the differential diagnosis of fever and rash is so long as to be overwhelming, it is greatly simplified by classifying the rash on the basis of its morphology. By distinguishing between vesicopustular eruptions, purpuric eruptions and erythematous eruptions, one can focus the differential diagnosis on a narrower list of diseases (Table 9-1). By limiting the differential diagnosis in this way, it is easier to use the clinical features of the diseases to differentiate one from another and arrive at the correct diagnosis (see Tables 9-2, 9-3 and 9-4).

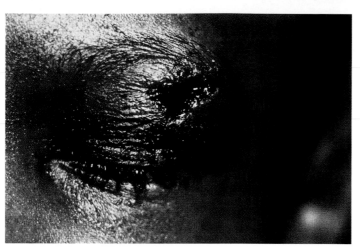

Figure 9-5

The cutaneous manifestations of infectious diseases are as diverse as the numerous organisms causing them. Some reaction patterns point to specific diagnoses, while other cutaneous reactions are nonspecific patterns that can be seen with many types of infection and different organisms. Swelling, erythema, and ulceration are nonspecific symptoms of infection that, in the patient shown in Figure 9-5, resulted from infection with ***Eikenella corrodens***.

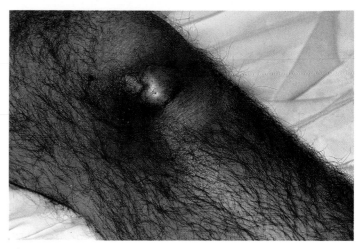

Figure 9-6

A variety of different cutaneous reaction patterns can result from infection with the same organism. *E. corrodens* was cultured from the pus-filled bulla on the knee of the patient in Figure 9-6. *Eikenella* infections often result in abscess formation, with skin lesions that are indolent and foul-smelling. Smaller pustules are nonspecific signs of limited local infections with organisms as diverse as *Staphylococcus aureus* and *Candida albicans*.

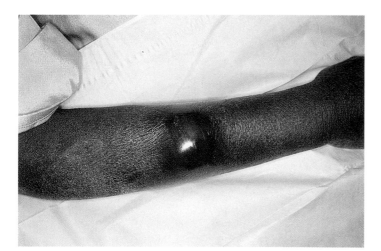

Figure 9-7

The source of infection can occasionally provide clues to the infecting organism. Infection resulting from direct inoculation by trauma or other means is often associated with a particular organism. The patient in Figure 9-7, for example, was bitten by a dog. The resulting abscess was caused by infection with ***Pasteurella multocida***. In contrast, human bites consist of a mixture of aerobic and anaerobic organisms.

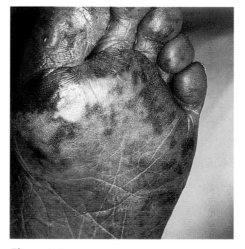

Figure 9-8

Overwhelming septicemia can be associated with **disseminated intravascular coagulation** (**DIC**), leading to widespread ecchymoses and petechiae. Formation of thrombi and emboli complicates this life-threatening condition. Consumption of coagulation factors leads to dangerous hemorrhage from many sites. Apart from bleeding in the skin, dermatologic stigmata of DIC include cutaneous infarcts and cyanosis. Figure 9-8 shows reticulated purpura of the foot in a patient with ***Bacteroides*** septicemia and DIC.

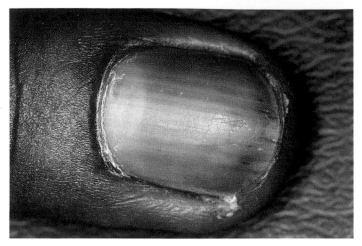

Figure 9-9

Subacute and acute bacterial **endocarditis** are associated with a wide array of cutaneous findings. Petechiae occur in 30–50% of patients. Crops of these nonblanchable, small purple macules can be seen on the conjunctiva, palate, buccal mucosa, and extremities. **Splinter hemorrhages** are linear red streaks frequently seen under the distal portion of the nail as a result of trauma. Splinter hemorrhages caused by endocarditis develop more proximally in the nail (Fig. 9-9). These slowly grow out over months as the nail grows.

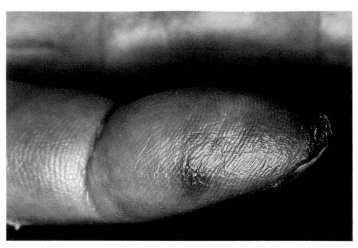

Figure 9-10

Osler's nodes occur in approximately 5% of patients with endocarditis and appear as crops of tender, red or purpuric nodules on the pads of the fingers and toes (Fig. 9-10). Occasionally, the thenar and hypothenar eminences are affected, and Osler's nodes can even develop on the arms. Lesions last hours to days and resolve without ulceration. Histologic examination of Osler's nodes in acute bacterial endocarditis reveals arteriolar microemboli with microabscess formation. In subacute bacterial endocarditis, septic emboli are not found, and skin lesions are caused by a vasculitis.

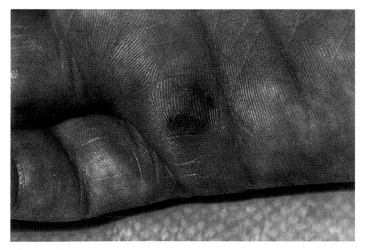

Figure 9-11

Janeway lesions are nontender erythematous or purpuric macules or nodules of the palms and soles in patients with acute bacterial endocarditis (Fig. 9-11). Less commonly, they can occur in patients with subacute bacterial endocarditis. Dermal microabscess formation with organisms has been demonstrated histologically in Janeway lesions, indicating that they arise from septic emboli. Lesions that are clinically and histologically identical to Osler's nodes and Janeway lesions have been found in patients with infected arterial catheters.

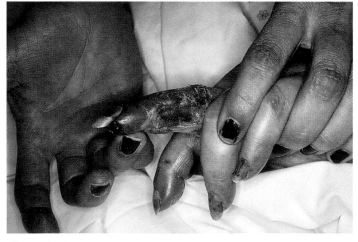

Figure 9-12

While subacute endocarditis can go on for many months and seldom results in septic emboli, acute bacterial endocarditis is rapidly progressive, and the spread of infectious material through the arterial circulation is more common. The patient shown in Figure 9-12 developed hemorrhagic necrosis and ulceration of several digits as a result of acute staphylococcal endocarditis.

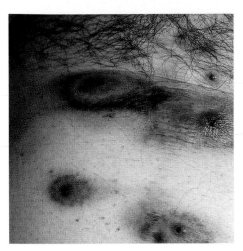

Figure 9-13

Staphylococcal bacteremia can give rise to a wide array of skin lesions. The patient shown in Figure 9-13 developed **purulent purpura** characterized by numerous large purpuric patches with central abscesses. Pustules, subcutaneous abscesses, deeper nodules that do not suppurate, and hemorrhagic infarctions can also occur. A Gram stain of aspirated material usually reveals Gram-positive cocci in clusters. When circulating exotoxins causes skin lesions, the organism is not found on Gram stain or on culture of those lesions.

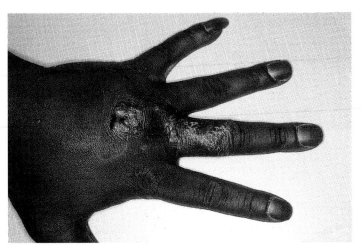

Figure 9-14

Botryomycosis refers to a rare, chronic staphylococcal infection of the skin or other organs. Introduction of a foreign body often initiates this infection. Pus extracted from skin lesions contains pinpoint white granules that consist of clusters of Gram-positive cocci in large numbers. Surgical debridement is usually curative but the patient in Figure 9-14 required many months of systemic antibiotics to clear his infection.

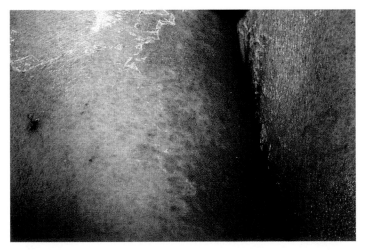

Figure 9-15

Toxic shock syndrome is a life-threatening disorder caused by exotoxin produced by certain strains of *Staphylococcus aureus*. While 85–90% of patients are menstruating women, in particular those who use super-absorbent tampons, other cases result from staphylococcal infections in soft tissue, bone, and other sites. The rash of toxic shock syndrome presents as diffuse erythema resembling sunburn (Fig. 9-15). Mucous membranes are erythematous and a "strawberry tongue" can occur. Swelling and erythema of the hands and feet are common, and desquamation of the palms (Fig. 9-16) and soles follows within

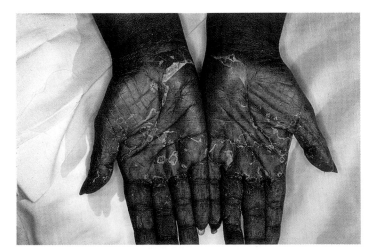

Figure 9-16

1–2 weeks. Diagnosis should be suspected in people with a constellation of signs and symptoms. Fever, rash, desquamation, and hypotension are diagnostic criteria. In addition, involvement of three or more organ systems is characteristic: myalgia or myositis with elevation of creatine phosphokinase levels; renal disease manifested by elevated blood urea nitrogen creatinine levels; toxic encephalopathy; liver disease with elevated liver function tests; and thrombocytopenia. Gastrointestinal symptoms are also common.

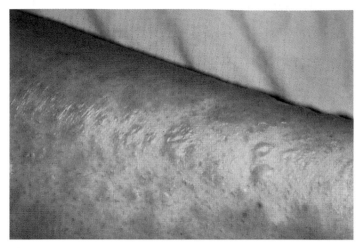

Figure 9-17

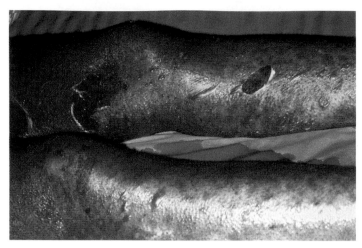

Figure 9-18

Staphylococcal scalded skin syndrome is a severe generalized rash caused by S. *aureus* phage group 2. The condition may develop as a result of a wound infection, from occult abscess, staphylococcal conjunctivitis, or another staphylococcal infection. The staphylococci elaborate a circulating exfoliative toxin that results in separation of the upper layers of epidermis with generalized formation of bullae and exfoliation remote from the primary infection. Consequently, culture of the skin fails to yield the causative organism. The primary lesion is a bulla (Fig. 9-17), which fills with clear fluid and ruptures rapidly. The skin is diffusely erythematous and tender; patients generally have fever.

The skin wrinkles and exfoliates in large sheets (Figs 9-18 and 9-19), leaving extensive areas of denudation. Loss of water and nutrients through the skin is problematic, particularly in infants. An impaired cutaneous barrier to loss of body heat makes temperature regulation difficult.

Differentiation from **toxic epidermal necrolysis** is critical, because the latter condition is caused by medications whereas staphylococcal scalded skin syndrome should be treated with antistaphylococcal antibiotics. Toxic epidermal necrolysis usually affects adults, and prominently involves the mucous membranes. It occurs over 2–3 weeks, and has a

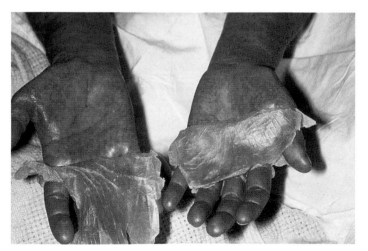

Figure 9-19

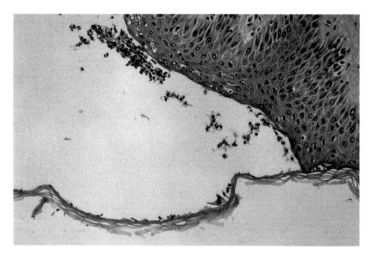

Figure 9-20

significant rate of mortality. In contrast, staphylococcal scalded skin syndrome typically occurs in children younger than 5 years old, it spares the mucous membranes, and lasts only for a few days. The mortality is low, and patients often recover even without antibiotic therapy.

Histologically the two conditions are easily distinguished by the location at which bulla formation occurs. In staphylococcal scalded skin

syndrome, separation develops in the upper layers of the epidermis. The bulla cavity in the latter condition usually contains free-floating, normal-appearing "acantholytic" cells (Fig. 9-20). In contrast, toxic epidermal necrolysis is characterized by separation at the basal layer of the epidermis with necrosis of epidermal cells.

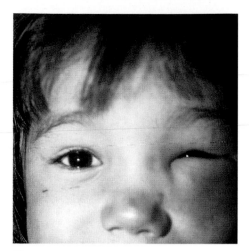

Figure 9-21

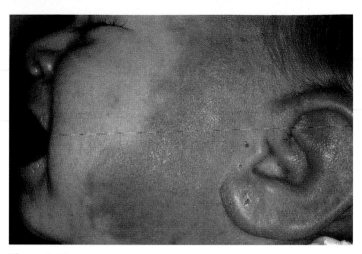

Figure 9-22

Erysipelas is a superficial infection of the skin involving the lymphatic vessels. Group A streptococci are most commonly responsible, although other organisms can rarely cause the infection. Bacteria typically enter through a small break in the skin. Common sites of entry include cutaneous ulcers, fissures caused by dermatophyte infections of the toe web spaces, umbilical stumps in neonates, or surgical scars. The responsible organism may originate in the patient's own respiratory tract or may be transmitted from other patients or

attendants. The bridge of the nose, cheeks, periorbital areas (Fig. 9-21), and lower extremities are common sites of involvement. Skin lesions are red, warm, sharply demarcated (Fig. 9-22), and often associated with high fever. The advancing border moves rapidly from day to day and, occasionally, vesicles and bullae develop. Although histologic examination shows invasion of the dermis and lymphatic vessels with streptococci, cultures of the skin surface or of aspirated tissue fluid only rarely yield Group A streptococci.

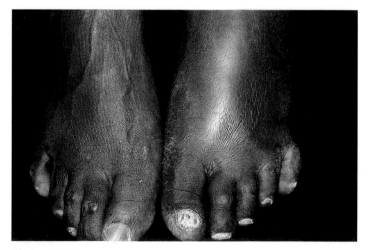

Figure 9-23

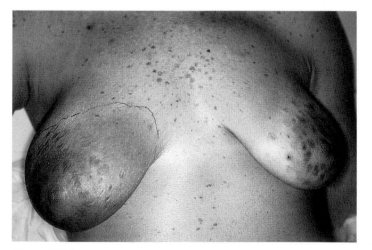

Figure 9-24

Erysipelas can be differentiated from **cellulitis** because cellulitis involves deeper subcutaneous tissues. Both *S. aureus* and Group A streptococcal infections commonly cause cellulitis, but other organisms are occasionally responsible, especially in immunosuppressed patients. Cellulitis often develops in a preexisting wound or following trauma. Affected skin is erythematous, warm, edematous, and tender but, in contrast to erysipelas, the border is not sharply demarcated. Figure 9-23

shows a patient with cellulitis of the left foot. Tinea pedis caused maceration of the toe web spaces, allowing entry of *S. aureus*. The patient seen in Figure 9-24 has a cellulitis of the breast, which is swollen, inflamed, and tender. In both cellulitis and erysipelas, subcutaneous abscesses may form. Extensive infection may lead to bacteremia and distant spread. Debilitated and immunosuppressed patients may succumb to the infection despite treatment with systemic antibiotics.

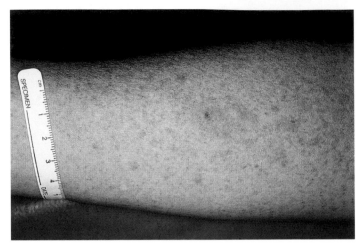

Figure 9-25

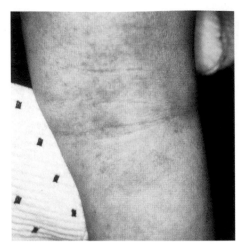

Figure 9-26

Scarlet fever is characterized by a diffuse erythematous eruption caused by Group A streptococcal infection. It usually occurs in children, but can affect adults. Bacteria causing a streptococcal tonsillopharyngitis elaborate an erythrogenic toxin that circulates, resulting in the characteristic rash. Scarlet fever begins with pharyngitis and fever, occasionally associated with nausea, vomiting, headache, and malaise. The pharynx is inflamed, and the tonsils are enlarged and covered with an exudate that may be yellow, gray, or white. Tender, anterior, cervical or submandibular lymphadenopathy is usually present. The tongue is covered by a white coating through which red papillae project, giving the appearance of a "white strawberry tongue". By the fifth day, the tongue appears beefy red with prominent papillae. Twenty-four to 48 h after the onset of pharyngitis, a generalized erythematous rash begins on the neck and spreads to the trunk and extremities (Fig. 9-25). The rash is characterized by minute erythematous punctate papules that may be easier to palpate than to see. Flushing of the cheeks with circumoral pallor is occasionally present. The rash may be more visible in the antecubital, popliteal, or axillary folds. Occasionally a linear petechial eruption known as Pastia's lines can be seen in these folds (Fig. 9-26). The rash lasts 5 days, or less in milder cases. As the rash fades, striking

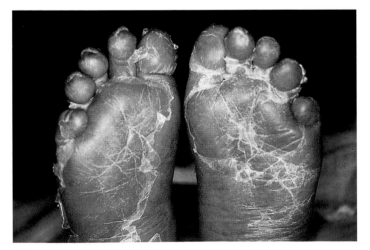

Figure 9-27

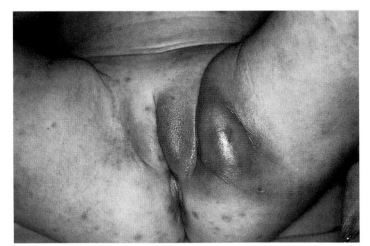

Figure 9-28

desquamation occurs and prominently involves the palms and soles (Fig. 9-27). Generalized lymphadenopathy and splenomegaly can occur. Diagnosis of scarlet fever is definitively established by demonstrating Group A streptococcal infection. Occasionally patients develop this disease following Group A streptococcal infection of nonpharyngeal sites.

The child in Figure 9-28 developed a scarlatiniform rash in association with a streptococcal groin abscess.

If untreated, scarlet fever lasts approximately 4–5 days followed by desquamation that may last a few weeks. Fever and constitutional symptoms respond rapidly to penicillin. Even without antibiotic treatment, the severity of scarlet fever has diminished over the years, and most cases seen today are mild and uncomplicated.

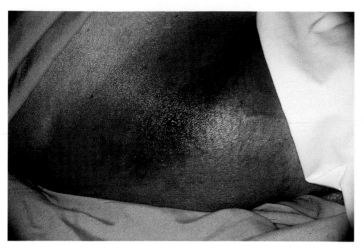

Figure 9-29

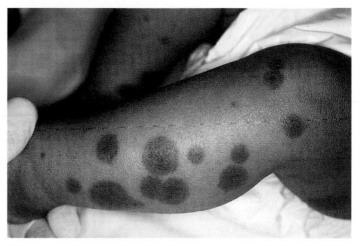

Figure 9-30

Pseudomonas **septicemia** generally occurs in patients who are debilitated and immunosuppressed. A variety of different cutaneous lesions occur, including hemorrhagic vesicles and bullae, gangrenous cellulitis, and ecthyma gangrenosum. The latter begins as a hemorrhagic vesicle that becomes necrotic, resulting in an ulceration that consists of a central black eschar surrounded by erythema (Fig. 9-29). The anogenital and axillary areas are most commonly involved.

Acute **meningococcemia** is characterized by the abrupt onset of fever, headache, and mental confusion, which can be followed rapidly by the development of a hemorrhagic rash, vomiting, and hypotension. Epidemics occur, particularly in crowded environments like military camps, but isolated cases should not be overlooked. Occasionally patients experience a prodrome consisting of an upper respiratory infection, headache, myalgias, nausea, and vomiting. When it occurs, the prodrome is often brief, mild, and easily overlooked. Petechial and purpuric skin lesions are most commonly seen and typically involve the trunk and extremities (Fig. 9-30), although any cutaneous surface can be affected. Lesions on the palms and soles are easily confused with the rash

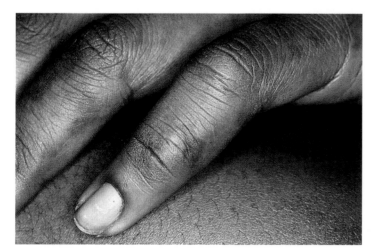

Figure 9-31

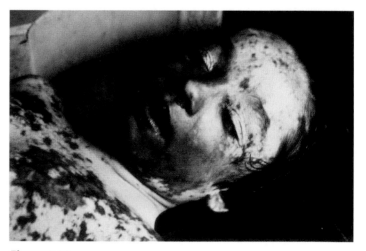

Figure 9-32

of Rocky Mountain spotted fever. Mucous membrane lesions frequently occur as well. When damage to cutaneous blood vessels is more extensive, hemorrhagic bullae can form, as shown on the finger of the patient in Figure 9-31.

When meningococcemia is severe, DIC occurs rapidly, resulting in extensive hemorrhage with widespread purpura (Fig. 9-32), hypo-

tension, and death. If untreated, the condition is usually fatal, but with treatment most patients recover. Diagnosis is usually made by finding evidence of meningococcal infection in the cerebrospinal fluid. *Neisseria meningitidis* is a Gram-negative diplococcus that can occasionally be seen on smear or culture of skin lesions. Blood cultures often reveal the causative organism as well.

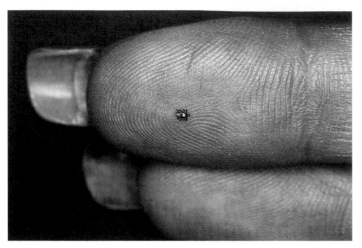

Figure 9-33

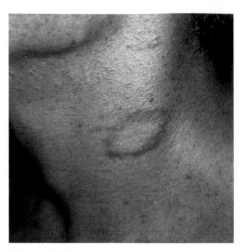

Figure 9-34

Although concentrated in areas such as the northeastern portion of the USA, **Lyme disease** is worldwide in its distribution. The causative organism, *Borrelia burgdorferi*, is transmitted by the *Ixodes dammini* tick or another closely related species. The tick can be as small as one or two pepper grains (Fig. 9-33) but becomes larger when engorged. Daily examination of household members is an important part of disease prevention in endemic areas. Transmission of Lyme disease may be prevented by simple removal of the tick within 18 hours of its attachment to a human host.

Erythema chronicum migrans appears at the site of a tick bite approximately 1–3 weeks later. The classic lesion begins as a macule or papule that rapidly enlarges, with central clearing, to form an annular patch (Fig. 9-34). If untreated, erythema chronicum migrans can last up to 1 year and lesions may attain a diameter in excess of 30 cm, but most clear within weeks or months. The appearance of erythema chronicum migrans is highly variable. Some lesions appear urticarial and never achieve central clearing. Others are so small they go unnoticed. Even a vesicular variant of erythema chronicum migrans has been described.

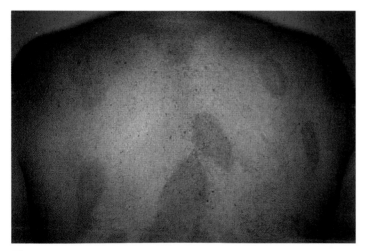

Figure 9-35

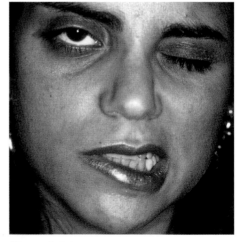

Figure 9-36

Lesions are often asymptomatic, but patients occasionally complain of burning or itching. The acute illness can be associated with systemic symptoms such as fever, chills, lethargy, malaise, and headache. Regional lymphadenopathy may be present. Hematogenous dissemination of spirochetes to multiple cutaneous sites can give rise to multiple annular patches of erythema chronicum migrans (Fig. 9-35).

Arthritis involving one or a few large joints may occur early in the course of Lyme disease but often begins a few weeks later. Bouts of arthritis can occur for months or years. Approximately 10% of patients develop a chronic erosive arthritis. Neurologic symptoms develop approximately 1–3 months after the onset of Lyme disease. In some patients, the tick bite may not be noticed, early signs of Lyme disease may be subclinical or overlooked, and the presenting symptom of Lyme disease may be a neurologic symptom such as Bell's palsy (Fig. 9-36). Cardiac involvement may become apparent several months after the start of Lyme disease. Heart failure from carditis, cardiac conduction abnormalities (including complete heart block), and electrocardiographic abnormalities have been reported.

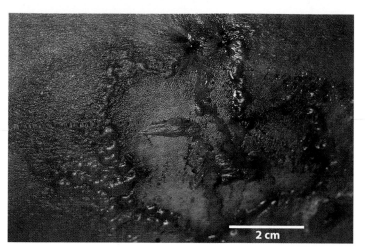

Figure 9-37

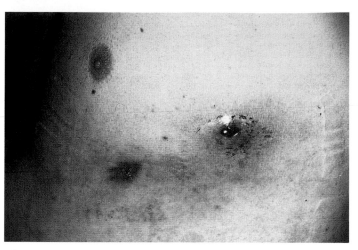

Figure 9-38

Necrotizing fasciitis refers to a rapidly progressive, life-threatening destruction of skin and subcutaneous tissues caused by a mixed infection of anaerobes and facultative organisms. Infection is usually preceded by surgical or traumatic wounds, abscesses, or cutaneous ulcers. Diabetic people or those debilitated by alcoholism or drug abuse may be predisposed to this disorder. The affected skin is warm, erythematous, painful, and swollen. Within 1–2 days hemorrhagic bullae form and rupture, leaving a well-demarcated area of gangrene (Fig. 9-37) extending down to fascia. Group A streptococci can cause a unique form of necrotizing fasciitis in patients who are otherwise healthy.

Actinomycosis is a rare infection characterized by formation of draining sinus tracts that create chronic cutaneous ulcers (Fig. 9-38). *Actinomyces israelii* infects skin after local trauma. Common sites of involvement are the lower face, neck, chest, and abdomen. Patients characteristically present with systemic symptoms such as fever, shaking chills, night sweats, and weight loss. Extension to underlying structures results in osteomyelitis. Local involvement of lymph nodes does not generally occur. Sulfur granules can be identified in sputum, bronchial aspirates, pus, and tissue, and a Gram stain shows Gram-positive beaded hyphae.

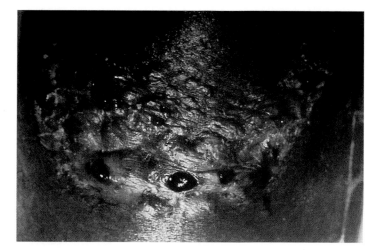

Figure 9-39

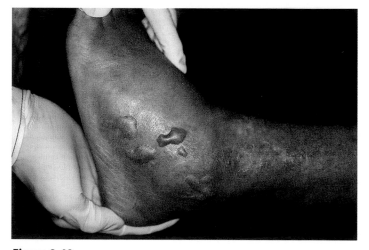

Figure 9-40

Nocardiosis is an acute infection caused by *Nocardia asteroides*, a Gram-positive, acid-fast organism. The site of primary infection is usually in the lungs, and pulmonary symptoms predominate. Chest radiographs reveals a pulmonary infiltrate and marked thickening of the pleurae. Skin lesions are characterized by multiple sinus tracts leading to the surface from underlying abscesses (Fig. 9-39).

Vibrio vulnificus infection can occur several days after sustaining minor trauma while swimming in sea or lake water, or while cleaning seafood. Infection develops into virulent cellulitis with lymphangitis and bacteremia. Patients with hepatic cirrhosis or (less commonly) other immunosuppressive conditions, can develop fever and hypotension secondary to *V. vulnificus* septicemia 1–2 days after eating raw oysters. Large hemorrhagic bullae break down to necrotic ulcers and erosions (Fig. 9-40). Leukopenia is common and DIC can occur.

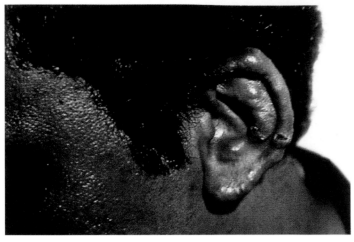

Figure 9-41

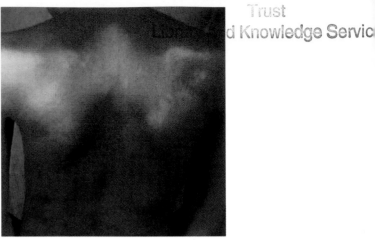

Figure 9-42

Leprosy is a mycobacterial infection that is common worldwide, affecting as many as 15 000 000 people, but some parts of the world are almost entirely spared. Most victims are in the tropics, with large concentrations in Africa, India, and Southeast Asia. The condition is caused by infection with *Mycobacterium leprae*, an acid-fast, Gram-positive organism. It is thought to be transmitted through mycobacteria in nasal discharge and through open cutaneous ulcers of people with lepromatous leprosy, as shown on the ear of a patient in Figure 9-41. Not surprisingly, family members living with a lepromatous person have a significant risk of acquiring the disease.

Once infected, symptoms generally do not occur for 2–3 years. Symptoms such as paresthesias and numbness may begin in the peripheral nerves without any other cutaneous manifestations. Once skin lesions of leprosy develop, their appearance and the course of the disease is determined by the individual's immunologic response to the infection. The earliest cutaneous lesions of leprosy are small, solitary, or multiple, hypopigmented macules that are often not associated with any neurologic symptoms. Lesions can grow to cover large areas (Fig. 9-42).

In patients who exhibit strong cell-mediated immunity against *M. leprae*, so-called **tuberculoid leprosy**, very few organisms may be

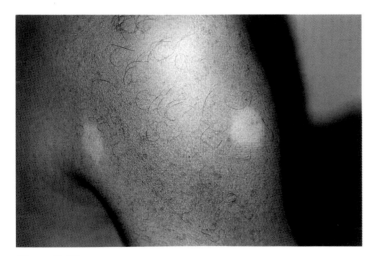

Figure 9-43

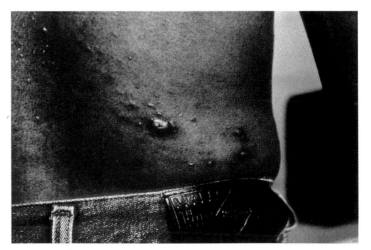

Figure 9-44

found but severe nerve damage can occur as a result of the intensity of the cell-mediated response. Lesions of tuberculoid leprosy are extremely variable in their appearance and extent. They may arise *de novo* or develop from indeterminate lesions. The classic tuberculoid lesion is a hypopigmented macule (Fig. 9-43) surrounded by a raised border.

At the other extreme, patients with **lepromatous leprosy** exhibit very little immune response against *M. leprae*, and thousands of organisms can be found in the dermis, peripheral nerves, and nasal mucosa. The

skin lesions of lepromatous leprosy may begin as macules, but eventually the dermis becomes diffusely infiltrated with organisms, and discrete nodules arise (Fig. 9-44). The ears and face are commonly affected and nodules can be single or multiple, in some cases coalescing to form large plaques. Some patients develop hypopigmented or erythematous macules, others develop diffuse thickening of the dermis. Peripheral nerves are tender and swollen. Hair loss, impaired sweating, and sensory loss can occur.

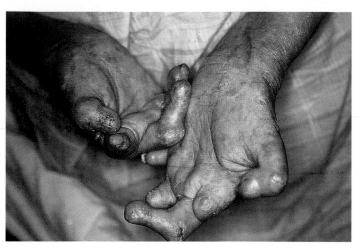

Figure 9-45

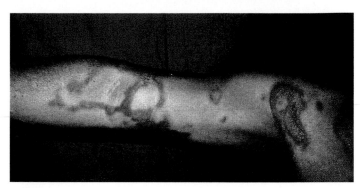

Figure 9-46A

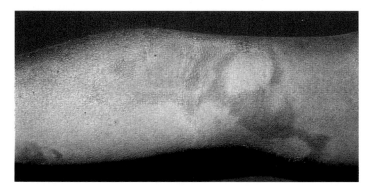

Figure 9-46B

Borderline leprosy refers to a broad range of diseases between the two extremes of tuberculoid and lepromatous leprosy. Cutaneous lesions are quite variable and are greatly affected by the degree of cell-mediated immunity that is mounted against the infection. Hypopigmented macules similar to those seen in tuberculoid leprosy are seen in some patients. Others will have plaques and nodules resembling those of lepromatous leprosy. As in tuberculoid and lepromatous forms, borderline leprosy is associated with neurologic impairment.

Tender, swollen, hard nerves can be seen or palpated and sensory impairment detected. Resulting muscle atrophy, paresis, paralysis, and neuropathic ulceration of extremities can result in crippling deformities (Fig. 9-45). This can be prevented by early treatment. The patient shown in Figure 9-46A has borderline leprosy. He was treated with rifampin and dapsone and his response after 6 weeks is shown in Figure 9-46B.

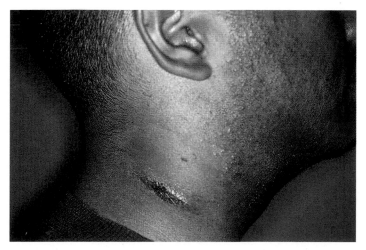

Figure 9-47

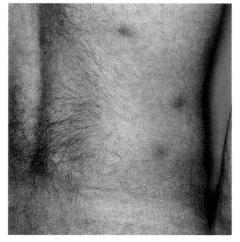

Figure 9-48

Despite the persistence of **tuberculosis**, skin involvement is rarely seen in most of the world. The patient shown in Figure 9-47 has scrofuloderma, a condition caused by breakdown of skin overlying a deeper focus of tuberculosis. The condition often occurs on the neck, jaw, or supraclavicular areas over involved lymph nodes. A nontender, firm, deep nodule forms. Liquifaction and cold abscess formation ensue with sinus tract formation and ulceration of the overlying skin. Other cutaneous forms of tuberculosis are rarely seen. These include primary inoculation of tuberculosis, which results in a chancre or wart-like lesion (tuberculosis verrucosa cutis); lupus vulgaris, which usually presents as a brown plaque on the head or neck; and metastatic tuberculous abscesses, which appear in immunosuppressed patients. **Miliary tuberculosis** represents widespread dissemination of *Mycobacterium tuberculosis* in the lungs and other organs. The patient in Figure 9-48 has miliary tuberculosis with multiple erythematous nodules in the skin. Acid-fast organisms can be identified in skin biopsies taken from the nodules. Miliary tuberculosis can also present with small erythematous or purpuric macules and papules in infants.

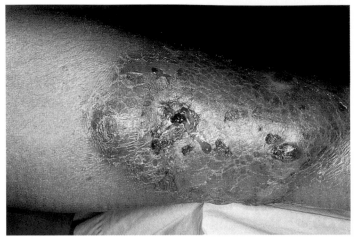

Figure 9-49

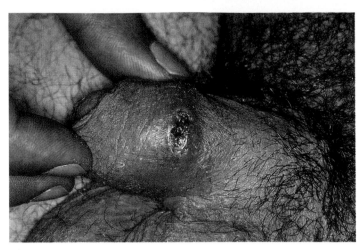

Figure 9-50

Atypical mycobacteria are ubiquitous in the environment, but infections with some of these organisms are often limited to immuno-suppressed patients. Occasionally infections have developed following surgical procedures. The patient shown in Figure 9-49 developed an atypical mycobacterial infection after injection of her own fat to augment the size of her lower legs. Person-to-person transmission generally does not occur with atypical mycobacteria. Post-traumatic wound infection with *Mycobacterium fortuitum* has been described.

Syphilis is caused by venereal transmission of the spirochete, *Treponema pallidum*. The earliest lesion of syphilis, the chancre, occurs 10–90 days after exposure. This lesion is a painless, indurated ulcera-tion that occurs at the site of inoculation, typically on the genitals (Fig. 9-50). Extragenital sites can be affected, occurring most commonly in the anus, rectum, mouth, or oral cavity. Chancres last for 1–6 weeks, and resolve even if untreated. Up to 30% of infected patients may be unaware of a chancre. Chancres on the cervix are often asymptomatic and therefore go unnoticed. Occasionally chancres can be inflamed and painful, and up to 25% of patients will have multiple ulcers. Nontender regional lymphadenopathy commonly occurs. Serologic tests may be negative early in primary syphilis, but usually become positive within several weeks. Dark-field examination of serum oozing from moist chancres usually reveal the causative organism.

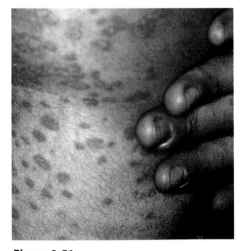

Figure 9-51

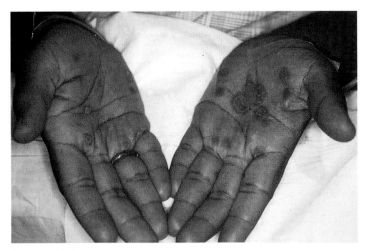

Figure 9-52

Secondary syphilis begins approximately 8 weeks after the appear-ance of the **chancre** and occasionally the two may overlap. Skin lesions can be quite varied. Papulosquamous lesions are most characteristic but macular, pustular, and nodular lesions have been described. Erythe-matous scaling macules resembling pityriasis rosea are shown in the patient with secondary syphilis in Figure 9-51.

Involvement of the palms and soles (Fig. 9-52) is characteristic of secondary syphilis, but often this finding is absent. Skin lesions of secondary syphilis contain viable *T. pallidum* and are therefore some-what contagious, although dry lesions are not as contagious as moist condyloma lata. Dark-field examination of serous fluid obtained from abraded dry lesions will usually reveal spirochetes.

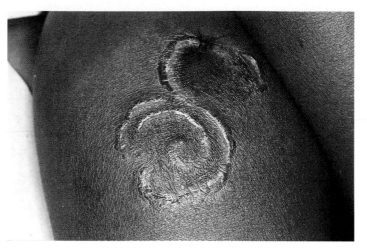

Figure 9-53

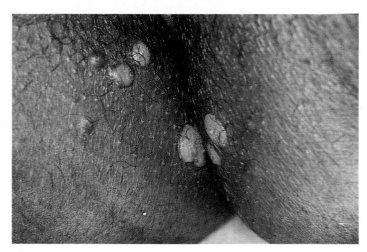

Figure 9-54

Occasionally lesions of secondary syphilis take on striking serpiginous or arcuate patterns (Fig. 9-53). Condyloma lata are moist papules covered with an exudate that is teeming with spirochetes. These

lesions have a predilection for the genitals and for intertriginous areas such as the perianal region (Fig. 9-54), submammary folds, and even toe web spaces. Mucous patches, another lesion of secondary syphilis, are

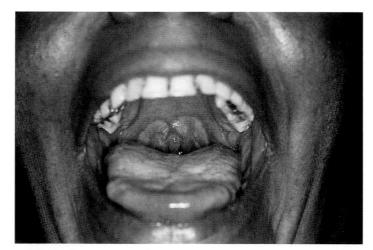

Figure 9-55

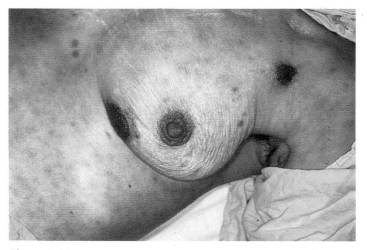

Figure 9-56

shown on the soft palate of a patient in Figure 9-55. These macerated spirochete-laden patches can be found anywhere on the oral mucosa and are occasionally found on genital mucous membranes as well.

Hematogenous spread of *T. pallidum* can affect almost any organ, resulting in a wide array of systemic manifestations in patients with secondary syphilis. Constitutional signs include fever, malaise, and weight loss. Lymphadenopathy and splenomegaly are common. Complications as diverse as glomerulonephritis, hepatitis, periostitis, and uveitis have been reported. Myalgias, arthralgias, deafness, syphilitic meningitis, and other central nervous system findings can occur as well.

Diagnosis is usually made by nontreponemal serologic tests—the Venereal Disease Research Laboratory (VDRL) test, the rapid plasma reagin (RPR) test, and the automated reagin test (ART). False-negatives can occur in patients with acquired immunodeficiency syndrome or as a

result of the prozone phenomenon. The fluorescent treponemal antibody absorption (FTA-Abs) test rarely gives false-negative results.

If untreated, the signs of secondary syphilis resolve spontaneously, and the disease enters a late stage. Only 25% of untreated patients will go on to develop signs of **tertiary syphilis**. The **gumma** is a deep, granulomatous tissue reaction to a few organisms. It begins as a deep, painless nodule or tumor with a predilection for sites of trauma. Gummata increase in size, causing necrosis and ulceration of the overlying dermis and epidermis (Fig. 9-56). These lesions of tertiary syphilis usually occur 3–7 years after secondary syphilis, but some people develop lesions as early as 1 year or as late as 30 years following secondary syphilis. Gummata develop independently of other signs of tertiary syphilis such as syphilitic aortitis, neurosyphilis, and late syphilitic involvement of bone.

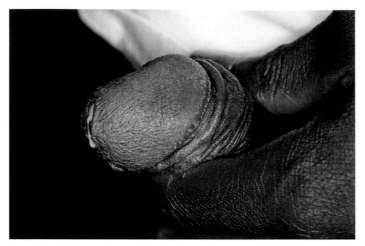

Figure 9-57

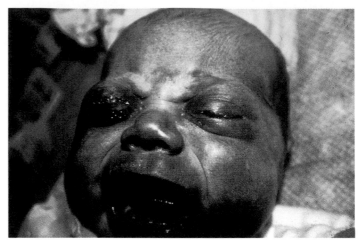

Figure 9-58

Gonorrhea is a sexually transmitted disease caused by *Neisseria gonorrhoeae*. Following a single exposure, approximately 25% of men and more than 50% of women will contract the disease. In men, acute symptoms begin approximately 2–10 days after exposure and consist of dysuria and purulent urethral discharge (Fig. 9-57). In women, dysuria and vaginal discharge or bleeding may develop from several days to several weeks following exposure. Approximately 15% of men and up to 50% of women have few or no symptoms and therefore go undiagnosed and untreated. This untreated reservoir of infected patients is responsible for the persistence of this treatable disease. While symptomatic proctitis and pharyngitis can occur as a result of rectal intercourse and

fellatio, asymptomatic colonization of the anorectal and pharyngeal areas is more common.

The disease can also be acquired by the newborn exposed to an infected birth canal during parturition. **Gonococcal ophthalmia neonatorum**—a purulent conjunctivitis—results (Fig. 9-58). When untreated, acute symptoms of gonorrhea subside, although patients remain contagious. In women, ascending infection causes pelvic inflammatory disease with symptoms that range from mild abdominal pain to a severely tender abdomen with fever. Chronic pain and infertility can result.

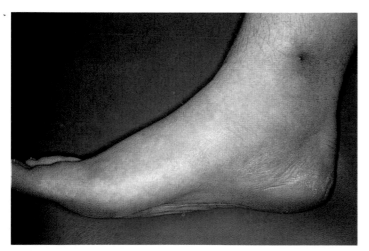

Figure 9-59

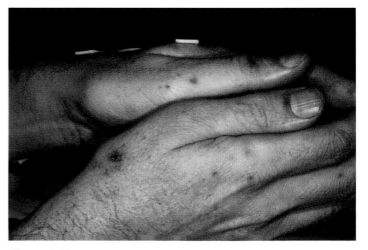

Figure 9-60

Gonococcal bacteremia occurs in up to 3% of patients, particularly females. The **arthritis–dermatitis syndrome** is the most common manifestation of disseminated gonococcemia. Arthralgias, arthritis, and tenosynovitis are common and may be associated with constitutional symptoms such as fever and chills. Discrete isolated skin lesions occur on the extremities, occasionally around swollen joints. Figure 9-59 shows a hemorrhagic pustule adjacent to the swollen ankle of a patient with disseminated gonococcemia. Skin lesions are scarce, numbering fewer than 20, and may present as papules, vesicles, pustules, or hemorrhagic or necrotic macules. The patient whose hands are shown in Figure 9-60 has lesions that are characteristic but more numerous than usual.

Rapid treatment of the dermatitis–arthritis syndrome is essential since joint destruction may result from this bacterial arthritis. Rare complications of gonococcemia include endocarditis and meningitis. Gonococcal peritonitis can lead to a perihepatitis with hepatic capsular fibrosis and adhesions.

Diagnosis of gonococcal infections is often made on clinical grounds, but definitive diagnosis can be made by growth of the organism on Thayer–Martin medium, or by identification of Gram-negative diplococcal organisms in skin lesions or in urethral discharge.

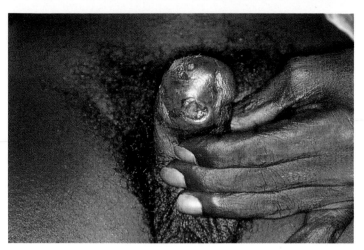

Figure 9-61

Patients have developed lesions of **chancroid** as early as 1 day and as late as 2 weeks after sexual exposure. Men contract the disease far more frequently than women, and many epidemics have been reported in areas where female prostitutes have been infected. The primary lesion occurs at the sight of inoculation on the genitals and begins as a macule or papule that quickly breaks down to a soft demarcated painful ulcer from 1–20 mm in diameter (Fig. 9-61).

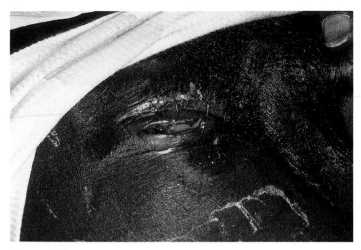

Figure 9-62

The ulcer base is very tender, bleeds easily, and is covered by a necrotic exudate. There are usually two to five ulcers present at the same time. Approximately 1 week after the genital lesion begins, a third to a half of patients develop enlarged, tender inguinal nodes that have been called buboes. Suppuration of the bubo often occurs, leaving a moist ulcer (Fig. 9-62).

Definitive diagnosis of chancroid can be made by identifying the causative organism, *Haemophilus ducreyi*, on a smear of serous exudate from the ulcer. Organisms can also be found on aspiration of a bubo.

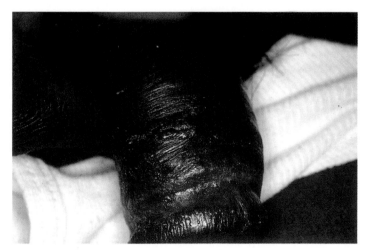

Figure 9-63

Lymphogranuloma venereum is a chlamydial disease transmitted by sexual contact. Genital, rectal, or pharyngeal infection can occur. Primary lesions occur within 30 days of exposure and consist of asymptomatic superficial erosions (Fig. 9-63) that heal within a few days without treatment. Days to weeks later, large tender inguinal nodes develop that may rupture, forming draining sinus tracts (Fig. 9-64). In patients

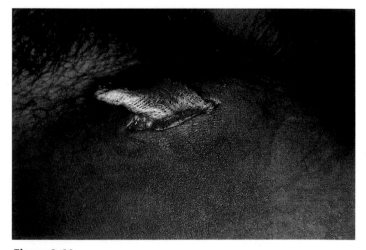

Figure 9-64

with rectal infection, proctocolitis and rectal stricture may occur. Meningoencephalitis and hepatosplenomegaly have been reported.

Diagnosis of lymphogranuloma venereum is often suspected on clinical grounds. Definitive diagnosis by culture is optimal but not widely available. Serologic tests, including the complement fixation test and microimmunofluorescence test, can confirm a suspected diagnosis of lymphogranuloma venereum.

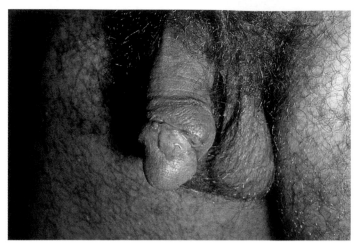

Figure 9-65

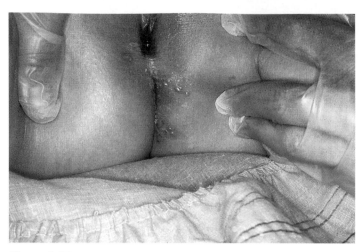

Figure 9-66

Granuloma inguinale is a sexually transmitted disease caused by a Gram-negative rod. The condition is rare in the US, but is more commonly seen in tropical and subtropical regions. Primary lesions involve the penis or scrotum in men and vulval, vaginal, or cervical mucosa in women. Skin lesions rapidly ulcerate and may involve large areas of genital skin and mucosa. Alternatively, ulcerated nodules may form (Fig. 9-65) or the condition may resemble expanding scar tissue. In a small percentage of patients, the disease may involve the gastrointestinal tract or bone.

Genital herpes is one of the most common sexually transmitted diseases, affecting more than 25 000 000 Americans. The vast majority of patients are asymptomatic and unaware of their infection. Nevertheless, in the absence of overt lesions patients can still be infectious. Even in patients with symptomatic outbreaks of genital herpes, asymptomatic viral shedding occurs without clinically overt lesions or symptoms. In people without antibodies to herpes viruses, severe primary infections usually occur within 2 weeks of exposure. Vesicular lesions can be widespread and debilitating. Apart from genital pain, patients may present with fever, tender inguinal lymphadenopathy, and signs of an aseptic meningitis with headache, stiff neck, and cerebrospinal fluid abnormalities. Many are unable to urinate. The patient shown in Figure 9-66 is a young girl who was sexually abused by her

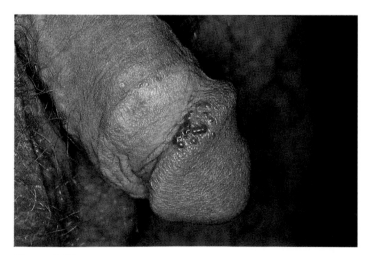

Figure 9-67

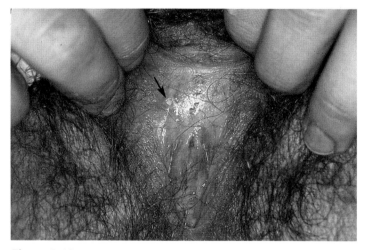

Figure 9-68

father. Widespread grouped vesicles were present over her buttocks, upper thighs, and genital area. In contrast, recurrent outbreaks of herpes simplex virus type 2 genital infection are characterized by localized areas of grouped vesicles (Fig. 9-67) that are not associated with major systemic symptoms.

Vesicles are preceded by a prodrome of itching or pain followed by the formation of erythematous macules and papules that subsequently develop into vesicles. These rapidly change to pustules, which break open to form ulcers and crusts before reepithelializing over 5–10 days. Vesicles and pustules break very quickly in women, who therefore frequently present with genital ulcers (Fig. 9-68) or fissures.

Apart from the social stigma associated with **genital herpes**, recurrent episodes are often asymptomatic or minimally painful, although some patients suffer from significant local pain or prodromal symptoms.

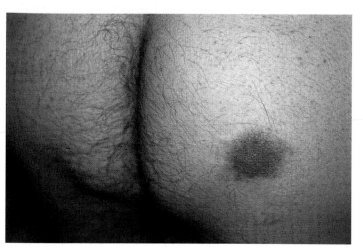

Figure 9-69

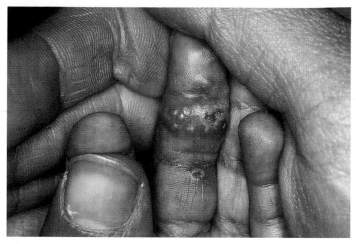

Figure 9-70

Most patients experience only three or four occurrences per year; however, a small but significant number of patients continue to have 10 or more annual recurrences for years after their initial episode. Following initial infection, herpes simplex virus remains latent in nerve root ganglia, eventually reappearing in the distribution of peripheral sensory nerves. Genital infection can therefore result in recurrences on the buttocks (Fig. 9-69), which occurs in approximately 10% of infected patients.

Herpes virus infections are associated with a number of complications. Autoinoculation can occur with both herpes virus types 1 and 2. **Herpetic whitlow** refers to a herpes simplex infection of the fingers. The patient in Figure 9-70 developed characteristic grouped pustules on her finger after touching her own herpes labialis. Dentists and physicians can develop herpetic whitlow after exposure to infectious oral or, less commonly, genital secretions. Irritated or abraded skin may increase the risk of infection. As in genital or labial herpes, whitlow begins with vesicles that progress to pustules, erosions, and

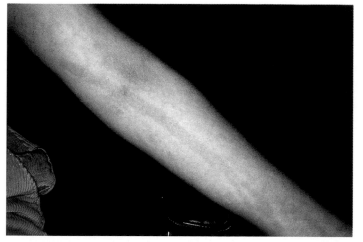

Figure 9-71

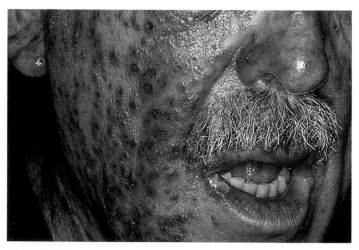

Figure 9-72

crusts before reepithelializing. The patient in Figure 9-71 developed herpetic whitlow because of autoinoculation of genital herpes. The herpetic whitlow recurred at monthly intervals and was associated with a viral lymphangitis presenting as a red streak along her arm. With each episode she developed enlarged, tender, axillary lymph nodes.

Neonatal herpes is perhaps the most feared complication of genital herpes. Neonates born to mothers with recurrent genital herpes have some degree of protection in the form of antiherpes antibodies that cross the placenta. Therefore, even if exposed to herpes during vaginal delivery, these infants have only a small risk of contracting neonatal herpes. In contrast, infants born to mothers who develop a primary episode of genital herpes late in pregnancy have a substantial risk of neonatal herpes with significant morbidity and mortality.

Patients with atopic dermatitis and other conditions that impair the skin's protective functions against viral infection are uniquely sensitive to the herpes simplex virus. Localized herpes labialis or herpes genitalis in these patients can become widespread, covering large portions of the body. The infection, called **eczema herpeticum**, can be life-threatening and is often associated with fever and generalized lymphadenopathy. Differentiation from other causes of vesicopustular rash and fever can be made by clinical features (Table 9-2). The patient in Figure 9-72 had severe atopic dermatitis. He developed widespread herpetic vesicles following an episode of herpes labialis. Tzanck smear of each vesicle revealed multinucleated giant cells, and culture was positive for herpes simplex virus type 1.

Table 9-2. Clinical and Laboratory Features of Acute Vesicopustular Eruptions Associated with Fever

Disorder	Clinical features	Laboratory
Herpes simplex	Vesicles on erythematous base become pustules, erosions and crusts; prodromal pain	Viral culture; Tzanck and Pap smears
Varicella	Vesicles on red base, lesions in different stages begin on trunk and spread to face and extremities	Tzanck prep; viral culture
Herpes zoster	Grouped vesicles on erythematous base in a unilateral dermatomal distribution: prodromal pain	Tzanck prep; viral culture
Kaposi's varicelliform eruption	Follows vaccination or herpes simplex infection in a patient with atopic dermatitis, Darier disease, or other dermatosis	Tzank prep; viral culture
Variola	Eradicated; started on face and extremities: all lesions in same stage	Tzank prep with Giemsa stain: electron microscopy; immunofluorescence; viral culture
Hand foot and mouth disease	Children: oral vesicles; oval vesicles on hands, feet and buttocks; 1 day prodrome of fever and abdominal pain	Viral culture; acute serum-neutralizing antibody titers (usually unnecessary)
Enterovirus infection	Occasional exanthem: associated symptoms variable	Viral culture; acute and convalescent titers
Rickettsial pox	Eschar at site of mite bite, erythematous papulovesicles, lymphadenopathy	Negative Weil–Felix; acute and convalescent complement-fixing antibody titers
Staphylococcal scalded skin syndrome	Staphylococcal infection: erythema followed by bulla formation; Nikolsky sign; desquamation of large sheets of skin	Bacterial cultures from primary site of infection (not skin); skin biopsy or peel

Modified from Fisher M, Katz S. Fever and rash. In: Lebwohl M (ed). Difficult Diagnoses in Dermatology. New York: Churchill Livingstone; 1988: 177.

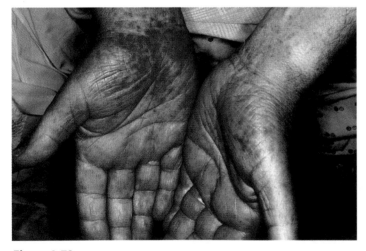

Figure 9-73

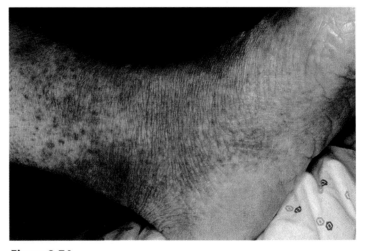

Figure 9-74

Rocky Mountain spotted fever is the most frequent and most severe rickettsial infection in the USA. The causative organism, *Rickettsia rickettsii*, is transmitted by a tick bite. Three to 12 days after the tick bite, there is an abrupt onset of fever, chills, headache, and myalgias. A distinctive rash appears approximately 4 days after the start of these systemic symptoms. Erythematous macules characteristically start on the wrists, ankles, and forearms. The rash then spreads centrally to the arms, legs, trunk, and face. After 2–4 days of the onset of rash, petechiae and purpura develop in the affected areas, characteristically beginning on the wrists and ankles (Figs 9-73 and 9-74). Small foci of gangrene may develop in acral areas and the scrotum or vulva is affected in many patients.

Because the mortality of Rocky Mountain spotted fever is high if untreated, early diagnosis and therapy are critical. Weil–Felix tests or other more specific complement fixation or indirect fluorescence antibody titers will show an increase from acute to convalescent serum specimens. More rapid diagnosis can be made by biopsy of skin lesions for immunofluorescence to identify the causative organism in the walls of cutaneous blood vessels. The latter test is performed by some commercial labs and can usually be completed within a few hours. To justify early treatment, clinical features can help distinguish Rocky Mountain spotted fever from other causes of purpuric rash and fever (Table 9-3).

Table 9-3. Approach to the Patient: Clinical and Laboratory Features of Acute Purpuric Eruptions Associated with Fever

Disorder	Clinical features	Laboratory
Atypical measles	History of killed vaccine (1963–1967); pneumonitis; erythematous macules and papules and petechiae begin on wrists and ankles	Acute and convalescent titers; giant cells in nasopharyngeal scrapings; chest x-ray
Echovirus 9	Upper respiratory, gastrointestinal, and neurologic symptoms	Acute and convalescent titers
Rocky Mountain spotted fever	Endemic areas; rash starts few days after fever; pink macules start on wrists and ankles and become purpuric	Direct immunofluorescence of skin biopsy; Weil-Felix, complement fixation tests
Epidemic typhus	Pink macules start in axillae become purpuric	Weil-Felix, complement fixation tests
Meningococcemia	Purpuric lesions occur on trunk and legs	Blood, spinal and nasopharyngeal cultures; Gram stain of purpuric lesions; counterimmunoelectrophoresis of cerebrospinal fluid
Allergic vasculitis	Purpuric lesions most prominent on lower extremities; arthritis	Urinalysis; stool guaiac; elevated erythrocyte sedimentation rate; skin biopsy and immunofluorescence
TORCHS	Neonatal purpura, "blueberry muffin baby"	*Toxoplasma* antibodies; rubella antibodies; IgM immunofluorescent test for cytomegalovirus; maternal and fetal VDRL; Tzanck prep; Gram stain; dark-field exam; viral and bacterial cultures; CBC
Gonococcemia	Arthritis; 5–20 lesions	Genitourinary, rectal, throat, blood, and synovial cultures
Staphylococcal sepsis	Intravenous drug abuse, other source of infection	Blood and skin culture; Gram stain of skin lesions
Pseudomonas sepsis	Burn patients, immunosuppressed patients: ecthyma gangrenosum, vesiculobullous lesions, gangrenous cellulitis and rose spot-like lesions	Blood and skin cultures; Gram stain of skin lesions
Subacute bacterial endocarditis	Heart murmur, petechiae, splinter hemorrhages, Osler's nodes, Janeway lesions	Blood cultures; Gram stain of skin lesions sometimes helpful

CBC: complete blood count; TORCHS: *toxoplasmosis, other, rubella, cytomegalovirus, herpes* simplex, *syphilis*; VDRL: Venereal Disease Research Laboratory test.
Modified from Fisher M, Katz S. Fever and rash. In: Lebwohl M (ed). Difficult Diagnoses in Dermatology. New York: Churchill Livingstone; 1988: 163.

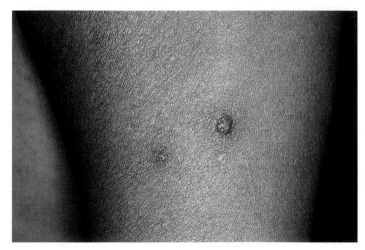

Figure 9-75

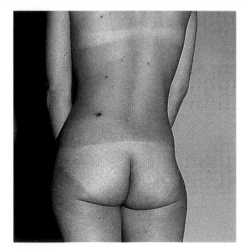

Figure 9-76

Rickettsialpox is a rickettsial disease characterized by high fever and a distinctive rash. It has been reported in the US and in Russia, but because this condition is usually not suspected and is self-limited, its diagnosis is probably often missed. *Rickettsia akari* is the causative organism and its vector is the mite of the house mouse. The disorder can occur in small epidemics, usually in urban areas. A papulovesicular lesion forms at the site 1–2 days after the mite bite. Several days later, high fever develops. It is associated with a vesicopustular eruption (Fig. 9-75) that is acneiform in appearance. Lesions are sparse but usually occur on the face, trunk, and extremities. Oral mucosal lesions

can occur as well. Perhaps the most characteristic finding is a large black eschar at the site of the original mite bite. The patient in Figure 9-76 had forgotten about the lesion on her back since the bite preceded her systemic symptoms by several days, but the diagnosis of rickettsialpox was not suspected until the black eschar on her back was seen.

The definitive diagnosis is made by demonstration of rising complement fixing or indirect fluorescence antibody titers. The Weil–Felix test is negative (Table 9.2). Therapy with systemic antibiotics markedly shortens the course of the disease.

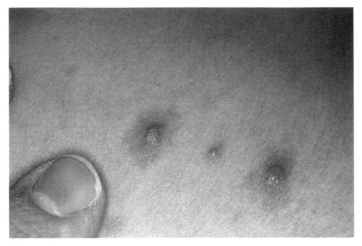

Figure 9-77

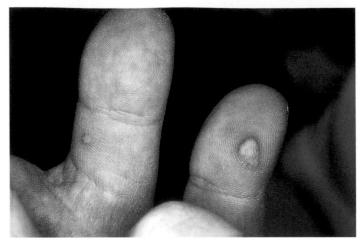

Figure 9-78

Varicella, commonly called chickenpox, is caused by the varicella zoster virus. Characteristics of this highly contagious disease include a short prodromal phase and a rash characterized by pruritic macules, papules, and vesicles that rapidly progress to pustules and crusts. Varicella most frequently strikes children, and serious systemic complications are rare. However, when varicella occurs in adulthood, in the neonatal period, or in immunosuppressed people, constitutional symptoms are often worse, the rash is more extensive, and severe com-plications such as pneumonia can occur. The average incubation period is approximately 2 weeks, though it can be 1–4 weeks. Patients are infectious for 1–2 days before the rash appears and until all lesions have crusted, about 5 days after the onset of the last crop of skin lesions. Transmission is either by direct contact with lesions or by inhalation of infected airborne droplets.

The primary lesion of varicella is the vesicle; it usually evolves from a pink macule that rapidly develops into a papule and then into a vesicle

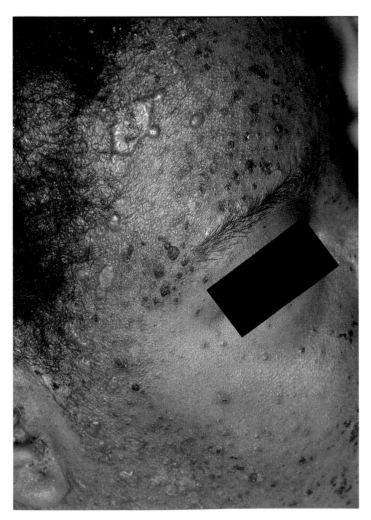

Figure 9-79

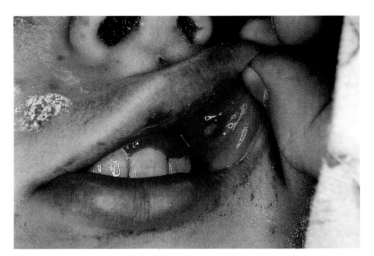

Figure 9-80

on an erythematous base (Fig. 9-77). This in turn quickly becomes a pustule (Fig. 9-78) and finally dries to form a crust. The entire evolution from macule to vesicle to crust may take less than 12 h. New crops of vesicles continue to arise for 4–5 days. This leads to the presence of lesions in all stages, so that in a given area one can find macules and papules adjacent to vesicles, pustules, and crusts (Fig. 9-79). The distribution of lesions is usually central with the greatest concentration of lesions occurring on the face and trunk. However, some lesions occur on the extremities, and occasional lesions may even occur on the palms and soles. Mucous membrane lesions are frequent and oropharyngeal vesicles or ulcers may be seen (Fig. 9-80). Severe pruritus commonly occurs. Fever is directly related to the severity of the rash. The most common complication of varicella is secondary bacterial infection and scarring of skin lesions. Varicella pneumonia may develop within the first week of the rash and affects approximately 15% of adults with varicella. Cough, hemoptysis, pleuritic chest pain, dyspnea, and cyanosis

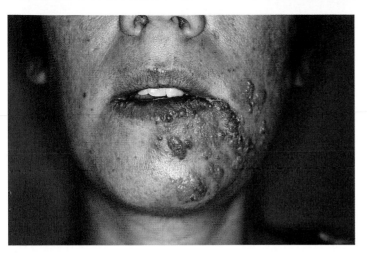

Figure 9-81

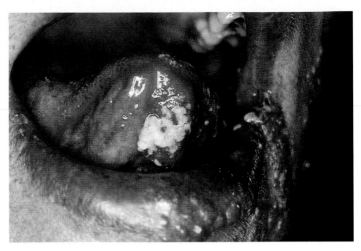

Figure 9-82

occur. Pulmonary involvement is more easily detectable by chest radiographs than by physical findings. Some patients may have a very mild course with only a few skin lesions.

Tzanck smear, performed by scraping the base of the vesicle onto a glass slide and staining for a few seconds with methylene blue, can confirm the diagnosis. When positive, this smear reveals the presence of numerous, multinucleated giant cells.

After a bout of varicella, the varicella zoster virus moves to sensory ganglia where it lies in a latent state for many years. Reactivation of this dormant virus results in **herpes zoster**, a vesicular eruption in a dermatomal distribution (Fig. 9-81) that corresponds to the dermatome

innervated by a single sensory ganglion. An outbreak of herpes zoster is often proceeded by a prodromal period of several days, during which skin lesions are not apparent but pain, itching, and paresthesias affect the involved dermatome. This prodrome can be so severe that patients have been mistakenly diagnosed with appendicitis, cholecystitis, myocardial infarctions, and other ailments before the diagnostic rash of herpes zoster emerged. The rash consists of grouped vesicles on erythematous bases concentrated in a distribution that is unilateral and dermatomal. Figure 9-82 showing a patient with herpes zoster involving the tongue, demonstrates that even mucosal lesions are unilateral.

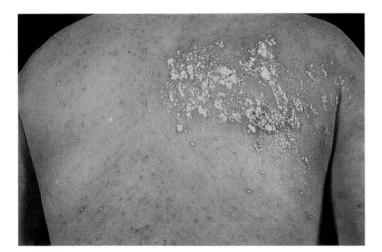

Figure 9-83

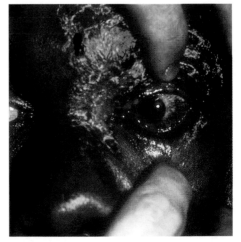

Figure 9-84

Before vesicles develop, lesions may appear as erythematous macules or papules. The vesicles are usually apparent in 1–2 days and form crusts within approximately 1 week (Fig. 9-83). The rash is contagious for up to a week after the onset of new lesions, and exposure to herpes zoster can result in varicella in patients who have not had chickenpox. One of the dreaded complications of herpes zoster occurs when the nasociliary branch of the ophthalmic division of the trigeminal nerve is involved. This results in lesions of herpes zoster on the nose and signals ophthalmic involvement. Conjunctivitis, keratitis, scleritis, ptosis, and other complications may develop (Fig. 9-84).

The most common complication of herpes zoster is postherpetic neuralgia, affecting more than 10% of patients, especially those more than 60 years old. The pain of postherpetic neuralgia can last for months, but in most patients it eventually resolves. Hematogenous dissemination of herpes zoster outside the affected dermatome results in a generalized vesicular eruption. Many patients will have a few vesicles outside the primary dermatome but these pose little risk to the patient, in contrast to widespread dissemination, which is associated with significant morbidity and mortality.

Table 9-4. Clinical and Laboratory Features of Acute Generalized Erythematous Eruptions Associated with Fever

Disorder	Clinical features	Laboratory
Erythema infectiosum	Children: "slapped cheeks"	
Measles	Cough, coryza, conjunctivitis, Koplik's spots	Sputum smears (Warthin-Finkeldey cells); acute and convalescent titers
Rubella	Tender lymphadenopathy, Forchheimer spots	Acute and convalescent titers
Roseola	Children; rash follows fever	
Viral exanthems	Occasional enanthem; associated symptoms variable	Stool and oropharyngeal cultures; acute and convalescent titers
Infectious mononucleosis	Pharyngitis, adenopathy, splenomegaly, supraorbital edema	Lymphocytosis with atypical lymphocytes; heterophil/monospot
Hepatitis B	Jaundice, urticaria, erythema multiforme, palpable purpura, and papular acrodermatitis can occur	Hepatitis B surface antigen; elevated liver function tests; rising anti-HBc and anti-HBs antibody titers
Scarlet fever	Pharyngitis, strawberry tongue, Pastia's lines, desquamation of palms and soles	Culture of nose or throat; elevated antistreptolysin O (ASLO), streptozyme hemagglutination
Toxic shock syndrome	Tampon use or bacterial infection, hypotension, desquamation of palms and soles, gastrointestinal symptoms, neurologic symptoms	Elevated liver function tests, creatine phosphokinase, blood urea nitrogen, and creatinine; abnormal urinalysis; *Staphylococcus aureus* cultured from vagina or other source
Kawasaki disease	Children; conjunctivitis, chapped lips, strawberry tongue, desquamation of palms and soles, cervical adenopathy; neurologic, gastrointestinal, and cardiovascular symptoms	Elevated platelets, white blood cells, and erythrocyte sedimentation rate; electrocardiographic abnormalities; infiltrates on chest x-ray
Drug reaction	History of drug ingestion	
Connective tissue diseases	Malar rash, discoid lesions, photosensitivity, mucosal ulcers, arthritis, muscle weakness, alopecia, Raynaud phenomenon	ANA, CPK, aldolase, BUN, creatinine, complement, rheumatoid factor, ESR, VDRL, urinalysis, skin biopsy and immunofluorescence
Erythema multiforme (toxic epidermal necrolysis, Stevens–Johnson syndrome)	Preceding infection or drug; target lesions, mucosal lesions; diffuse erythema and erosions (TEN)	Skin biopsy; skin peel and Tzanck prep for toxic epidermal necrolysis
Secondary syphilis	Preceding chancre; condylomata lata, symptoms variable	VDRL, FTA; dark-field exam of nonintraoral lesions
Lyme disease	Endemic areas; preceding tick bite; annular lesions, arthritis, myocarditis, neuropathy	Lyme disease serology; spirochetes on silver stain of skin biopsy

ANA, antinuclear antibodies; BUN, blood urea nitrogen; CPK, creatine phosphokinase; ESR, erythrocyte sedimentation rate; FTA, fluorescent titer antibody; HBc, hepatitis B core antigen; HBs, hepatitis B surface antigen; VDRL, Venereal Disease Research Laboratory Test.
Modified from Fisher M, Katz S. Fever and rash. In: Lebwohl M (ed). Difficult Diagnoses in Dermatology. New York: Churchill Livingstone; 1988: 135.

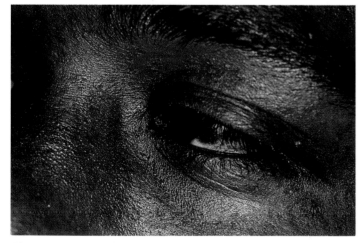

Figure 9-85

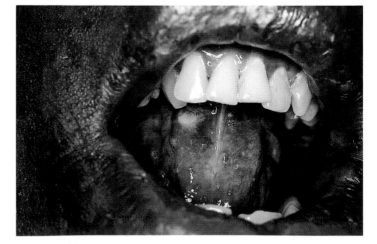

Figure 9-86

Measles is a highly contagious childhood illness that is common worldwide. Attempts at vaccination in the US have been partially successful but sporadic outbreaks still occur. Differentiation of measles from other causes of erythematous rash and fever can often be made by clinical features (Table 9-4). Following an incubation period of approximately 10 days, patients experience 3–4 days of prodromal symptoms consisting of fever, conjunctivitis (Fig. 9-85), and upper respiratory tract symptoms, including cough and coryza. Characteristic

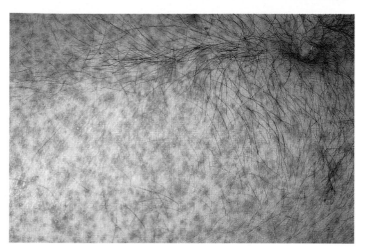

Figure 9-87

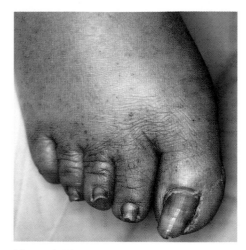

Figure 9-88

oral lesions called Koplik spots develop 1–2 days before the rash. These are pinpoint white papules surrounded by erythematous macules on the oral mucosa (Fig. 9-86). Erythematous macules and papules then develop on the head, most characteristically in the ears. These spread downward, involving the neck, trunk, and extremities. Erythematous macules and papules are discrete in some areas but form confluent patches in other areas (Fig. 9-87). Pruritus is not a striking symptom. Some patients develop generalized adenopathy. Most symptoms fade within 7 days of the onset of the rash. Complications of measles include encephalitis, thrombocytopenic purpura, and secondary bacterial pneumonia. Subacute sclerosing panencephalitis is a late—but rare—complication of this viral infection.

Atypical measles occurs in patients who are immunized with the killed-measles vaccine that was administered in the 1960s. The condition occurs following exposure to the measles virus and is characterized by a prodrome of fever, cough, headache, and myalgia lasting for 2–3 days. A rash consisting of purpuric macules starts on the feet (Fig. 9-88) and spreads to the rest of body. It is often associated with x-ray evidence of pneumonia, occasionally with pleural effusion. The rash is easily mistaken for Rocky Mountain Spotted fever, but the presence of cough in an individual who would have been a child in the early-to-middle 1960s should suggest the possibility of atypical measles. Definitive diagnosis can be made by demonstrating a rise in antibody titers to the measles virus.

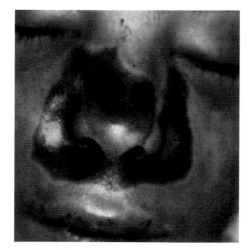

Figure 9-89

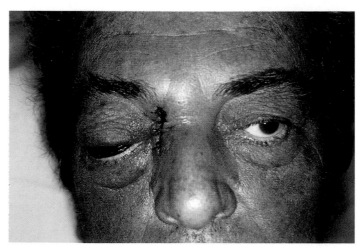

Figure 9-90

Mucormycosis is a rapidly destructive fungal infection that can be caused by a number of different organisms such as *Mucor, Rhizopus, Absidia, Mortierella* and *Basidiobolus*. Many patients with mucor have diabetes, and the condition specifically occurs in the setting of diabetic ketoacidosis. Mucor also develops in immunosuppressed patients, including those receiving systemic corticosteroids, antimetabolites, or other immunosuppressive agents, and in patients with leukemia. Infection usually begins in the eyes, nose, or sinuses. Pain and erythema are followed by purulent discharge with grossly disfiguring swelling. Rapidly progressive necrosis and gangrene ensue (Fig. 9-89) and are

accompanied by fever and leukocytosis. With ocular involvement, proptosis can occur (Fig. 9-90). Because the causative fungi are common contaminants, culture alone may not suffice for diagnosis. Definitive proof of mucormycosis is established by demonstrating fungal invasion of tissues. However, the rapidity with which this infection progresses requires that treatment be undertaken once the diagnosis is suspected. Systemic antifungal therapy and surgical debridement result in significantly increased survival rates.

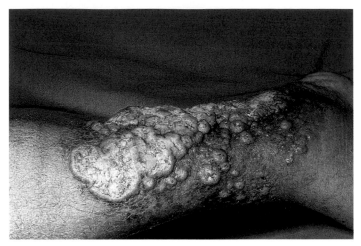

Figure 9-91

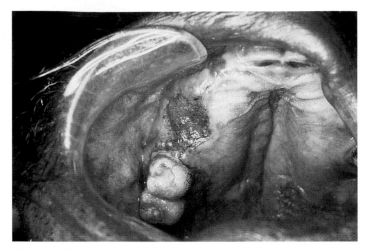

Figure 9-92

Blastomycosis is a chronic fungal infection that typically affects male farmers and laborers over the age of 50 years. It is seen in Africa and in North and South America, especially in southeastern US. Infection usually begins in the lungs and is followed by hematogenous spread to the skin, bones, and genital tract. Several types of skin lesions can be seen, including large ulcers, which characteristically have elevated verrucous borders, as seen on the leg of the patient shown in Figure 9-91.

The central ulceration heals with an atrophic scar. More superficial ulcers can also occur, and ulceration of the oral or nasal mucous membranes occurs in about 25% of patients (Fig. 9-92). Other affected individuals present with indurated subcutaneous nodules with overlying pustules.

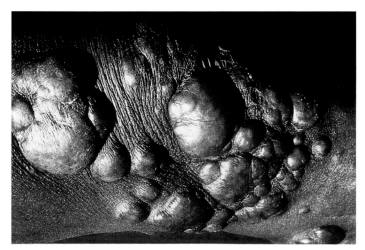

Figure 9-93

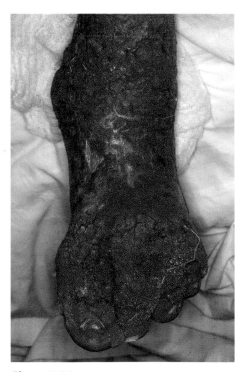

Figure 9-94

Approximately 50% of patients have abnormal chest radiographs or positive sputum cultures. A third have bone lesions that occasionally extend to subcutaneous tissue, resulting in abscess formation with local tenderness. The clinical presentation of infected people can be quite variable. The patient in Figure 9-93 developed numerous indurated skin-colored nodules caused by *Blastomyces dermatitides*. Diagnosis is made by culture of skin lesions, sputum, urine, or pus. On microscopic examination with 10–20% potassium hydroxide, budding cells with thick walls can be seen. The causative organism grows in culture on either blood agar plates or fungal media. Blastomycosis responds to systemic antifungal therapy and surgical debridement and drainage of abscesses.

Mycetoma, also known as Madura foot, is a chronic infection of the skin, subcutaneous tissue, and bone of the foot, although other sites can occasionally be infected. Several species of actinomycetes and a number of fungi have caused this infection, which is most commonly seen in India, Africa, and South America. Skin lesions are characterized by massive hyperkeratosis with marked swelling, thickening, and sinus tract formation that are grossly deforming but not very painful (Fig. 9-94). Radiographs show features of osteomyelitis. Sinus tracts drain visible granules that are composed of colonies of fungal hyphae. Treatment with antibiotics and surgical debridement are often unsuccessful, and amputation may be necessary.

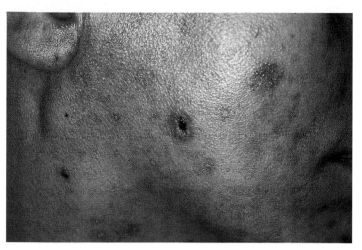

Figure 9-95

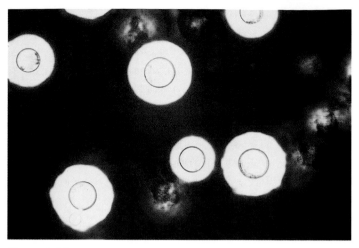

Figure 9-96

Cryptococcal infection of the skin occurs in approximately 10–15% of people with systemic **cryptococcosis**. This chronic infection is acquired by inhalation of the yeast *Cryptococcus neoformans*. The organism is found in pigeon excreta and nests, and air-conditioning vents contaminated with pigeon excreta are the source of infection sometimes. Although the lungs are the primary site of infection, most patients do not complain of cough or other pulmonary symptoms. Chest radiographs, however, can reveal striking abnormalities despite the absence of symptoms. Skin lesions often begin as erythematous papules or nodules that may break down to form ulcers (Fig. 9-95).

Most patients with cryptococcosis present with meningitis. Symptoms develop insidiously with the gradual development of headache or confusion over a period of months. Diagnosis is made by identification of the organism from skin lesions, sputum, urine, or, most commonly, cerebrospinal fluid. India ink preparations reveal budding encapsulated yeast forms (Fig. 9-96). In the presence of central nervous system symptoms, cryptococcal infection should be suspected—especially in patients with immune defects such as diabetes or AIDS.

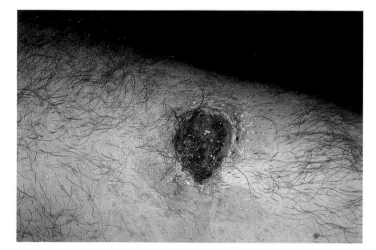

Figure 9-97

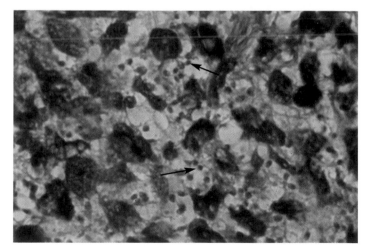

Figure 9-98

Leishmaniasis is a protozoan infection transmitted by the bite of a sandfly. Millions of cases occur worldwide, but most cases in the USA and Europe occur in travelers from the Middle East or South America. Visceral leishmaniasis has recently emerged as an important opportunistic infection in patients with AIDS, but this protozoan infection is often limited to the skin in cutaneous leishmaniasis, or to mucous membranes in mucosal leishmaniasis. Skin lesions of cutaneous leishmaniasis begin as erythematous papules, which develop shortly after the bite of a sandfly. The papule enlarges to 2 cm or more and eventually becomes crusted and ulcerated (Fig. 9-97). Cutaneous ulcers last for months to years.

Diagnosis can be made by histologic examination of skin biopsy specimens or by Giemsa staining of aspirates taken from the periphery of ulcers. These show amastigotes, called Leishman–Donovan bodies, inside macrophages (Fig. 9-98). While touch preparations are most easily performed, diagnosis can also be confirmed by culture using Novy–MacNeal–Nicolle (NNN) medium. Most recently, polymerase chain reaction (PCR) has been used to identify leishmaniasis in fixed tissue specimens.

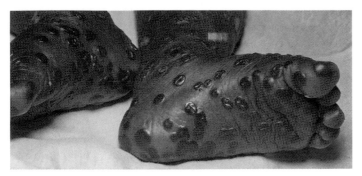

Figure 9-99

Aggressive worldwide vaccination programs resulted in the successful eradication of **smallpox** by 1980. Recent concern about bioterrorism has raised the possibility that stored variola virus could be used as a weapon. These concerns have led to new vaccination programs, specifically in Israel and the United States. Smallpox is spread through inhalation of the virus or contact with secretions. Twelve to 13 days following exposure, patients develop a prodrome consisting of fever, malaise, and backache lasting three to four days. This is rapidly followed by the development of numerous vesicles that may begin on the palms and soles (Fig. 9-99), but rapidly spread in a centrifugal pattern. Smallpox can be differentiated from varicella in that the latter condition is characterized by lesions in various stages of development with crusts next to vesicles or pustules. In contrast, lesions of smallpox are more homogeneous, as shown on the face, trunk and extremities of an

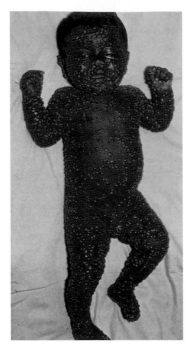

Figure 9-100

infected infant (Fig. 9-100). On biopsy of vesicles of smallpox, ballooning degeneration and cytoplasmic inclusion bodies are seen within keratinocytes.

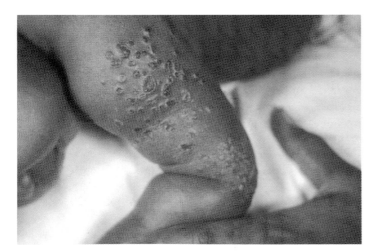

Figure 9-101

Live **vaccinia** virus is used to vaccinate against smallpox. Regional lymphadenopathy, fever and malaise can occur following vaccination. Spread of the virus from the vaccination site can occur, as shown on the arm of an infant in Figure 9-101. Vesiculation at the primary inoculation site on the arm is expected, but because live vaccinia virus is used, care must be taken to avoid autoinoculation or to avoid inoculating others. In patients who are immunosuppressed or have underlying skin disorders such as atopic dermatitis, the vaccinia virus can disseminate, resulting in vesicles over large parts of the cutaneous surface. Patients are febrile and debilitated. Mortality of 5% has been reported historically. Treatment with vaccinia immune globulin may be beneficial.

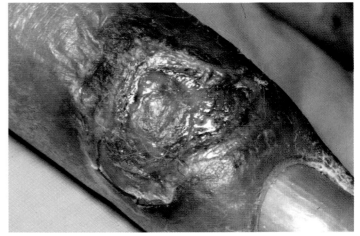

Figure 9-102

Anthrax, another potential agent of bioterrorism, is caused by *Bacillus anthracis*, a gram positive rod-shaped bacterium. Traditionally, there is a low disease rate following exposure to anthrax, and cutaneous anthrax accounts for 95% of cases, usually manifesting as an eschar-covered ulcer on exposed areas of skin following direct contact with infected animals. Hands and fingers are most commonly affected (Fig. 9-102). In contrast, inhalational anthrax is rapidly progressive and frequently fatal. At least 23 cases of anthrax occurred as a result of bioterrorism in the United States in 2001, including the patient whose photograph is shown in Figure 9-102.

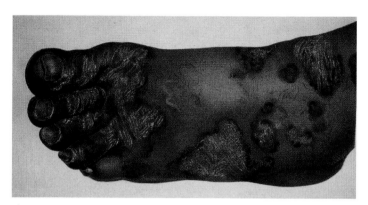

Figure 10-1

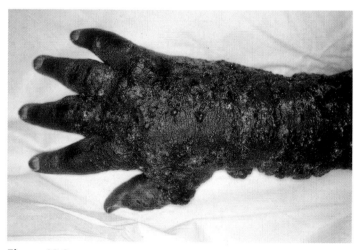

Figure 10-2

Sarcoma idiopathicum multiplex hemorrhagicum pedis dextri.

Kaposi M. Handatlas der Hautkrankheiten fur Studirende und Arzte; 1900.

Moritz Kaposi originally described a sarcoma that primarily affected elderly Mediterranean men and was not associated with clinically apparent immunosuppression (Fig. 10-1). Like acquired immunodeficiency syndrome (AIDS)-related Kaposi sarcoma, classic **Kaposi sarcoma** is characterized by purple macules, papules, plaques, and nodules. Histologically, the two forms of Kaposi sarcoma are similar, but classic Kaposi sarcoma is very slowly progressive, often remaining confined to the lower extremities for years. By contrast, AIDS-related Kaposi sarcoma often develops explosively, and lesions are frequently widespread. Figure 10-2 shows the hand of a patient infected with the human immunodeficiency virus (HIV). The hand is covered with ulcerated nodules of Kaposi sarcoma.

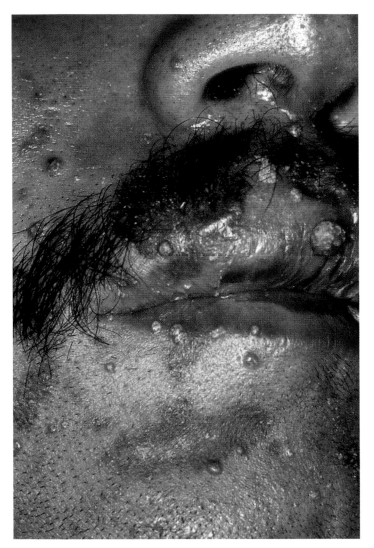

Figure 10-3

The patient shown in Figure 10-3 has numerous cutaneous stigmata of **AIDS**. The umbilicated white papules on and around the lips, on the nose, and on the right malar area, are lesions of molluscum contagiosum. The verrucous papule on the upper lip is a wart, and the purple patches on and beneath the lips are lesions of Kaposi sarcoma.

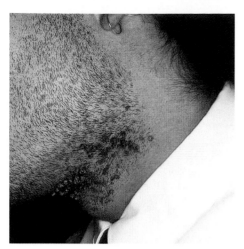

Figure 10-4

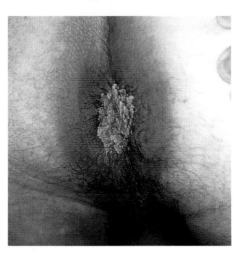

Figure 10-5

Numerous skin lesions associated with AIDS or with related opportunistic infections occur in most patients. Human papillomavirus infection produces warts on the hands, feet, face, and genitals, which can reach considerable size. Simple warts, which in the normal host would be easily treated, grow in size and number, and spread over the entire cutaneous surface. In patients with advanced disease, the aim of treatment is to control growth and spread of warts, since lasting "cure" of warts in HIV-infected patients is often difficult to achieve unless the HIV infection is controlled. The patient in Figure 10-4 presented with hundreds of warts on the face and neck.

Condyloma acuminata are found in over 25% of patients with AIDS and can be extensive in both size and number (Fig. 10-5). Treatment by any means may be associated with temporary reduction in wart mass, but condylomata usually recur within a short time. Carcinomas have been documented within perianal condylomata in homosexual men, and human papillomavirus DNA has been identified in squamous cell carcinomas.

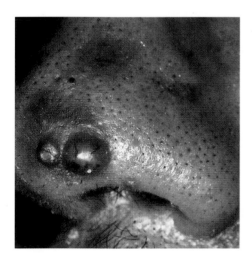

Figure 10-6

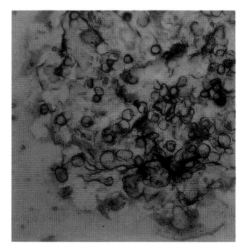

Figure 10-7

Molluscum contagiosum is a self-limited infection often seen in the normal pediatric population. Adults frequently acquire this infection through sexual contact, and lesions commonly develop in the genital region. In the AIDS population, lesions become widespread, attaining relatively large sizes of 1–2 cm in diameter (Fig. 10-6). Lesions occur in unusual locations, and treatment can be frustrating as molluscum often recurs in AIDS patients. Even after extensive treatment with fulguration

or cryotherapy, new sites usually develop. Because some lesions of cutaneous cryptococcosis can resemble molluscum, definitive identification of the causative organism should be sought, even in characteristic umbilicated white papules. Lesions of molluscum that are scraped and smeared onto a glass slide can be stained with methylene blue to reveal characteristic molluscum bodies (Fig. 10-7).

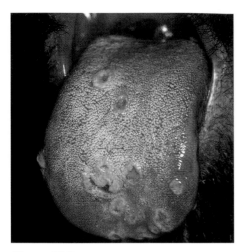

Figure 10-8

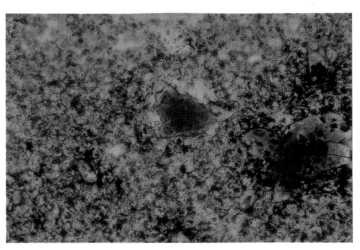

Figure 10-9

Herpes simplex virus infection in immunocompetent patients is generally self-limited and discrete, but in AIDS patients the same viruses produce lesions that are chronic and erosive, often failing to resolve without therapy. Herpes simplex infections evolve into large erosions and ulcerations (Fig. 10-8) from which the virus can easily be cultured or identified by Tzanck smears. Tzanck smears are performed by scraping an ulcer or the base of a vesicle onto a glass slide. Multinucleated giant cells can be seen by staining the slides with methylene blue, Wright's stain, or Giemsa stain (Fig. 10-9). Ulcers most commonly occur on the genitals and in the perianal area, but any site

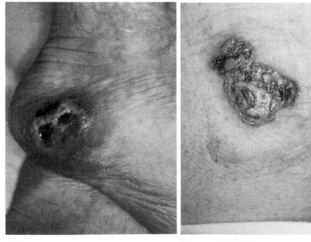

Figure 10-10A   **Figure 10-10B**

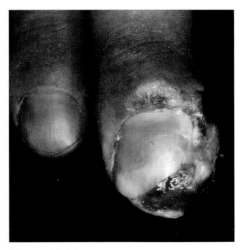

Figure 10-11

can be infected, including feet, hands, and trunk. The patient in Figure 10-10A had an ulceration of the heel of the foot for 6 months before a correct diagnosis of chronic herpes simplex infection was established. The patient often sat with his heels touching his buttocks; the infection was undoubtedly transmitted by direct contact with the chronic erosive herpes infection on his buttock (Fig. 10-10B). Chronic erosive herpes infections were recognized as a sign of progression to AIDS even before serologic assays for HIV were available. There are reports of AIDS patients developing chronic herpetic whitlow of the digits. The patient in Figure 10-11 had a chronic ulcer of the finger that was first misdiagnosed as a mycobacterial infection and later as a deep fungal infection. Ultimately, viral culture revealed herpes simplex virus. Oral acyclovir therapy has been successful in treating most herpes infections. However, acyclovir resistance has been reported in some patients with AIDS; these patients can be successfully treated with intravenous foscarnet.

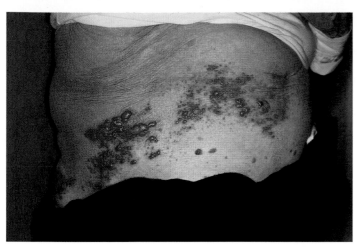

Figure 10-12

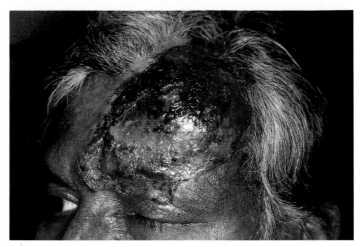

Figure 10-13

Typical appearing **herpes zoster**, characterized by grouped vesicles in a dermatomal distribution, can be the first sign of HIV infection. This should not be surprising, since herpes zoster is known to appear in the setting of other diseases associated with immunosuppression, such as Hodgkin disease, non-Hodgkin lymphomas, and leukemias. As in the general adult population, the extent of herpes zoster can vary from a small patch of grouped vesicles to large areas of extensive hemorrhage, necrosis, or bulla formation (Fig. 10-12). However, some patients with

AIDS develop chronic nonhealing herpes zoster that persists for months, causing severe pain and scarring. The man in Figure 10-13 developed a severe cranial herpes zoster infection that continued to erode and ulcerate for months. By contrast, the AIDS patient shown in Figure 10-14 developed a limited herpes zoster infection characterized by a few grouped vesicles in a dermatomal distribution on the abdomen. These continued to fester for months as new ulcerations developed within the same dermatome.

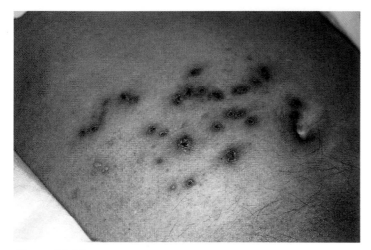

Figure 10-14

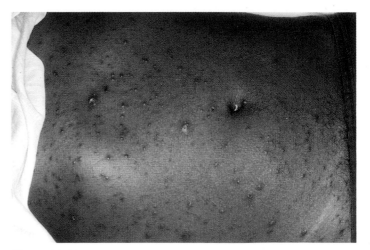

Figure 10-15

HIV-infected patients with herpes zoster can be successfully treated with acyclovir. However, as occurs in herpes simplex infections in people with AIDS, acyclovir resistance has developed in some HIV-seropositive patients with varicella zoster virus infections. Fortunately, resistance to acyclovir has been uncommon. Recurrences of herpes zoster are much more frequent in HIV-infected individuals, and

recurrent varicella has occurred in patients with AIDS. In individuals who are severely immunosuppressed, herpes zoster often disseminates. Widespread erythematous papules, vesicles, and crusts develop and in some instances resemble varicella (Fig. 10-15). The presence of some lesions in a dermatomal distribution, however, helps to distinguish disseminated zoster from chickenpox.

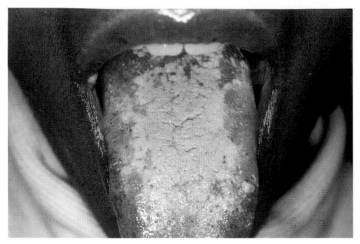

Figure 10-16

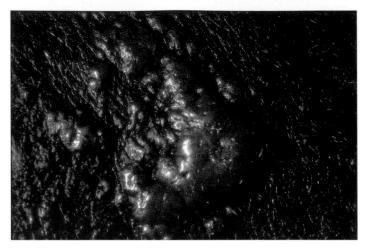

Figure 10-17

Monilial infections of the groin, inframammary areas, axillae, and perianal area are frequent in the general population but unquestionably increased in patients with AIDS. Oral thrush that is refractory to treatment commonly develops in HIV-infected patients (Fig. 10-16). In contrast to oral hairy leukoplakia, which cannot be wiped off, the white patches of oral thrush easily rub off, leaving a red base. Yeast often infects the throat and esophagus as well. When candidiasis occurs in the esophagus, it is considered an opportunistic infection meeting clinical criteria that were originally established to document progression of HIV infection to AIDS.

Cryptococcosis is another common opportunistic infection in patients with AIDS. Skin findings can develop even in the absence of central nervous system or pulmonary symptoms. Cutaneous lesions vary in appearance, ranging from umbilicated papules resembling molluscum contagiosum to keloid-like plaques, as shown in the patient in Figure 10-17. Although widespread hematogenous dissemination can occur, systemic symptoms may be mild or absent. Symptomatic cutaneous cryptococcal infection may therefore precede clinically apparent involvement of multiple organs. Skin lesions are present in 10% of patients with cryptococcal infection and occasionally lead to the

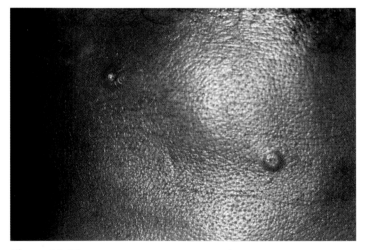

Figure 10-18

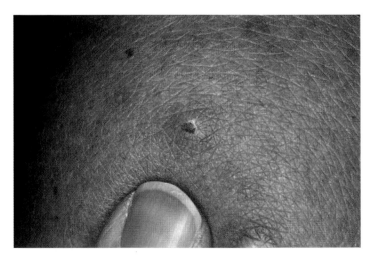

Figure 10-19

diagnosis. The patient in Figure 10-18 developed umbilicated papules on the forehead. These were felt to be typical lesions of molluscum contagiosum until a skin biopsy revealed cryptococci. The causative organism, *Cryptococcus neoformans*, is a yeast-like fungus that reproduces by budding and is surrounded by a polysaccharide capsule. Mucicarmine stains allow visualization of the capsule; the organism can also be seen with methenamine silver or periodic acid-Schiff stains. Diagnosis is usually made by identifying cryptococci in tissue or cerebrospinal fluid, but the organism can grow on appropriate fungal culture media. Occasionally the organism is grown from blood cultures.

Infection with *Histoplasma capsulatum* in patients with normal immune systems rarely results in disseminated disease. In patients with AIDS, however, disseminated **histoplasmosis** is common. Cutaneous manifestations of disseminated histoplasmosis vary considerably. Mucosal ulcerations are often present, including ulceration of the nasal mucosa. Erythematous maculopapular eruptions and acneiform eruptions have been described. As in disseminated cryptococcosis, patients have been reported with umbilicated papules resembling molluscum contagiosum. The patient shown in Figure 10-19 presented with ulcerated papules that grew *H. capsulatum* on culture. The course of disseminated histoplasmosis can be severe, with recurrent fevers, weight loss and, ultimately, death.

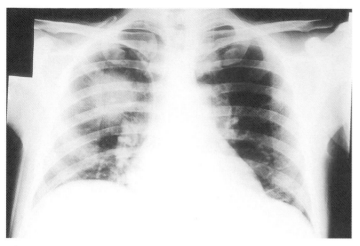

Figure 10-20

Aspergillus species are ubiquitous in nature but rarely cause cutaneous disease. Bronchial infection resulting in a "fungus ball" can occur, but in the normal host the infection is usually contained, and patients may be asymptomatic. In immunosuppressed patients, however, hematogenous dissemination of *Aspergillus* can occur, and local invasion of adjacent tissues is possible. The HIV-infected patient whose radiograph is shown in Figure 10-20 presented with a solitary cutaneous ulceration on the back caused by invasion from the fungus ball in the right upper lobe of his lung.

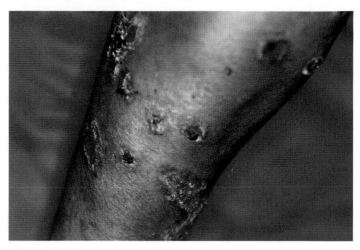

Figure 10-21

Sporotrichosis is a cutaneous fungal disease that rarely results in systemic manifestations. The causative organism, *Sporothrix schenckii*, grows in soil and on vegetation and is transmitted by accidental implantation into the skin. Ulceration develops at the site of implantation, and lymphatic spread of the organism results in linear cutaneous nodules. The HIV-infected patient in Figure 10-21 presented with multiple leg ulcers from which *S. schenckii* was cultured. Patients with AIDS can develop widespread cutaneous lesions, as well as hematogenous dissemination to multiple organs, culminating in death.

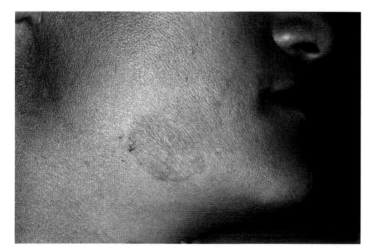

Figure 10-22

Dermatophytosis is common in the general population but may be increased in patients with AIDS. Common cutaneous infections such as tinea pedis have been found more frequently in patients who are seropositive for HIV compared to those who are seronegative. Onychomycosis and tinea cruris are also common in HIV-infected patients. AIDS can predispose to dermatophyte infection that is more severe or widespread, or that occurs in atypical locations or unusual forms. The patient in Figure 10-22 was thought to have nummular eczema until scrapings revealed hyphal forms consistent with tinea faciale.

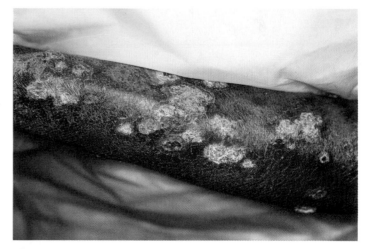

Figure 10-23

Bacterial infections in people with AIDS are more frequent, severe, or chronic than those seen in people with normal immune function. *Staphylococcus aureus* is a particularly common pathogen that has been identified in bacterial folliculitis and in an intertriginous rash occurring in AIDS patients. The latter condition can involve the axillae and resembles moniliasis. Subcutaneous abscesses have also been reported. The patient shown in Figure 10-23 developed multiple ulcers covered with thick crusts on the scalp and extremities. Cultures repeatedly grew *S. aureus* but a number of Gram-negative organisms were grown intermittently. Treatment with intravenous antibiotics was ineffective.

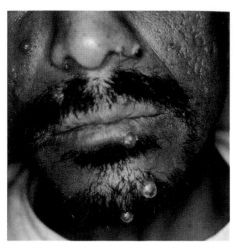

Figure 10-24

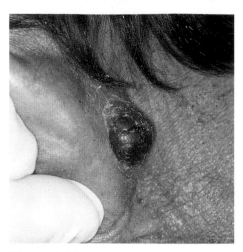

Figure 10-25

Bacillary angiomatosis, also known as epithelioid angiomatosis, is an unusual vascular response in the skin of AIDS patients. This condition is caused by infection with an organism whose identity has been the subject of intense investigation. Histologically, the nodules of bacillary angiomatosis are characterized by vascular proliferation, and vessels are lined by atypical endothelial cells. Systemic symptoms include fevers, chills, and night sweats. Bony lesions may occur, and chronic disease is associated with weight loss. Treatment with oral antibiotics can result in marked improvement. Patients present with skin lesions that may be solitary or widespread. These purple papules and nodules are occasionally mistaken for Kaposi sarcoma or pyogenic granulomas (Figs 10-24 and 10-25). Biopsy of nodules may reveal small bacilli that are visible with Warthin–Starry stains. Early investigators suspected that the causative organism was the cat scratch bacillus, *Afipia felis*, because it is also a Warthin–Starry-positive bacillus, and because many patients with bacillary angiomatosis report a history of cat scratch or cat bite. More recently, however, *Rochalimaea henselae*, a Gram-negative, Warthin–Starry-positive bacillus, has been identified in lesions of bacillary angiomatosis.

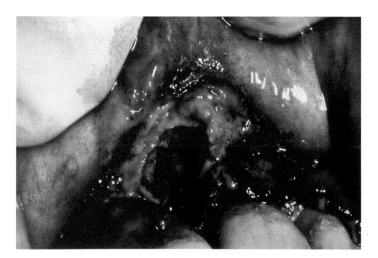

Figure 10-26

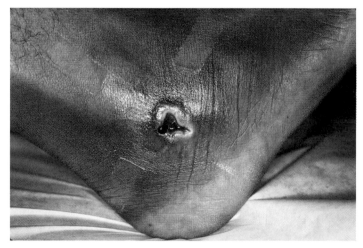

Figure 10-27

Infection with *Mycobacterium avium intracellulare* (MAI) is common in patients with AIDS, but most do not develop symptomatic skin disease. Because of bacteremia and widespread dissemination of MAI, this organism is usually an incidental finding in skin lesions. Occasionally, however, patients develop deep cutaneous ulcerations, especially over draining infected nodes or MAI osteomyelitis. Figure 10-26 shows gingival destruction in a patient with AIDS and aggressive MAI infection. The patient died after mycobacterial invasion of the maxillary sinus.

Mycobacterium haemophilum is a rare cause of infection, and virtually all reported patients have been immunosuppressed. It is, therefore, not surprising that disseminated *M. haemophilum* infection develops in patients with AIDS. Swelling and tenderness of wrists, ankles, and knees have been reported. Skin lesions present as painful, erythematous or violaceous nodules and plaques, or as tender ulcerations. *M. haemophilum* has also been identified in a patient presenting with a subcutaneous abscess. The patient in Figure 10-27 developed a lateral malleolar ulcer from which *M. haemophilum* was cultured. On skin biopsy, acid-fast bacilli may be seen, and cutaneous granulomas develop in some patients.

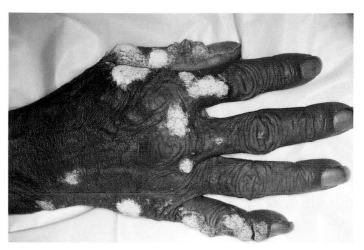

Figure 10-28

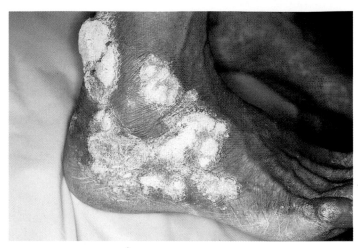

Figure 10-29

In populations where HIV infection is prevalent, outbreaks of **scabies** are common. Not surprisingly, both typical and unusual manifestations of scabies infection have been reported in AIDS patients. The causative organism, *Sarcoptes scabiei* var. *hominis*, is usually transmitted by skin-to-skin contact, and sexual transmission is often responsible. In the normal host, the rash of scabies has a predilection for the web spaces of the fingers and the volar surfaces of the hands and wrists. Characteristically there is involvement of the buttocks, the genitals in men, and the nipples in women. The pathognomonic lesion of scabies is the burrow, a linear lesion less than 1 cm in length. The burrow contains the adult female mite, which can often be seen on microscopic examination

of scrapings of the burrow. Severe pruritus is characteristic and, because of the incidence of pruritic dermatoses in patients with AIDS, a diagnosis of scabies should be considered and a topical scabicide applied if any question exists. Norwegian scabies is a rare form of the infection that occurs in patients with AIDS and was previously reported in immunosuppressed patients as well as patients with Down syndrome. It is characterized by thick scales loaded with thousands of mites. The average patient with scabies has fewer than 12 adult female mites. In Norwegian scabies, patients may harbor more than 1 000 000 mites, creating a highly contagious environment. The patient shown in Figures 10-28 and 10-29 presented with thick hyperkeratotic scales on

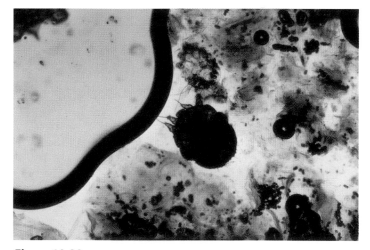

Figure 10-30

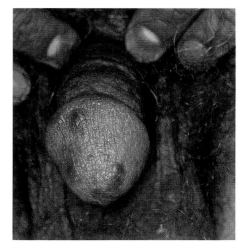

Figure 10-31

the dorsa of the hands, the feet, and the extensor surfaces of the elbows and knees. In Norwegian scabies, thick scaling of the elbows and knees may simulate psoriasis, and dystrophic changes of the nails can be reminiscent of psoriasis. This form of scabies is very difficult to clear despite repeated use of scabicidal treatments.

Because of the unusual appearance of Norwegian scabies, its diagnosis is often missed. The causative mite can usually be found by examining scrapings of cutaneous scales with the microscope under low power

(Fig. 10-30). **Nodular scabies** is thought to represent an immunologic response to the mite, since these pruritic nodules can persist for months after scabies has been successfully treated. The histology of nodular scabies can resemble that of a cutaneous lymphoma. The most common site of involvement is the scrotum. Although an immunologic etiology has been suggested for nodular scabies, this condition can occur in AIDS patients, as it did in the patient shown in Figure 10-31.

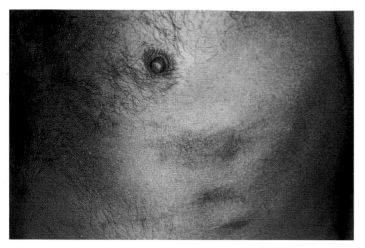

Figure 10-32

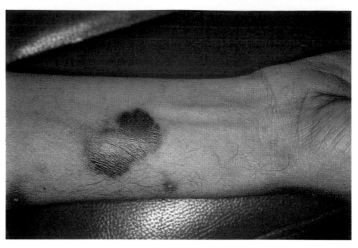

Figure 10-33

Once a rare disease, classic **Kaposi sarcoma** was most commonly described in elderly Jewish Ashkenazi or Italian men. A second "endemic" form of Kaposi sarcoma affected indigenous black Africans. A role for immunodeficiency in the development of Kaposi sarcoma was suspected before the advent of AIDS because immunosuppressed patients developed the disease. Patients with lymphomas and kidney transplant patients on immunosuppressive drugs occasionally developed widespread, rapidly progressive Kaposi sarcoma. When immunosuppressive therapy was stopped, however, the skin lesions frequently regressed.

AIDS patients with Kaposi sarcoma present a very different clinical picture from that found in elderly Mediterranean men, but they share features with immunosuppressed patients and equatorial Africans. Classic Kaposi sarcoma begins on the feet or legs and progresses very slowly. In some AIDS patients, the disease can be quite aggressive, with hundreds of lesions developing within a short time. In other HIV-infected patients, Kaposi sarcoma can progress slowly, gradually resulting in more cutaneous lesions.

AIDS-related Kaposi sarcoma may vary substantially in its appearance. Patients present with macules, patches, papules, plaques, nodules, or tumors. Lesions can be solitary or multiple and range from purple to brown (Figs 10-32 and 10-33). The patient in Figure 10-33 has a typical-appearing patch of Kaposi sarcoma on the forearm; nearby, a

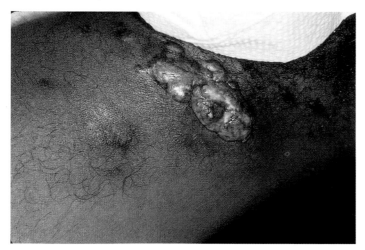

Figure 10-34

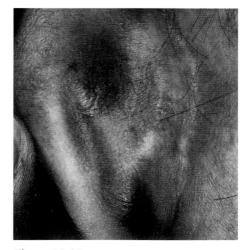

Figure 10-35

smaller patch is also seen. Some lesions grow quickly and ulcerate, while others remain small. The patient shown in Figure 10-34 initially presented with a solitary patch of Kaposi sarcoma but went on to develop multiple patches, nodules, and tumors, including an ulcerating groin tumor. Unlike classic Kaposi sarcoma, which typically involves the lower extremities, AIDS-related Kaposi sarcoma can affect any part of the body, including a number of unusual sites. Involvement of the nose is common. The patient shown in Figure 10-35 presented with two characteristic purple nodules of Kaposi sarcoma behind the ear. Penile Kaposi sarcoma has been reported in a number of AIDS patients as well.

Misdiagnosis of Kaposi sarcoma is frequent. Occasionally lesions resemble harmless nevi or dermatofibromas. Alternatively, they may resemble vascular lesions, such as angiomas or venous varicosities. Other misdiagnoses include vasculitis, purpura, or hematomas.

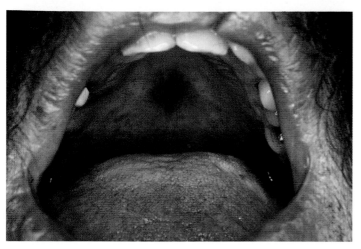

Figure 10-36

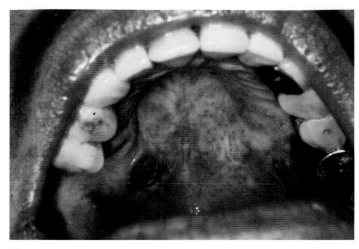

Figure 10-37

AIDS-related Kaposi sarcoma frequently involves mucous membranes. Oral mucosal involvement is commonly seen, and it too can vary in appearance. The patient in Figure 10-36 has an asymptomatic purple patch on the palatal mucosa. By contrast, Kaposi sarcoma shown in the patient in Figure 10-37 appears as an ulcerating nodule involving the palatal mucosa. Although Kaposi sarcoma of the gastrointestinal mucosa is common, gastrointestinal bleeding rarely occurs.

Most patients with AIDS-related Kaposi sarcoma succumb to opportunistic infections. The lesions of Kaposi sarcoma are seldom life-threatening and may only be cosmetic problems for some patients with AIDS. Nevertheless, patients with rapidly progressive pulmonary Kaposi sarcoma have been seen. The rapid destruction of pulmonary parenchyma can result in respiratory insufficiency. Recent evidence has strongly associated all types of Kaposi sarcoma with human herpes virus 8.

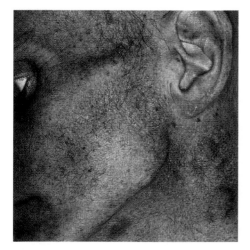

Figure 10-38

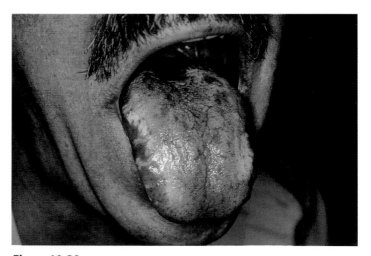

Figure 10-39

Kaposi sarcoma responds to treatment with local radiation therapy, cryotherapy, and intralesional injection with vinblastine. A number of systemically administered chemotherapy agents have been used with variable success. The patient shown in Figure 10-38 was treated with intravenously administered chemotherapy. Partial clearing can be seen within the centers of some of the lesions of Kaposi sarcoma on his neck.

Oral hairy leukoplakia is a lesion that has been found on the lingual mucosa of HIV-infected patients. The lateral surfaces of the tongue are the most characteristic sites of involvement, and the lesion consists of a white plaque composed of multiple adjacent linear white papules that give the plaque a "hairy" appearance (Fig. 10-39). The lesions resemble oral candidiasis, but unlike thrush, oral hairy leukoplakia cannot be rubbed off. Coexisting candidal infection of the mouth has been found in a high proportion of patients with oral hairy leukoplakia, suggesting a fungal etiology. Some investigators have attributed the condition to human papillomavirus or to Epstein–Barr virus infection.

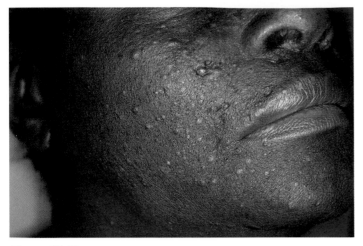

Figure 10-40

Eosinophilic pustular folliculitis is a term applied to a pruritic AIDS-related dermatitis that has a nonspecific appearance. Histologically it is characterized by an eosinophilic and neutrophilic infiltration of hair follicles. Occasional pustules, follicular papules, and urticarial papules develop (Fig. 10-40). Lesions can be generalized, but the face, upper trunk, and proximal extremities are most commonly affected. Skin lesions and pruritus are recalcitrant to topical corticosteroids or topical and systemic antibiotics, but ultraviolet B phototherapy is effective. Although the condition, also called HIV-associated eosinophilic folliculitis, is not life-threatening, pruritus is usually severe. Patients may have peripheral leukocytosis and eosinophilia.

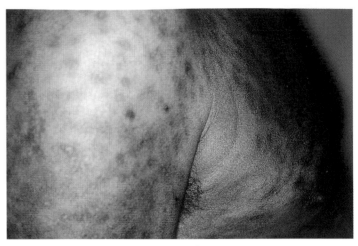

Figure 10-41

Several chronic papular eruptions have been noted in patients infected with HIV. Pruritus has been the most consistent symptom. Some patients present with discrete skin-colored papules that have been labeled **papular eruption of AIDS**. Others simply present with thick, scaling, excoriated papules caused by repeated scratching. The patient in Figure 10-41 had a chronic pruritic eruption consisting of erythematous papules and excoriations with postinflammatory hyperpigmentation on the trunk and extremities. Skin biopsy revealed a nonspecific, superficial, perivascular, mononuclear infiltrate. The patient responded to treatment with ultraviolet B.

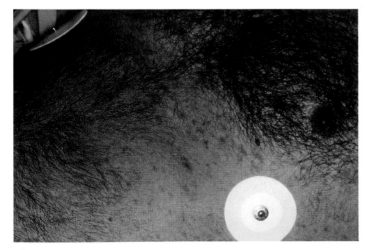

Figure 10-42

In patients who are first exposed to human immunodeficiency virus, a rash can occur before they become seropositive. The rash may be associated with systemic symptoms including malaise, fever, lymphadenopathy, arthralgias, myalgias, and sore throat. In one well-studied case, this constellation of symptoms developed 10 weeks after sexual exposure to an HIV-infected individual. The acute rash of HIV has been described as vesicular, pustular, or roseola-like, but is usually reported as erythematous macules (Fig. 10-42). Oral mucosal lesions

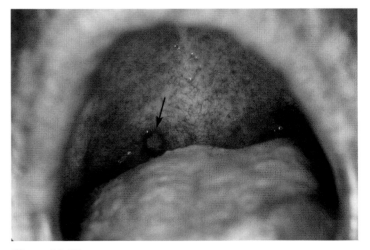

Figure 10-43

have been described. The patient shown in Figures 10-42 and 10-43 developed an erythematous macule with central erosion on the palate (Fig. 10-43). Skin lesions usually disappear over approximately 2 weeks. On skin biopsy, a nonspecific perivascular dermal lymphohistiocytic infiltrate has been described with sparing of the epidermis. The number of reported cases with an acute HIV exanthem is small, suggesting that most patients who acquire this infection do not experience these early symptoms.

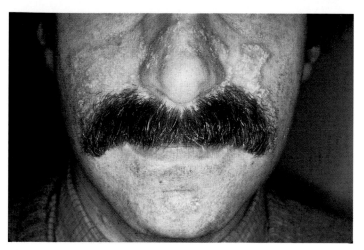

Figure 10-44

Seborrheic dermatitis was one of the earliest cutaneous eruptions to be associated with AIDS. It consists of erythema and scaling or crusting of the scalp, eyebrows, beard, nasolabial folds, malar areas (Fig. 10-44) and postauricular areas. The axillae, chest, groin, and back can be affected as well. While this eruption is common in the non-HIV population, patients with AIDS often develop more severe seborrheic dermatitis. Treatment with topical steroids or topical antifungal preparations is temporarily effective in most patients.

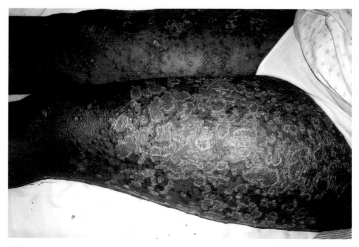

Figure 10-45

Severe **psoriasis** has been reported in patients with AIDS, but the question of whether this condition is more common or severe in HIV-infected patients is controversial. The patient in Figure 10-45 first developed psoriasis after HIV seroconversion. His skin lesions became progressively worse as his immunodeficiency developed. In treating AIDS patients with psoriasis, it is clear that significant immunosuppressive treatment such as methotrexate should be avoided. Phototherapy, though controversial, does not produce clinically significant immunosuppression and is often effective. Oral retinoids can be

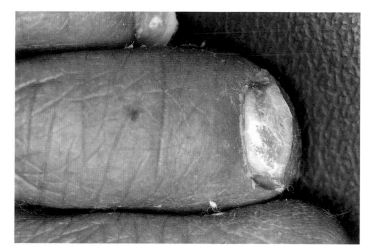

Figure 10-46

effective and use of zidovudine has been reported to produce dramatic clearing of resistant psoriasis in isolated cases, but has failed in others. The prevalence of onychomycosis in patients with HIV infection is clearly increased over its prevalence in the general public. In one series, over 20% of HIV-infected individuals had onychomycosis. In HIV-infected patients with abnormal looking nails, the prevalence of onychomycosis was 50%. White, superficial onychomycosis and proximal subungual onychomycosis (Fig. 10-46) are uncommon in the general population, but are well recognized in patients with HIV infection. Their presence should alert the clinician to the possibility of HIV infection.

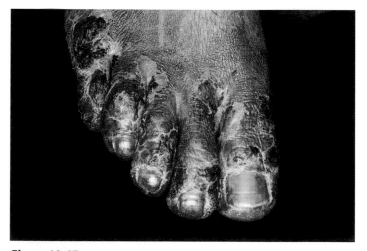

Figure 10-47

Reiter syndrome, which is rare in the non-AIDS population, has been reported in a significant number of HIV-infected individuals. The characteristic clinical features of Reiter syndrome have been described in these patients, including arthritis, urethritis, conjunctivitis, uveitis, balanitis circinata, mucosal ulcers, and keratoderma blennorrhagicum (Fig. 10-47). The latter is a psoriasiform eruption of the palms and soles. In some patients Reiter syndrome develops at the same time as AIDS. Considering the rarity of Reiter syndrome in the general population, its association with HIV infection may not be coincidental.

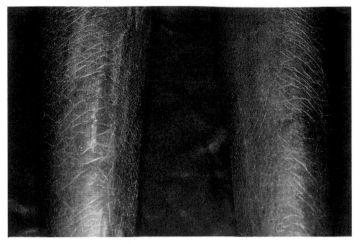

Figure 10-48

Acquired ichthyosis, which is characterized by dry skin, geometrically shaped, large, plate-like scales and an absence of inflammation, is commonly found on the lower legs of HIV-infected patients (Fig. 10-48). Although ichthyosis vulgaris commonly begins on the lower legs in children, its development in an adult is uncommon. Even before the era of AIDS, the recognition of acquired ichthyosis suggested the possibility of an underlying malignancy, specifically Hodgkin disease. Non-Hodgkin lymphomas and other malignancies also occur in patients with acquired ichthyosis.

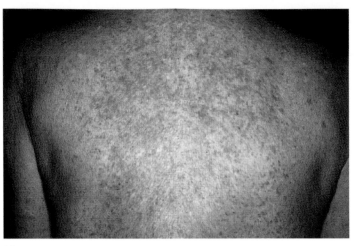

Figure 10-49

HIV-infected individuals have a higher than expected incidence of drug reaction to trimethoprim–sulfamethoxazole, a drug that is commonly prescribed for the prevention and treatment of *Pneumocystis carinii* pneumonia. The rash simulates other drug reactions and consists of generalized, pruritic, erythematous macules and papules that develop within 12 days of beginning treatment (Fig. 10-49). In some patients the rash resolves despite continued therapy, but many patients have to discontinue the offending drug. Readministration of trimethoprim–sulfamethoxazole results in recurrence of the rash in some, but not all, patients.

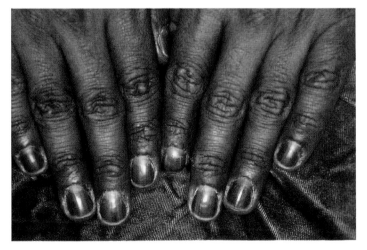

Figure 10-50

Hypersensitivity reactions to a number of drugs are reported in patients infected with HIV. In addition to **trimethoprim–sulfamethoxazole**, other antibiotics, anticonvulsants, and nonsteroidal antiinflammatory drugs have been associated with an increased incidence of cutaneous drug reactions. **Zidovudine (AZT)**, one of the most widely prescribed drugs for patients with AIDS, is associated with unusual pigmentation of the nails. Hyperpigmentation begins at the proximal fingernails and eventually moves out to involve the entire nail (Fig. 10-50). Toenails can be affected as well.

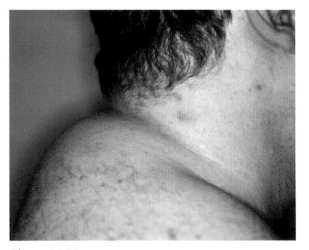

Figure 10-51

Antiretroviral therapy frequently results in abnormalities of fat distribution. **Protease inhibitors** frequently cause lipoatrophy, resulting in sunken cheeks and a wasted appearance. Lipohypertrophy or fat accumulation occurs in the dorsal–cervical region, abdominal area, and breasts, resulting a "buffalo-hump" appearance (Fig. 10-51), and enlargement of the abdomen or breasts. Concomitant increases in cholesterol and triglyceride levels and insulin resistance can occur.

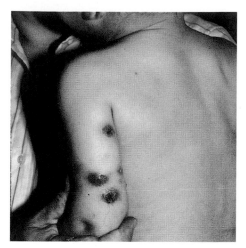

Figure 10-52

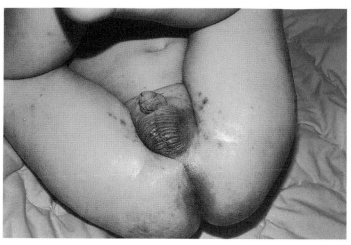

Figure 10-53

Non-AIDS immunodeficiency diseases are frequently associated with cutaneous manifestations. **Chronic granulomatous disease** is a rare disorder in which phagocytosis occurs normally, but leukocytes are unable to generate hydrogen peroxide and free oxygen radicals that kill bacteria and fungi. Patients are therefore susceptible to severe, persistent, and recurrent infections that lead to the development of granulomas. Recurrent furunculosis (Fig. 10-52) is common, and bacterial infections can occur in other organs, including lungs, lymph nodes, bones, and gastrointestinal tract. In infancy, many patients develop an atopic dermatitis-like rash. Moniliasis often develops in the diaper area (Figure 10-53). Aphthous stomatitis, perirectal abscesses, and a variety of mucocutaneous infections can occur. The disorder is usually inherited in an X-linked recessive pattern so that most affected individuals are male. Diagnosis is made by the nitroblue tetrazolium (NBT) dye test. The dye cannot be reduced to a blue–black color by leukocytes of patients with chronic granulomatous disease. Female

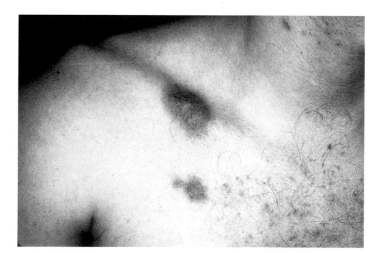

Figure 10-54

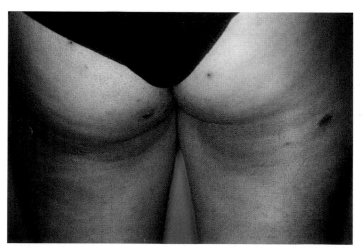

Figure 10-55

carriers can also be identified with this test. Annular erythematous patches resembling lesions of discoid lupus have been described in heterozygous female carriers of the gene for chronic granulomatous disease. The patient in Figure 10-54 is a man with chronic granulomatous disease who developed truncal annular lesions identical to those described in females. These began during his adolescence and have continued to develop. Most recently, daily home treatment with subcutaneously administered interferon has been shown to reduce the incidence of infection in individuals with this disorder.

Job syndrome, first described in red-haired, fair-skinned women, is a rare disorder of chemotaxis associated with markedly increased levels of immunoglobulin E. Patients develop recurrent furunculosis (Fig. 10-55) and recurrent respiratory tract and bone infections. "Cold abscesses" are chronic, and recurrent, huge, noninflammed, staphylococcal abscesses that are neither red, warm, nor tender. In addition to *S. aureus*, *Haemophilus influenzae* is a common pathogen. Mucocutaneous candidal infections may occur as well. Peripheral eosinophilia is occasionally present, and many patients suffer from a cutaneous eruption resembling atopic dermatitis.

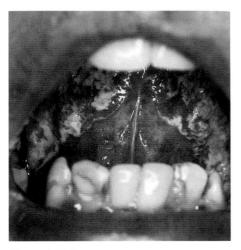

Figure 10-56

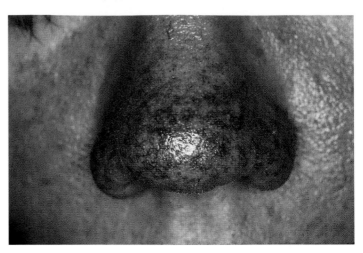

Figure 10-57

Chronic mucocutaneous candidiasis refers to a group of disorders that share a propensity to severe refractory candidal infections of the skin and mucous membranes. The disorders are distinguished by different inheritance patterns and varying immunologic defects. Autosomal recessive, autosomal dominant, and sporadic inheritance patterns have been described. While some forms of chronic mucocutaneous candidiasis begin in adolescence or adulthood, many begin in infancy or early childhood. Oral thrush (Fig. 10-56) produces white patches on the tongue or oral mucosa. The patches can be discrete or can become confluent covering large areas of mucosa. Candidal esophagitis or laryngitis can occur as well. Perlèche refers to an angular cheilitis caused by *Candida albicans*. The oral commissures are red,

inflamed, macerated, and fissured. Other mucous membranes can be involved including the perianal, penile, and vulvovaginal areas. Candidal infections are associated with burning, itching, redness, and maceration. In the case of vaginal candidiasis, white patches are present on the vaginal mucosa, and a thick white vaginal discharge loaded with *C. albicans* may occur.

An unusual characteristic of some cases of chronic mucocutaneous candidiasis is the occurrence of thickly crusted, hyperkeratotic candidal granulomas. These most commonly occur on the face, scalp, and digits. Early involvement of the nose can be associated with telangiectasia and thus mimic rhinophyma (Fig. 10-57). Invasion of the nails by *C. albicans*

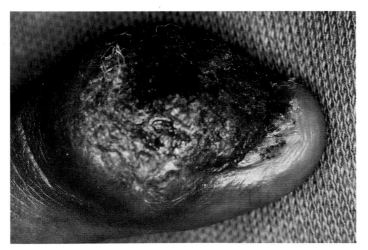

Figure 10-58

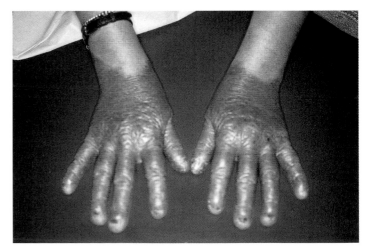

Figure 10-59

results in marked thickening and hyperkeratosis. The distal finger tips may be swollen and the paronychial areas are inflamed (Fig. 10-58). A variety of endocrinopathies have been described in association with chronic mucocutaneous candidiasis. Specifically, congenital polyendocrinopathy occurs, consisting of hypoparathyroidism, hypothyroidism, hypoadrenalism, and vitiligo. Diabetes and various autoimmune syndromes such as alopecia totalis and thyroiditis have also been reported in patients with chronic mucocutaneous candidiasis. A number of specific defects in cell-mediated immunity have been

described. Anergy specifically to *C. albicans* antigen can occur in some patients, while others are anergic to all skin test antigens. Selective immunoglobulin A deficiency can be associated with this disorder.

In addition to difficulty in clearing candidal infections, one group of patients also has a propensity for dermatophyte infections. The patient in Figure 10-59 had typical stigmata of chronic mucocutaneous candidiasis associated with extensive, severe dermatophytosis of the hands and feet. Humoral immunity is unaffected, and patients do not develop disseminated, life-threatening candidiasis.

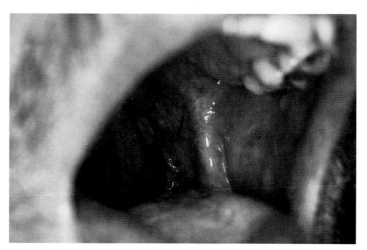

Figure 10-60

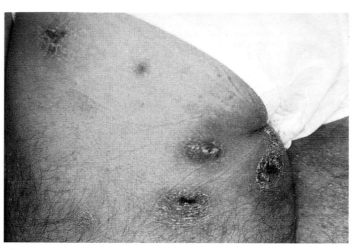

Figure 10-61

Cyclic neutropenia is a rare disorder that usually begins in childhood but occasionally begins in adulthood. The main problem is a marked reduction of circulating neutrophils that occurs approximately every 28 days. When the neutrophil count drops, patients develop fever, oral ulcers, and gingivitis. The oral ulcers resemble ordinary aphthous stomatitis (Fig. 10-60), except that they recur with cyclical drops in neutrophil count. Cervical lymphadenopathy is common, and some patients have developed recurrent furunculosis (Fig. 10-61). Symptoms last only 4–8 days, resolving as the neutrophil count rises, only to return after an interval of approximately 21 days. Platelets, reticulocytes, and other white blood cells fluctuate at similar intervals as well. Definitive diagnosis requires the demonstration of a cyclical reduction in neutrophils with total and differential white blood counts repeated every 3 days for 1 month. The primary abnormality in this disorder appears to be a defect of bone marrow stem cells. Granulocyte colony-stimulating factor has successfully improved symptoms by stimulating production of neutrophils.

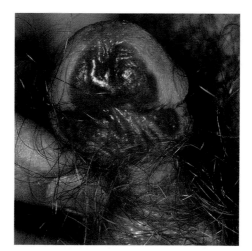

Figure 10-62

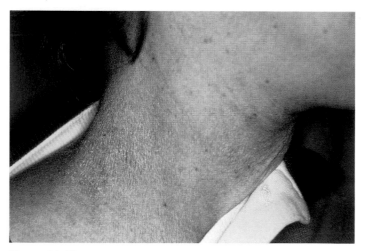

Figure 10-63

The different types of agammaglobulinemia have in common a reduction in antibody formation. Diagnosis of agammaglobulinemia is made by demonstration of reduced immunoglobulins on immunoelectrophoresis. Affected patients are susceptible to recurrent bacterial infections, including severe furunculosis. The patient shown in Figure 10-62 had recurrent monilial infections of the genitals. The frequency and severity of viral infections is not increased. Apart from infection, several systemic associations of the agammaglobulinemias occur, including chronic diarrhea resembling sprue, a chronic non-infectious arthritis, and hypersplenism. An increased incidence of lymphomas occurs in these patients. Some patients develop recurrent neutropenia, which may be associated with aphthous ulcers. A variety of noninfectious cutaneous manifestations can occur in patients with agammaglobulinemia, including an atopic dermatitis-like rash (Figure 10-63). Of interest, several other skin diseases in which the immune system plays a role can develop in people with agammaglobulinemia. For example, angioedema, rhus dermatitis, and drug eruptions can occur.

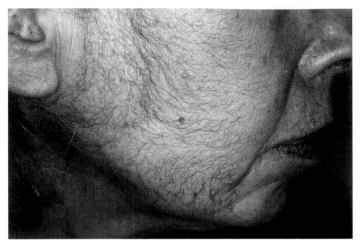

Figure 10-64

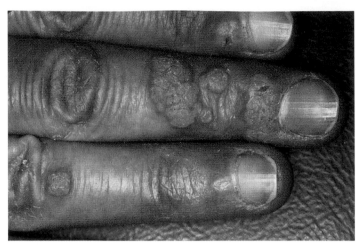

Figure 10-65

Clinical immunodeficiency states can result from neoplastic processes or from immunosuppressive or chemotherapeutic medications. Susceptibility to cutaneous or systemic infection can result in nonspecific skin changes. Several immunosuppressive medications also have distinctive cutaneous side effects. **Cyclosporine**, for example, is used extensively to prevent transplant rejection. In addition, it has been used in a number of skin diseases such as pyoderma gangrenosum. **Hypertrichosis** is a common cutaneous side effect. The woman shown in Figure 10-64 was treated with cyclosporine for severe psoriasis and

developed a marked increase in facial hairs. Patients treated with cyclosporine or azathioprine have also been prone to cutaneous viral infections, including molluscum contagiosum and warts. The patient in Figure 10-65 underwent liver transplantation and was subsequently treated with oral steroids, azathioprine, and cyclosporine. Multiple warts are noted on the fingers.

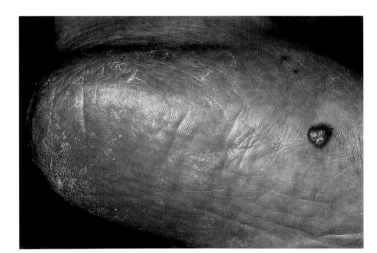

Figure 10-66

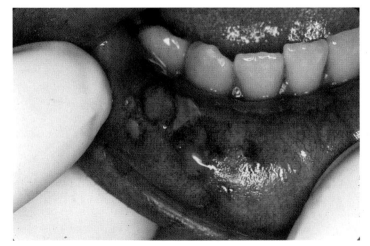

Figure 10-67

Kaposi sarcoma has been noted in patients treated with **azathioprine** and steroids. The purple patches, papules, and plaques of this vascular neoplasm are histologically indistinguishable from other forms of Kaposi sarcoma. When the immunosuppressive drugs are reduced or discontinued, the lesions of Kaposi sarcoma can regress or disappear. The patient shown in Figure 10-66 was treated with azathioprine and prednisone for bullous pemphigoid. He developed lesions of Kaposi sarcoma on the feet. The lesions cleared upon tapering of his immunosuppressive medications.

Cyclophosphamide, a derivative of nitrogen mustard, is a suppressor of B-cell function. It is used for its immunosuppressive properties in many of the same autoimmune conditions that are successfully treated with azathioprine. A number of cutaneous adverse affects can occur, including reversible alopecia similar to that seen in patients treated with other chemotherapy agents. Hyperpigmentation of the skin or nails can also occur. The patient shown in Figure 10-67 developed oral mucosal ulcers associated with a reduction in white blood cell count while receiving cyclophosphamide. Similar oral ulcers can occur with many chemotherapeutic or immunosuppressive agents currently in use.

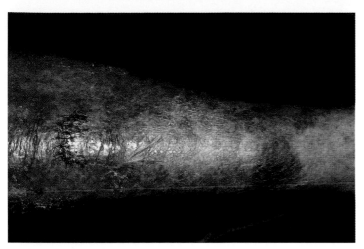

Figure 10-68

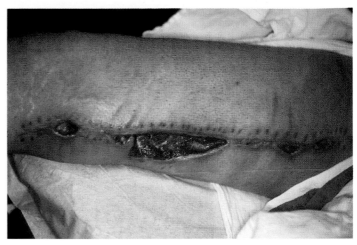

Figure 10-69

Corticosteroids, the oldest of the currently used immunosuppressive drugs, are potent suppressors of inflammatory processes and have been used for disorders as diverse as arthritis and poison ivy. Considering their powerful immunosuppressive properties, it is not surprising that they are effective against autoimmune diseases. Like cyclosporine and azathioprine, they are also used to prevent transplant rejection. Short-term use of systemic steroids is not likely to result in clinically significant immunosuppression or major cutaneous findings. One exception may be monilial infection in diabetic patients whose blood sugars are increased by systemic steroids.

The cutaneous stigmata of chronic steriod use are diverse and reflect the skin findings of iatrogenically induced Cushing syndrome. Steroid

purpura (Fig. 10-68) is common with long-term use of systemic steroids and results from increased vascular fragility. It is characterized by purple discoloration that is most noticeable on the arms and legs and can take months to resolve. Cutaneous atrophy leaves the skin thin and shiny, resulting in marked fragility. The skin is easily torn by minor trauma. The laceration on the leg of the patient in Figure 10-68 took many weeks to heal despite suturing. The patient subsequently developed P. *carinii* pneumonia as a result of his steroid-induced immunosuppressed state. Although the latter condition is most commonly seen in patients with AIDS, the patient was seronegative for HIV. Poor wound healing in patients on chronic steroid therapy can lead to dehiscence of surgical wounds. The patient in Figure 10-69 was

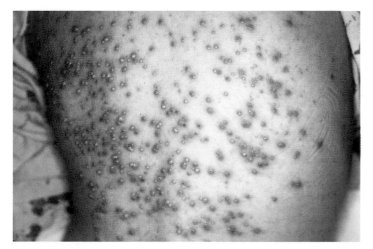

Figure 10-70

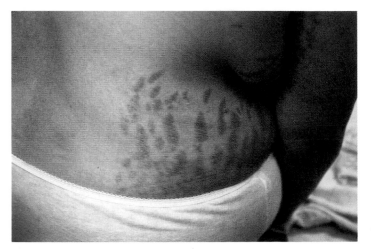

Figure 10-71

treated with steroids for systemic lupus erythematosus and underwent coronary artery bypass surgery. The wound over the saphenous vein donor graft site dehisced in several locations shortly thereafter.

Steroid acne is another common complication of prolonged therapy with corticosteroids. The 8-year-old girl shown in Figure 10-70 was

treated for Crohn's disease with high-dose systemic steroids. She developed severe steroid acne with multiple pustules and erythematous papules on the face, chest and back. Steroid-induced striae, shown in the patient in Figure 10-71, are irreversible.

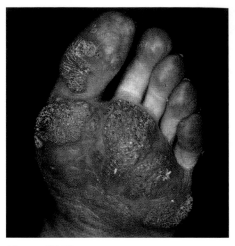

Figure 10-72

Susceptibility to cutaneous and systemic infection is a major drawback to chronic steroid therapy. The patient shown in Figure 10-72 had long-term therapy with high doses of systemic steroids for systemic lupus erythematosus. She developed many of the cutaneous stigmata of Cushing syndrome, namely, purpura, telangiectasia, and striae. In addition, she developed truncal obesity, "moon facies" and a "buffalo hump". One of her most troubling complications of steroid therapy, however, was the development of extensive plantar warts (Fig. 10-72) covering large areas of both feet.

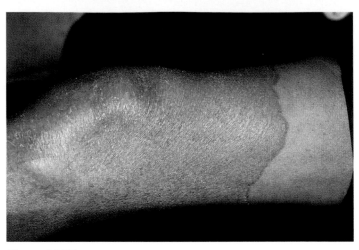

Figure 10-73

Advances in organ transplantation have resulted in large numbers of individuals surviving kidney, liver, lung, heart and other major organ transplant procedures. Because these individuals are on combinations of potent immunosuppressive agents, they are susceptible to malignancies and infections. The patient shown in Figure 10-73 survived liver transplantation, but now has extensive tinea corporis, a common infection in transplant recipients. The most common organism involved is *Trichophyton rubrum*, the same as that most commonly responsible for dermatophyte infections in nonimmuno-compromised individuals.

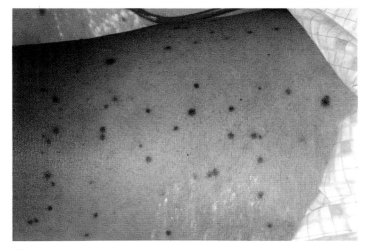

Figure 10-74

Immunosuppression caused by neoplasia or by chemotherapy for neoplastic diseases can make patients susceptible to cutaneous infection. Both common and uncommon cutaneous infections can occur. Candidal sepsis complicates neutropenia resulting from bone-marrow invasion by neoplastic cells or bone-marrow toxicity of chemotherapy agents. Although systemic candidal infection can be life-threatening in these patients, the first manifestation of candidal sepsis often appears in the skin in discrete foci from which candidal organisms can be cultured. Potassium hydroxide preparations of simple scrapings may reveal budding yeast and pseudohyphae.

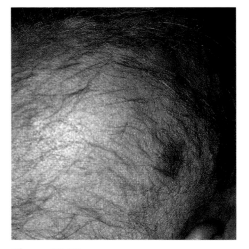

Figure 10-75

The patient shown in Figure 10-74 became neutropenic following chemotherapy. He developed fevers, and numerous purpuric macules, papules, and vesicles on the trunk and extremities that revealed candidal organisms. Atypical infections can also develop in the setting of chemotherapy or neoplasia-induced immunosuppression.

The child shown in Figure 10-75 became neutropenic after treatment of acute promyelocytic leukemia. *Candida krusei* was subsequently identified in blood cultures. While the patient was treated with intravenous amphotericin, numerous scalp nodules developed. On biopsy of the scalp nodules, *C. krusei* was again identified.

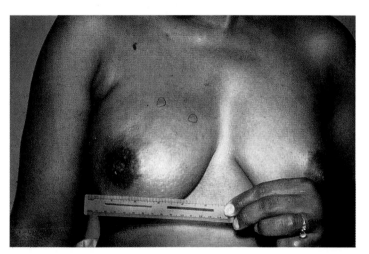

Figure 11-1

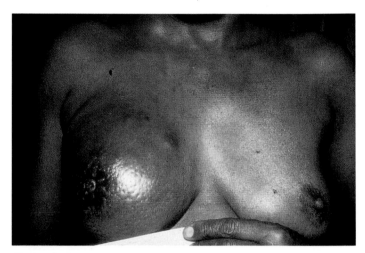

Figure 11-2

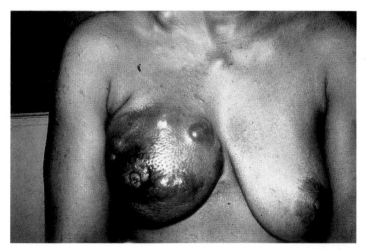

Figure 11-3

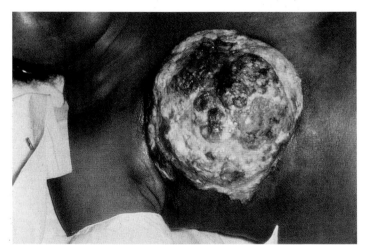

Figure 11-4

Progression of an untreated breast carcinoma. The patient in Figure 11-1 presented with an enlarged breast in August of 1958. Treatment was refused, and blockage of lymphatic vessels by tumor resulted in a peau d'orange appearance of the breast 4.5 months later (Fig. 11-2). The patient developed indurated nodules and areas of necrosis in the affected breast 8 months after the initial presentation (Fig. 11-3), which progressed to auto-amputation of the breast (Fig. 11-4).

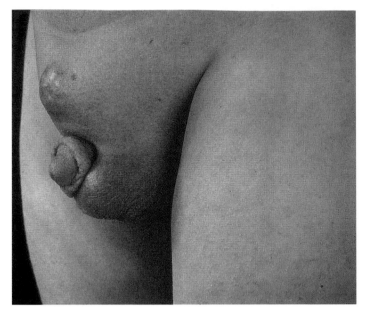

Figure 11-5

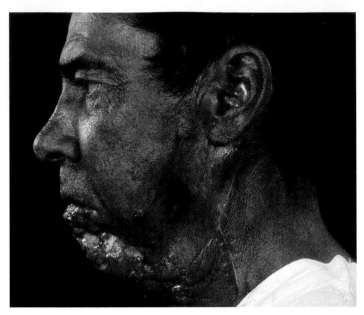

Figure 11-6

Cutaneous metastases are quite varied in their clinical presentation. The route by which tumors metastasize ultimately determines their distribution and appearance. Invasion of adjacent tissues, spread by lymphatic vessels, and hematogenous dissemination are the three main ways cutaneous metastases spread. When a malignancy reaches the skin by invasion of adjacent tissues, the source of the primary tumor is apparent in most cases. In other instances histologic examination can confirm the nature of the tumor. The child shown in Figure 11-5 had a rhabdomyosarcoma, the most common soft tissue sarcoma of children. Cutaneous metastases are rare, but occasionally dermal nodules develop as shown in Figure 11-5. In other patients, subcutaneous masses can occasionally be palpated even if they are not visible.

Oropharyngeal carcinomas commonly spread by local invasion, resulting in metastases to the skin of the face and neck. The patient in Figure 11-6 has a carcinoma of the floor of the mouth with cutaneous metastases. Early in its course this tumor spreads to adjacent areas, including the skin, gingiva, and periosteum of the mandible. With deep invasion the tongue may become fixed. Later in its course, carcinoma of the floor of the mouth is associated with lymphatic metastases.

When dissemination occurs via lymphatic vessels, cutaneous metastases usually involve skin in the region of the primary tumor and often occur later in the course of the malignancy. Thus, breast carcinoma, which spreads via lymphatic vessels, often involves skin of the anterior chest wall and axilla. Similarly, oral cavity malignancies

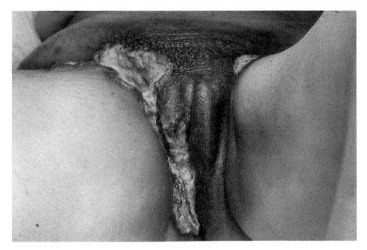

Figure 11-7

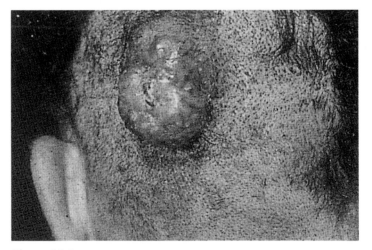

Figure 11-8

often present with cutaneous metastases in the submandibular area. The patient in Figure 11-7 had a **carcinoma of the urinary bladder**, which spread to a lymph node in the groin, resulting in ulceration and destruction of adjacent tissues.

Hematogenous dissemination of malignancies can result in solitary or multiple cutaneous lesions. The patient in Figure 11-8 had an **osteosarcoma** that metastasized to the scalp. Renal carcinoma and carcinoma of the lung characteristically spread hematogenously and often first

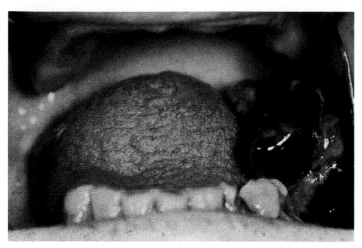

Figure 11-9

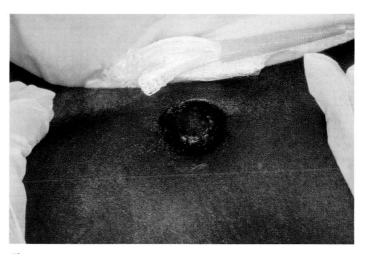

Figure 11-10

present with cutaneous metastases. In other instances, recurrence of a treated primary tumor may first be found in the skin. On occasion, distant metastases may appear years after discovery of the primary tumor.

The appearance of cutaneous metastases is usually not as useful as the location of the metastasis in determining the source of the primary tumor. Cutaneous metastases can resemble the primary tumor in color and consistency. Subcutaneous **leiomyosarcomas** (Fig. 11-9), for example, are vascular in nature, resembling angioleiomyomas. Their blue color is derived from the numerous thin-walled blood vessels within the tumor.

Lung cancers account for the largest number of cutaneous metastases in men. Histologic examination of cutaneous metastases in patients with lung cancer reveals adenocarcinoma in up to 30% of patients and squamous cell carcinoma in another 30 percent. Most commonly, an undifferentiated carcinoma containing a dense infiltrate of "oat cells" is found. Hematogenous dissemination is the usual mode of spread and tumors usually appear on the chest wall or upper extremities, but metastases can develop at any site. As with most other tumors, the clinical appearance of individual metastases is generally not helpful in determining the site of origin. The patient in Figure 11-10 presented with

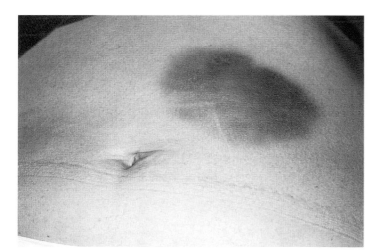

Figure 11-11

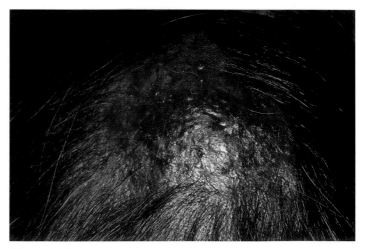

Figure 11-12

an ulcerated tumor of the lower back which proved to be a metastatic lung carcinoma. By contrast, the patient in Figure 11-11 first presented with an abdominal mass with overlying purpura. The mass was originally thought to represent an epidermoid cyst and attempts were made to incise and drain its contents. Biopsy revealed a cutaneous metastasis of a large cell carcinoma of the lung.

Although disseminated tumor cells can spread to any mucocutaneous surface, certain sites have a predilection for metastases. Surgical scars are

a common site of tumor recurrence, and metastases can develop in scars remote from the primary malignancy. The scalp also has a higher incidence of metastasis from a number of tumors, including the breast, lung, and genitourinary tract. The patient in Figure 11-12 had a **breast carcinoma** that metastasized to the scalp. Tumors of the scalp may ulcerate, resulting in a scarring alopecia that has been called alopecia neoplastica.

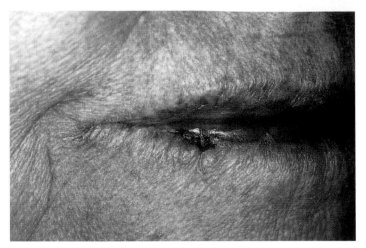

Figure 11-13

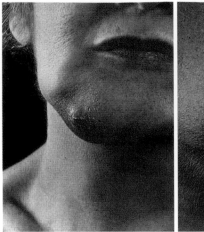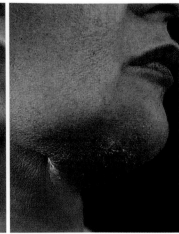

Figure 11-14A   **Figure 11-14B**

Head and neck tumors have a rich supply of blood vessels and lymphatic vessels, giving them ample opportunity to metastasize to remote body sites. Nevertheless, squamous cell carcinomas of the oral cavity commonly metastasize to skin of the face and neck. Squamous cell carcinomas of the exposed vermilion border of the lower lip are the most common malignancy of the oral cavity (Fig. 11-13). The upper lip is seldom involved, although this can be a site for basal cell carcinoma, and the lateral commissure is usually spared. Despite the possibility of local tissue invasion, bone involvement, and lymphatic spread, high cure rates are obtained with radiation therapy or surgery.

By contrast, squamous cell carcinomas of the tongue have an extensive vascular and lymphatic supply, resulting in early metastasis.

Lingual malignancies usually involve the anterior two-thirds of the tongue.

Carcinomas of the floor of the mouth spread quickly to gingiva and mandibular periosteum. Although examination and palpation of the area is easily performed, by the time diagnosis is made the disease is already advanced in most patients. Clinically apparent metastases to lymph nodes are present in approximately 40 percent, and occult metastases occur in a higher percentage of patients. Lymphatic drainage to the submandibular and deep cervical nodes is common, but submental nodes are usually spared. Mandibular involvement can be palpated. The patient in Figure 11-14 has an oral squamous cell carci-

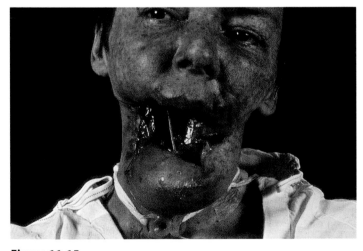

Figure 11-15

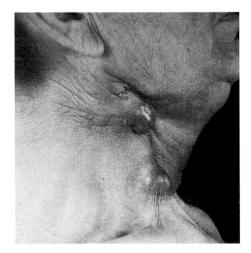

Figure 11-16

noma with fistula formation. In the patient in Figure 11-15, total destruction of the mouth and jaw resulted from an aggressive oral carcinoma.

Carcinoma of the larynx often presents with symptoms early in its course and consequently is frequently diagnosed at an earlier stage.

When untreated, tumors of the larynx invade the thyroid cartilage and adjacent soft tissue of the neck. Early in its course, carcinoma of the larynx is amenable to radiation therapy, with high cure rates. Later on, a combination of radiation therapy and surgery may be necessary. The patient in Figure 11-16 has an advanced carcinoma of the larynx with two nodules extending to the skin of the neck.

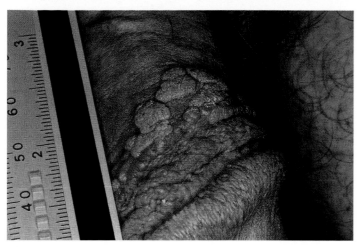

Figure 11-17

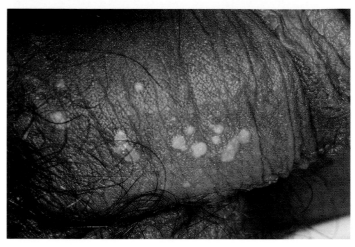

Figure 11-18

Sexually transmitted **human papillomavirus** (**HPV**) infection has reached epidemic proportions in the 1990s. There is compelling evidence to implicate at least some types of HPV in cervical cancer and other malignancies. Condylomata acuminata, the characteristic lesions of sexually transmitted HPV infection, typically present as verrucous cauliflower-like papules on the external genitalia (Fig. 11-17). Condylomata acuminata are highly contagious, with transmission occurring in 25–65% of patients after a single sexual exposure. Warts can develop from weeks to years after exposure.

Subclinical lesions can occasionally be visualized with magnification after application of acetic acid. Vinegar-soaked gauze applied for only a few minutes to the external genitalia can result in "acetowhitening" of HPV-infected skin (Fig. 11-18). Using colposcopy after soaking with vinegar, most male sexual partners of women with cervical intra-

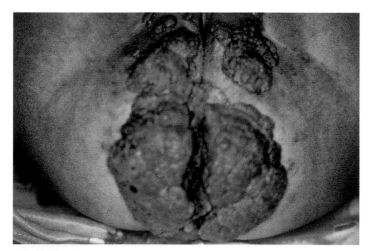

Figure 11-19

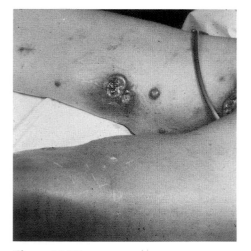

Figure 11-20

epithelial neoplasia can be shown to have evidence of HPV infection. The utility of acetowhitening of condylomata is limited by the occurrence of both false-positive and false-negative findings, but this technique can be useful with a little experience.

Extension of HPV infection to nonmucosal groin skin can result in hyperkeratotic verrucous papules, and rarely patients develop giant condylomata acuminata (Fig. 11-19). Nuclear atypia can be present, and these condylomata can become invasive and are called verrucous carcinoma or **giant condylomata of Buschke and Lowenstein**.

More than 50 HPV types have been described, but types 16, 18, and 31 are most prominently associated with malignancies. In particular, cervical, vulvar, and penile carcinomas have been associated with HPV infection, as has squamous cell carcinoma of the anus. It has been suggested that most, if not all, anogenital cancers contain HPV DNA. Long before the association between HPV infection and malignancy was known, the patient in Figure 11-20 had a destructive **vulvar carcinoma** with cutaneous metastases on the thigh. Examination of old preserved tissue samples has repeatedly shown HPV DNA in anogenital tumors biopsied years previously.

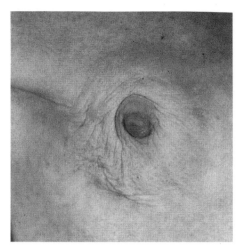

Figure 11-21

The skin overlying a **breast carcinoma** has been likened to an orange peel, the so-called peau d'orange. Blockage of lymphatic vessels by tumor cells results in local lymphedema and swelling. The peau d'orange appearance is created by nonpitting edema with depressions over follicular openings. Although cutaneous metastases are uncommon, breast carcinoma accounts for more than two-thirds of metastases to the skin in women. Cutaneous manifestations of breast cancer can be quite varied. Patients will often present with distortion or dimpling (Fig. 11-21) of the affected breast. Asymmetry of the breasts in size or

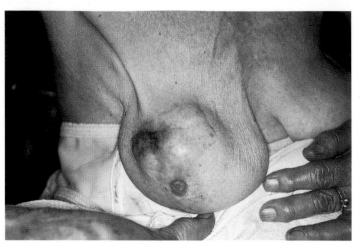

Figure 11-22

shape may be a sign of underlying breast carcinoma, although this is more commonly a normal variant unless recent in onset.

Occasionally tumors are very slow growing. The patient in Figure 11-22 presented with an enlarging breast mass that had been present for many years. She finally agreed to treatment when the overlying skin became ulcerated. She remained free of detectable disease for several years following mastectomy.

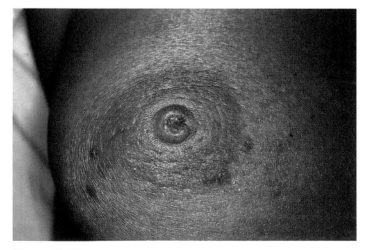

Figure 11-23

Paget disease of the nipple occurs in less than 4% of people with breast cancer. Patients often complain of itching or burning that is refractory to treatment with topical steroids, a feature that differentiates it from common eczematous dermatoses. Paget disease can extend to the areola but always involves the nipple (Fig. 11-23). It is always associated with an underlying ductal carcinoma of the breast, and the tumor can be palpated in two-thirds of patients.

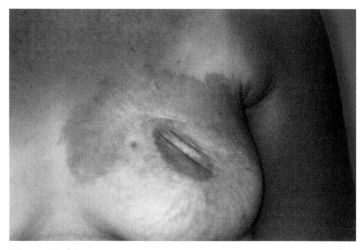

Figure 11-24

Inflammatory carcinoma of the breast, also called carcinoma erysipelatoides, affects only 1% of those with breast cancer but is distinctive in its appearance. It is caused by tumor cells invading dermal lymphatic vessels and subcutaneous tissue. The affected breast may appear enlarged and the overlying skin is red, warm, and indurated. The border is well demarcated and has been likened to the sharply demarcated border of erysipelas (Fig. 11-24). Skin biopsy reveals cancer cells blocking lymphatic vessels with little dermal inflammation.

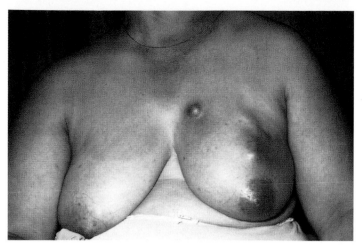

Figure 11-25

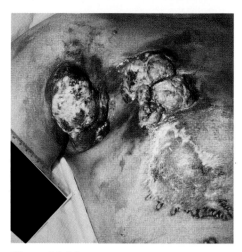

Figure 11-26

Unfortunately, the disease is often advanced at the time inflammatory breast carcinoma is detected. Metastasis rarely occurs by hematogenous spread, but more commonly follows lymphatic vessels, resulting in distinctive cutaneous patterns. The most common site of cutaneous metastasis is the anterior chest wall, and nontender indurated nodules are the commonest presentation (Fig. 11-25).

Once the primary tumor is removed, cutaneous metastases can occur after many years. Metastatic breast carcinoma often develops in the scar of a previous mastectomy (Fig. 11-26). The skin and subcutaneous tissue of the chest can be so extensively infiltrated that chest wall movement is restricted by the thick tumor, interfering with breathing. Cutaneous metastases of breast carcinoma can present as papules, nodules, or plaques that may be skin colored, erythematous, or violaceous. They are usually indurated, if not rock hard, and can ulcerate. The tumors may be fixed to underlying tissues or may be freely moveable.

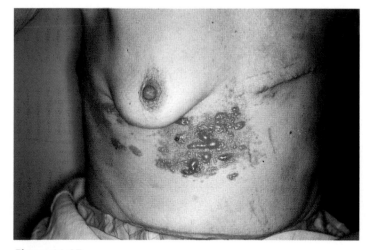

Figure 11-27

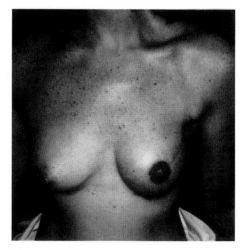

Figure 11-28

Herpes zoster is known to occur in patients with breast cancer within several months of radiation therapy if the radiation port includes the spinal cord. For the patient in Figure 11-27, the development of herpes zoster signaled the presence of a second carcinoma in the remaining breast. Vesicles and bullae are present in a dermatomal distribution extending from the back to the anterior abdomen and chest, stopping at the midline.

The surgical management of breast carcinoma has improved substantially over the years. Patients who previously would have been treated with radical mastectomies are often cured surgically with much smaller lumpectomies. For those undergoing more extensive surgery, plastic surgical reconstruction of the breast can restore a normal appearance. The patient in Figure 11-28 underwent mastectomy for a carcinoma of the left breast. The reconstructed breast is quite normal in appearance.

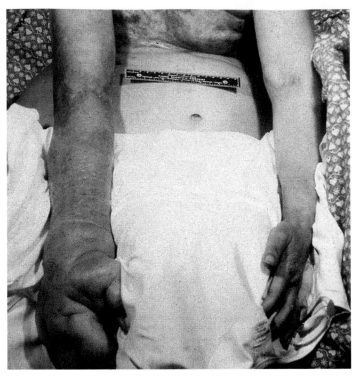

Figure 11-29

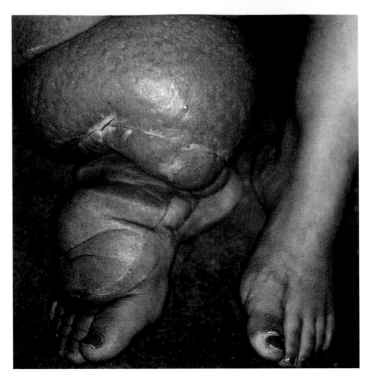

Figure 11-30

Lymphedema is a common sequel to treatment for breast carcinoma. Surgical removal or radiation fibrosis of lymph nodes results in obstruction of lymphatic flow in the upper extremities. Failure of lymphatic drainage results in swelling caused by accumulation of tissue fluid. The affected extremity can become grossly enlarged (Fig. 11-29). Lymphedema can also result from obstruction of lymphatic vessels or lymph nodes by tumors or destruction of lymphatic pathways by infections including filariasis.

Lymphedema is not always secondary to destructive processes. **Milroy disease** is a congenital, autosomal dominantly inherited disorder characterized by lymphedema. **Lymphedema praecox** (Fig. 11-30) primarily affects females, beginning between the ages of 9 years and 25 years. Initially, edema may be pitting and may disappear with elevation. As it becomes chronic, the overlying skin becomes more indurated and the edema becomes nonpitting. With any form of lymphedema, limbs can become grossly enlarged and deformed, a condition that has been descriptively called **elephantiasis**.

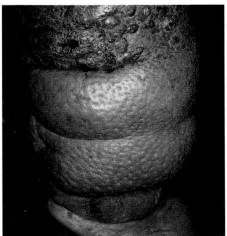

Figure 11-31

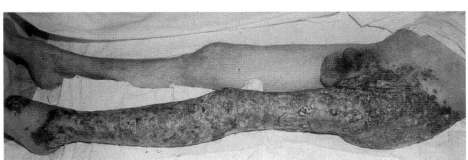

Figure 11-32

Persistent lymphedema can lead to the **Stewart–Treves syndrome** (Fig. 11-31). The syndrome is characterized by the development of cutaneous angiosarcomas in areas of chronic lymphedema. This frequently fatal tumor may appear as erythematous or violaceous papules and nodules on the affected skin. These tumors can eventually ulcerate. The vascular nature of angiosarcomas is apparent from the blue color of the tumors in Figure 11-31.

The term **hemangioendothelioma** has been used to refer to entirely different vascular tumors that can be benign or malignant. The similarity to angiosarcomas is shown in Figure 11-32. The patient's entire leg is infiltrated by painless vascular nodules of the dermis and subcutaneous tissues. The vascular proliferation extends from the distal portions of the patient's foot to the ipsilateral buttock, also involving the genitalia and suprapubic skin. Spindle cell hemangioendothelioma behaves like a low-grade angiosarcoma with histologic features of a cavernous hemangioma and Kaposi sarcoma.

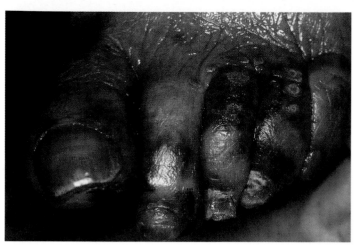

Figure 11-33

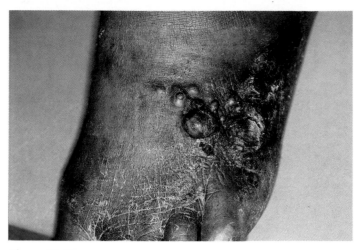

Figure 11-34

Kaposi sarcoma, as first described in 1872, differs significantly from the condition associated with acquired immunodeficiency syndrome (AIDS). **Classic Kaposi sarcoma** is a disease that most commonly strikes elderly Jewish Ashkenazi or Italian males. Despite the preponderance of Kaposi sarcoma in particular populations, multiple familial cases seldom occur, and the role of genetics in this disorder is therefore unclear. Classic Kaposi sarcoma initially presents on the feet as blue macules. To begin with lesions may be unilateral, but eventually both feet are involved. Macules that are poorly defined at first (Fig. 11-33) may slowly grow to form papules, nodules or plaques.

In contrast to AIDS-associated Kaposi sarcoma, the course of classic Kaposi sarcoma is usually indolent, with new lesions developing over years. Eventually numerous blue papules can develop on the feet, and these may eventually form verrucous papules or may ulcerate (Fig. 11-34).

Classic Kaposi sarcoma is associated with pedal edema which may be present even before skin lesions are apparent. Edema may be pitting at first, but eventually swelling becomes permanent and nonpitting. Papules of classic Kaposi sarcoma can become confluent to form plaques involving an entire extremity. Large chronic ulcers involving significant portions of the lower extremities lead to substantial mor-

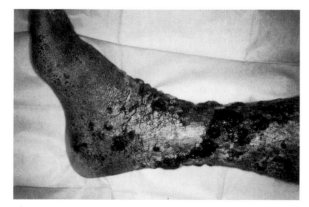

Figure 11-35A

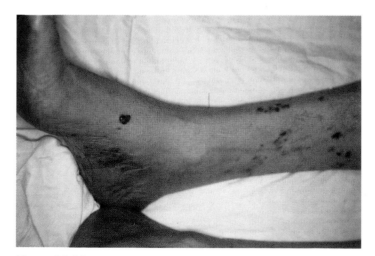

Figure 11-36

bidity (Fig. 11-35A). The cutaneous barrier to infection is lost, and patients are often treated for repeated bouts of cellulitis.

Classic Kaposi sarcoma can develop in the gastrointestinal tract and is frequently seen on the oral mucosa. Gastrointestinal bleeding can occur, but is uncommon. At autopsy, Kaposi sarcoma can be found in other organs, but it rarely causes symptomatic disease except in the legs. Spread to other cutaneous sites can occur, however, as shown on the hands of the patient in Figure 11-35B. A more aggressive course often occurs in AIDS-associated Kaposi sarcoma, endemic Kaposi sarcoma of black Africans, and Kaposi sarcoma associated with iatrogenic immunosuppression.

Diagnosis of Kaposi sarcoma is made by skin biopsy. The patient in Figure 11-36 presented with symmetric, palpable, purpuric papules and plaques of the lower extremities. Although a diagnosis of leukocytoclastic vasculitis was entertained, the patient proved to have classic Kaposi sarcoma.

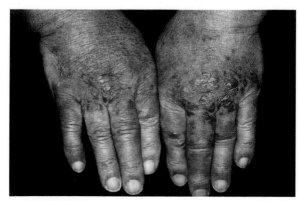

Figure 11-35B

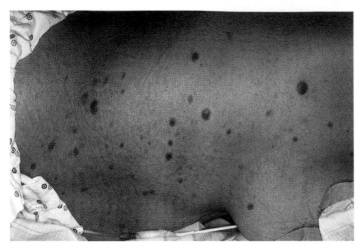

Figure 11-37

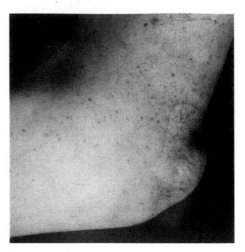

Figure 11-38

Acute myeloid leukemia (**AML**), the most common acute leukemia in adults, can present with a number of cutaneous manifestations. These can be related to the malignancy itself or may result from complications of the leukemia. Bone-marrow infiltration, resulting in neutropenia, renders patients prone to infection. Moreover, aggressive treatment of AML with chemotherapeutic agents or radiation therapy results in destruction of bone marrow. It is in this setting that the infectious complications of the disease are most commonly seen. Identification of the organism responsible for bacterial or fungal sepsis is occasionally made

by microscopic examination or culture of skin lesions. Broad-spectrum antibiotic prophylaxis against bacterial infections, and administration of antifungal drugs has also made cutaneous drug reactions a common occurrence in this group of patients.

Leukemic infiltrates of the skin are rarely the earliest finding and more commonly occur after the diagnosis has been made. Patients can present with a variety of skin lesions, including macules, papules, nodules that can be hemorrhagic or erythematous; tumors that may become necrotic, or ulcerations. The patient in Figure 11-37 suddenly

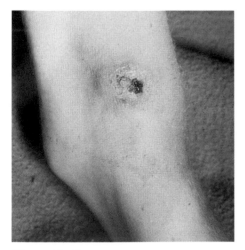

Figure 11-39

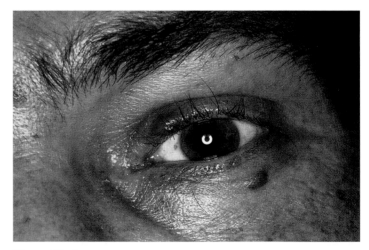

Figure 11-40

developed dozens of indurated erythematous papules on the back as the first sign of recurrence following complete remission. A patient with AML who presented with a tumor on the elbow is shown in Figure 11-38, and another patient with an ulcerated plaque on the arm is shown in Figure 11-39.

The periorbital region is a site commonly prone to infiltration by leukemic cells in patients with AML. The patient in Figure 11-40 developed a purpuric papule that was thought to be a stye on the upper eyelid margin. A second purpuric papule then developed on the lower lid. Biopsy revealed leukemic cells in the dermis.

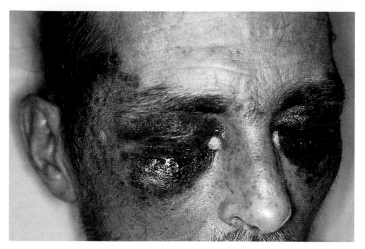

Figure 11-41

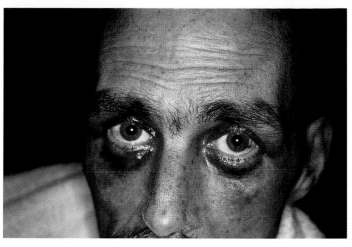

Figure 11-42

Involvement of bone marrow in **acute myeloid leukemia** results in thrombocytopenia, and those platelets that are seen in the peripheral circulation may be hypogranular and functionally defective. Leukemic infiltrates in the skin may therefore appear hemorrhagic. The patient in Figure 11-41 was thrombocytopenic and developed purpuric papules on the temples, eyelids and malar areas. These papules and plaques became confluent to form ecchymotic plaques on the upper and lower lids. The

plaques consisted of leukemic cells combined with extravasated red blood cells. Treatment of AML in this patient resulted in restoration of the bone marrow, normal circulating platelets, and improvement of the periorbital plaques (Fig. 11-42).

Increasing blast counts in the peripheral circulation can result in impaired blood flow, especially at levels greater than 100 000 cells/ml. This causes local hypoxemia with endothelial cell damage and hemor-

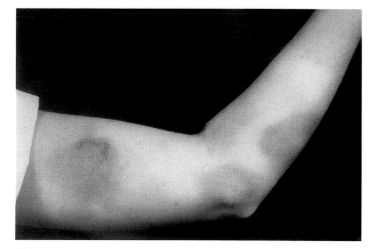

Figure 11-43

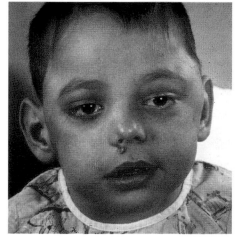

Figure 11-44

rhage into various organs including the skin. Hemorrhage also accompanies the **disseminated intravascular coagulation** (DIC) that often occurs with treatment of acute progranulocytic leukemia. DIC can also develop in patients with other acute leukemias as well as other malignancies. The coagulation abnormalities associated with DIC lead to significant bleeding into the skin and life-threatening hemorrhage in other organs. Ecchymoses not related to trauma are shown on the arm of a patient with AML in Figure 11-43.

Bitemporal infiltration is shown in a child with AML in Figure 11-44. **Chloroma**, a green tumor that is specific for AML, usually occurs in children or adolescents. The green color of these tumors is due to myeloperoxidase and fades upon exposure to air. It may be the earliest manifestation of this leukemia. Periosteum is infiltrated by leukemic cells most commonly in the skull. Scalp tumors result, and proptosis can develop when the orbit is affected. Growth of chloromas leads to pressure on bone and nerves and can be life-threatening.

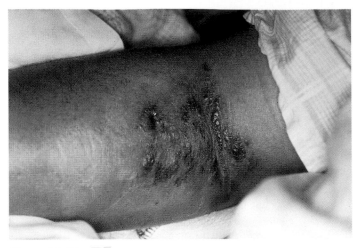

Figure 11-45

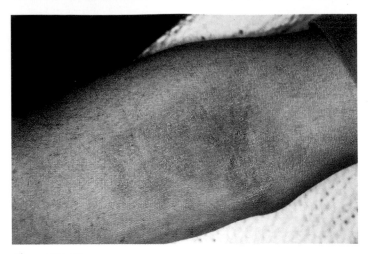

Figure 11-46

Complications of aggressive therapy have been reduced by improvements in prevention and management of infectious diseases and improvements in hyperalimentation and supportive care. These improvements, coupled with advances in chemotherapy and bone-marrow transplantation, have prolonged the survival of people with **acute myeloid leukemia**. The once dismal prognosis of this malignancy has improved considerably, with complete remissions achieved in up to 80% of patients, some of whom are cured of their disease. The patient in Figure 11-45 had AML, presenting with purpuric papules and plaques,

some of which were ulcerated. The hemorrhagic nature of the lesions was attributed to thrombocytopenia due to extensive replacement of normal bone marrow by leukemic cells. The skin lesions resolved with chemotherapy (Fig. 11-46), and the cutaneous hemorrhage improved as the patient's platelet count increased.

Because cutaneous involvement in AML can be quite variable in its presentation, a variety of therapeutic modalities may have to be used. Tumors may become so large or necrotic that surgical removal may be necessary. The goal of surgery in these instances is to alleviate local

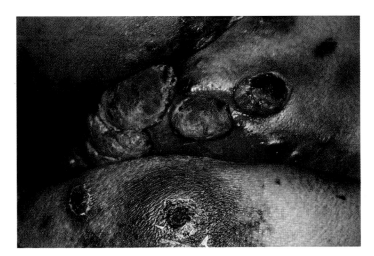

Figure 11-47

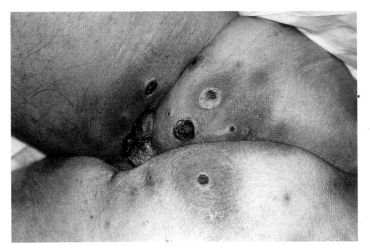

Figure 11-48

symptoms caused by tumor mass or removal of necrotic tumor that may be a focus of infection. Regardless of size, the presence of skin lesions infiltrated by leukemic cells provides a visible model for following the effectiveness of chemotherapeutic agents. The response of leukemic cells throughout the body to chemotherapy is likely to parallel the cutaneous

response to those agents. In Figure 11-47 large, necrotic, ulcerated tumors are shown on the buttocks of a patient with AML. The patient had a partial response to therapy, with shrinkage of the tumor as shown in Figure 11-48.

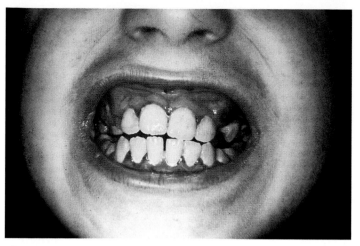

Figure 11-49

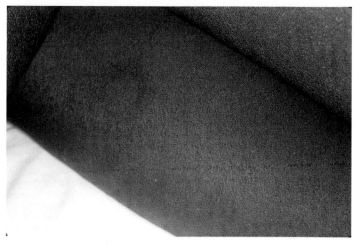

Figure 11-50

Acute monocytic leukemia is characterized by striking oral lesions. Gingival hyperplasia can be so extensive that gums entirely cover the teeth. Affected gums bleed and ulcerate easily. Purple macules, papules and tumors can develop on the gums (Fig. 11-49), as well as on the oral mucosa or on the skin. Gingival symptoms are so common that they may be the patient's first complaint, leading to diagnosis of this malignancy.

Skin lesions may be more common in monocytic leukemias than in other leukemias. While frequently present at diagnosis, they may be the first sign of disease, developing even while bone marrow biopsies are normal. As in other leukemias involving the skin, the site and morphology of the lesion can be quite variable. The patient in Figure 11-50 had acute monocytic leukemia and developed deep tender inflamed nodules with adjacent hemorrhage on the thighs. Histologic examination revealed a panniculitis with a leukemic infiltrate in the subcutaneous fat.

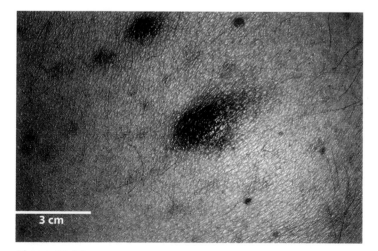

3 cm

Figure 11-51

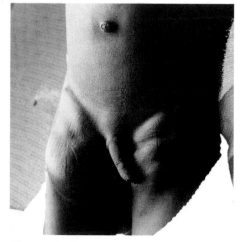

Figure 11-52

Cutaneous invasion is less common in the lymphocytic leukemias, but can occur. Skin lesions are nonspecific morphologically and therefore require biopsy to verify the diagnosis of leukemia cutis. Cutaneous infiltrates of the lymphocytic leukemias may be present at initial diagnosis or can develop later in the course of the disease. When first examined by a physician, the patient in Figure 11-51 had dozens of indurated erythematous nodules on the back, chest, and upper arms. Biopsy revealed a dermal leukemic infiltrate, and **chronic lymphocytic leukemia** was diagnosed.

Lymph node enlargement is one of the most common findings on physical examination. **Lymphadenopathy** may be localized or generalized. Affected nodes are firm, nontender, freely moveable, and range in size from a few millimeters in diameter to tumors larger than grapefruits. Occasionally lymph nodes develop in atypical locations such as the thorax or sacral region. Adjacent nodes can become confluent to form large masses in the neck, axillae, or femoral–inguinal areas. The child in Figure 11-52 has massive inguinal lymphadenopathy, a manifestation of his **acute lymphocytic leukemia.**

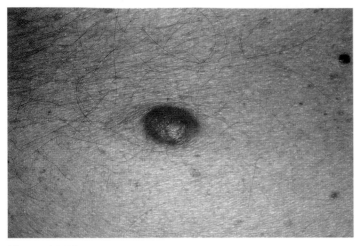

Figure 11-53

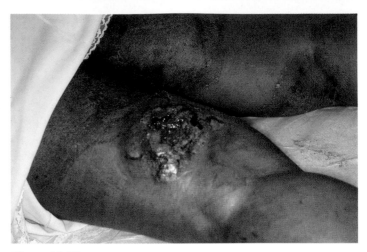

Figure 11-54

Lymphomas usually arise in tissues of lymphoid origin. On occasion, however, they develop in extranodal sites, including the skin. The patient in Figure 11-53 presented with recurring crops of erythematous papules and nodules on the trunk. Biopsy revealed a dermal infiltrate consisting of patches of normal appearing lymphocytes. In the absence of a more characteristic presentation, the differential diagnosis of **lymphoma cutis** must be considered and includes five conditions beginning with the letter **L**, all characterized by patchy lymphocytic infiltrates in the dermis: well-differentiated lymphocytic **L**ymphoma, polymorphous **L**ight eruption, discoid **L**upus erythematosus, Jessner's **L**ymphocytic infiltrate, and **L**ymphocytoma cutis.

To help establish a diagnosis of lymphoma cutis, fresh tissue can be sent for immunoglobulin and analysis of T-cell receptor gene rearrangements. Monoclonality of the surface immunoglobulins and of immunoglobulin or T-cell receptor genes supports a diagnosis of lymphoma cutis. The patient in Figure 11-53 went on to develop more characteristic signs of non-Hodgkin lymphoma with lymph node involvement. The patient in Figure 11-54 was thought to have a facticial ulcer on the posterior thigh and was subsequently misdiagnosed as having pyoderma gangrenosum. Only after repeated skin biopsies was a diagnosis of non-Hodgkin lymphoma made.

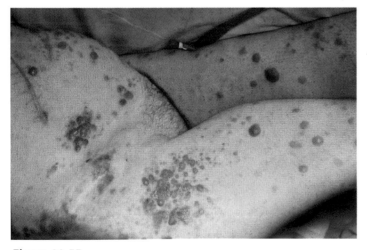

Figure 11-55

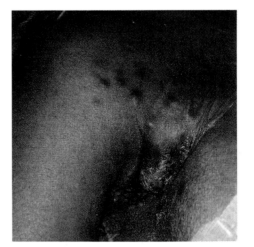

Figure 11-56

Diffuse non-Hodgkin lymphomas can result in widespread disease, including skin lesions. Cutaneous disease is particularly common in patients with diffuse large cell and high-grade lymphomas, but uncommon in patients with follicular lymphomas. The clinical presentation of skin lesions in patients with lymphomas varies considerably. Patients have presented with large cell lymphomas of the skin, which can be extensive despite the absence of lymph node involvement or visceral disease. The patient in Figure 11-55 developed widespread erythematous papules and nodules caused by diffuse large cell lymphoma. This contrasts with the cutaneous ulcer overlying involved axillary nodes and nearby erythematous nodules shown in a patient with a large cell lymphoma in Figure 11-56.

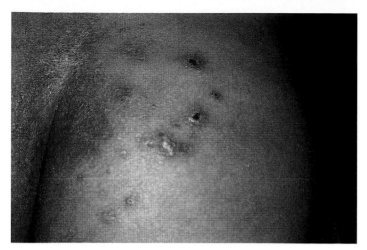

Figure 11-57

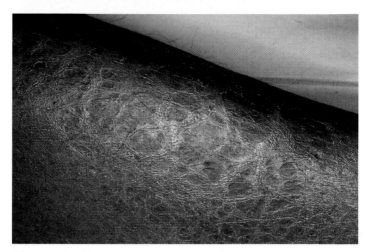

Figure 11-58

Specific cutaneous lesions are much less frequent in **Hodgkin disease** than in non-Hodgkin lymphomas. Papules, nodules, plaques, and ulcerations can develop, but are uncommon. The nonspecific lesions of Hodgkin disease are much more common. **Generalized pruritus**, for example, may be one of the earliest symptoms, and patients may present with generalized excoriations or prurigo nodularis ("picker's nodules") from repeated scratching (Fig. 11-57).

Acquired ichthyosis is a cutaneous manifestation of malignant disease that is strongly associated with Hodgkin disease. Skin changes resemble those of ichthyosis vulgaris, with large fishlike scales most prominent on the anterior aspects of the lower legs (Fig. 11-58). Unlike ichthyosis vulgaris, which begins in childhood, acquired ichthyosis develops in adults. It may precede other features of Hodgkin disease by months or days, or may develop after the diagnosis of Hodgkin disease has been made. Treatment of the malignancy may result in resolution of the skin changes. Acquired ichthyosis can develop in association with non-Hodgkin lymphomas, mycosis fungoides, multiple myeloma, and a number of solid tumors. Most recently, it has been reported in people with AIDS.

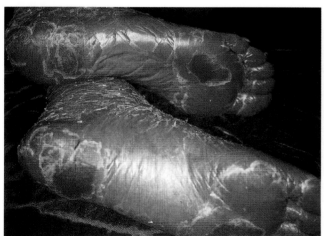

Figure 11-59

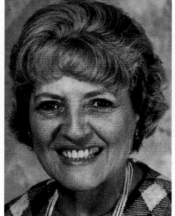

Figure 11-60A

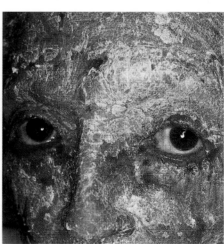

Figure 11-60B

Exfoliative dermatitis is another cutaneous manifestation of malignant disease that has been tied to Hodgkin disease. It can precede diagnosis of Hodgkin disease by years, can appear after diagnosis of the malignancy, or may develop simultaneously. It is characterized by a generalized angry red erythroderma with extensive scaling. Nails become thick with subungual hyperkeratosis and can eventually fall off. Hair loss is common, and hyperkeratosis of the palms and soles can occur (Fig. 11-59). The protective functions of the skin are lost. Patients experience difficulty with temperature control and often complain of chills. Hypothermia can develop. Loss of fluid can give rise to hypotension and renal failure. Protein loss through the skin and electrolyte imbalances are potential complications.

Exfoliative dermatitis is most commonly caused by drug reactions, psoriasis, or other dermatologic conditions. It is more commonly associated with mycosis fungoides and Hodgkin disease than with non-Hodgkin lymphomas or solid tumors, but it can be seen in association with a number of malignancies. The dramatic impact of exfoliative dermatitis is demonstrated in the patient shown in Figure 11-60. Figure 11-60A was taken a few years before the patient developed an exfoliative erythroderma. Her skin condition remained severe (Fig. 11-60B) for more than 1 year until a diagnosis of non-Hodgkin lymphoma was made.

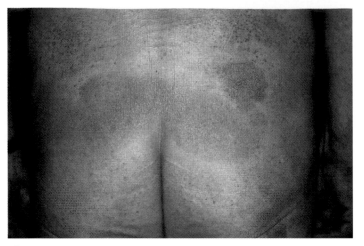

Figure 11-61

Cutaneous T-cell lymphoma (CTCL) encompasses a number of diseases resulting from clonal proliferation of T cells. Mycosis fungoides and related disorders including Sézary syndrome, cutaneous reticulum cell sarcoma, and dermal T-cell lymphoma are included. Lesions begin as scaling erythematous patches that can be pruritic (Fig. 11-61). The buttock, upper thighs, trunk, and intertriginous areas are often involved early in the course of the disease. Lesions in this **patch stage** are often misdiagnosed as chronic eczema, atopic dermatitis, chronic contact dermatitis, or psoriasis. Definitive diagnosis often takes up to 10 years following the onset of skin lesions. Diagnosis is made by light microscopic examination of skin biopsies stained with hematoxylin and

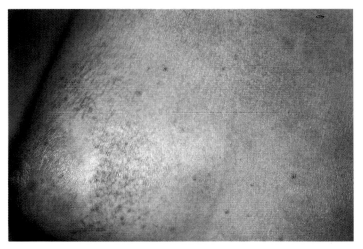

Figure 11-62A

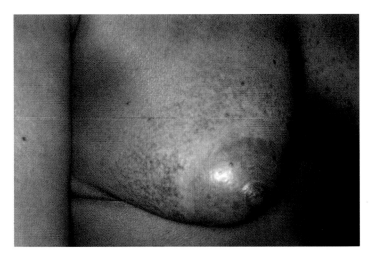

Figure 11-62B

eosin. Unfortunately, biopsies are often nonspecific, and repeated biopsies over months or years may be necessary. The patient in Figure 11-62A was first diagnosed with **large plaque parapsoriasis**, a condition that often progresses to CTCL. The skin lesions are identical to those of patch stage CTCL, and it is likely that many patients with large plaque parapsoriasis have an early stage of CTCL. Poikilodermatous changes characterized by cutaneous atrophy, telangiectasia (Figure 11-62B) and hyper- or hypopigmentation (Figure 11-62C) can predominate in the patch stage of this lymphoma.

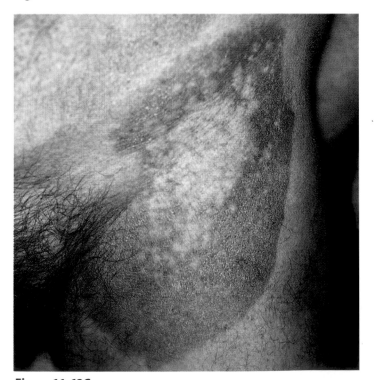

Figure 11-62C

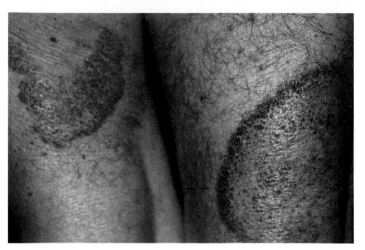

Figure 11-63

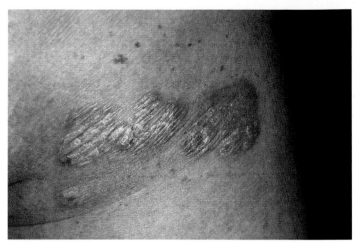

Figure 11-64

Months or years after the onset of skin lesions, patients progress to the **plaque stage** of CTCL. Patches may thicken into plaques, or plaques may develop in previously uninvolved skin. Lesions are palpable, well-defined, scaling plaques that are usually red or purple and are variable in size. Patches or plaques may regress spontaneously or clear in the center, leaving an elevated annular scaling border resembling tinea corporis (Fig. 11-63). Alternatively, plaques may be elevated throughout and may resemble psoriasis (Fig. 11-64). Itching can be severe in some people, while others are asymptomatic.

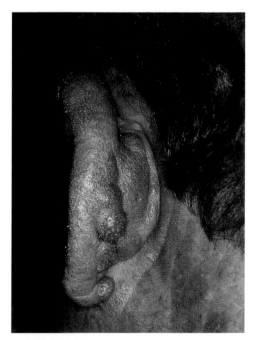

Figure 11-65A

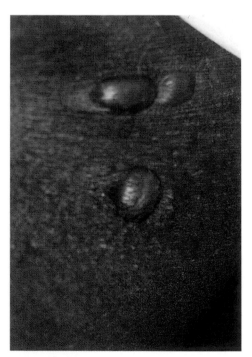

Figure 11-65B

In large series of selected patients, mean survival from histologic diagnosis has been 5 years, with survival averaging less than 9 years from the onset of skin lesions. In the patch and plaque stages, however, survival is extremely variable, with many patients living more than 20 years. In fact, lifespan is not reduced in most patients with patch stage mycosis fungoides, and most die of unrelated causes.

Eventually plaques can ulcerate or form nodules, the so-called **tumor stage** of CTCL. Occasionally tumors or ulcers arise *de novo*, presumably arising either from subclinically involved skin or cutaneous metastases. Tumors commonly occur on the face, buttocks, or in intertriginous (Figs 11-65A and 11-65B) or flexural sites such as the axillae, groin, antecubital fossae and inframammary area of females.

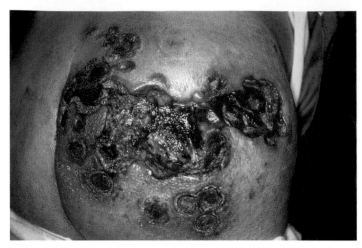

Figure 11-66

Ulcers caused by breakdown of tumors of **CTCL** are often large, deep, necrotic, and secondarily infected (Fig. 11-66). Nodules may be skin-colored, red, or violaceous, and these also frequently ulcerate. As in the patch and plaque stages, tumors can occasionally resolve without treatment, but the patient's prognosis is generally poor in the tumor stage, with a median survival of less than 3 years.

In advanced disease, CTCL can metastasize widely. Lymph node enlargement is often the first sign of extracutaneous spread. Affected nodes should be biopsied. Routine light microscopy often reveals only dermatopathic lymphadenopathy, although more sophisticated means show that a high proportion of these nodes are infiltrated by malignant cells. Hematogenous spread to spleen, liver, lungs, bone marrow, gastrointestinal tract, kidney, and heart is common, but involvement of these organs is often asymptomatic and detected only at autopsy. Sepsis originating in the skin is the ultimate cause of death in many patients with CTCL who are immunosuppressed in the course of the disease.

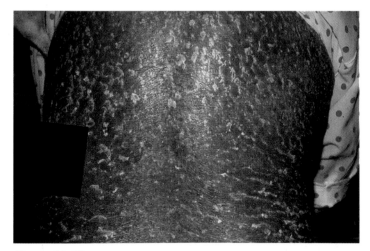

Figure 11-67

The erythrodermic form of CTCL, also called the **Sézary syndrome**, is characterized by generalized angry, red scaling skin (Fig. 11-67). There is thick hyperkeratotic scaling and fissuring of the palms and soles, and with longstanding disease nails become dystrophic. Eyelid ectropion is common. Erythroderma can develop in people with other forms of CTCL, or can occur *de novo*. Cutaneous barriers to fluid loss and infection are compromised. Patients may succumb to shock or, more commonly, to sepsis.

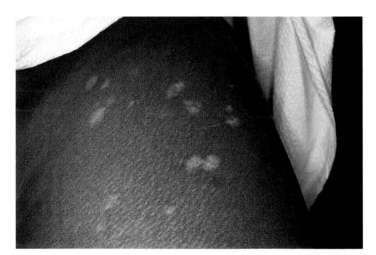

Figure 11-68

Hypopigmented mycosis fungoides is a variant of patch stage CTCL. The condition most commonly affects black, Hispanic, or dark-skinned white people, but it can occur in fair-skinned whites. Skin lesions are characterized by hypopigmented patches and macules that can be generalized or localized, affecting the trunk, extremities or face (Fig. 11-68). Lesions can be pruritic but are often asymptomatic and brought to the attention of physicians only because of the cosmetic problems they create. The prognosis of this condition can be good, with most patients surviving decades after the onset of skin lesions.

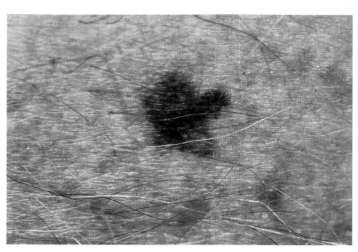

Figure 11-69

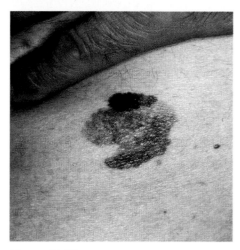

Figure 11-70

The incidence of malignant **melanoma** is increasing faster than that of almost any other malignancy, especially among young adults. Malignant melanoma can occur at any age over 20 years, with the exception of lentigo maligna melanoma, which occurs mostly in the elderly. Melanoma is rare in childhood, although it can occur in this age group in association with congenital nevi. Risk is greatest for fair-skinned whites who tan poorly and burn easily, and have blue eyes and blond or red hair. The death rate from melanoma is higher in individuals living in sunny climates closer to the equator. The most common sites in women are the lower legs and back, while men develop melanomas on the back more often than any other site. When this tumor occurs in blacks and

Asians, it is more common on the palms and soles. Since excision before deep invasion by the tumor still provides the best chance of cure, early recognition of melanoma is critical.

The most common type of melanoma, superficial spreading melanoma, represents 70% of all cases. There are several clinical features that readily allow differentiation of superficial spreading melanoma from benign melanocytic nevi.

Melanomas typically have irregular borders with sharp angles or notches (Fig. 11-69). The pigment variegation can be striking (Fig. 11-70), including brown, black, red, blue, gray, and white (areas of depigmentation). Lesions can be flat or elevated, but the development of an

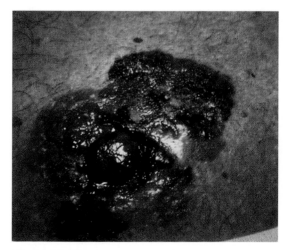

Figure 11-71

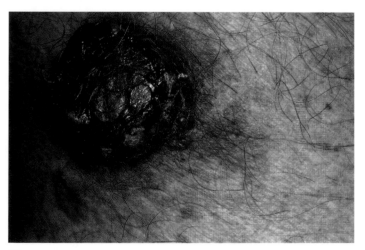

Figure 11-72

asymmetrical nodule within a pigmented lesion should raise the physician's suspicion (Fig. 11-71).

Nodular melanoma, the second commonest type, accounts for approximately 15% of cases of melanoma. It presents as a dark brown or

black papule or nodule that is elevated throughout (Fig. 11-72). While pigmentation can be variable, especially around the periphery of nodular melanomas, these tumors are often uniformly pigmented dark black, brown, or blue, making diagnosis more difficult. Unlike superficial spreading melanoma that evolve over long periods, nodular

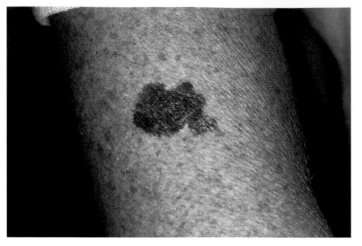

Figure 11-73

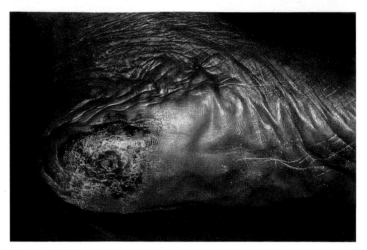

Figure 11-74

melanomas can grow rapidly over just months. This diagnosis should be suspected in any suddenly appearing dark papule or nodule, especially one that is changing.

Lentigo maligna most commonly develops in elderly individuals after their fifth or sixth decade of life, appearing on sun-exposed, sun-damaged skin. The vast majority of these tan, brown or black lesions occur on the head and neck or on the upper extremities and have very irregular borders and marked variegation of pigmentation (Fig. 11-73). Early lesions of lentigo maligna are flat and have a latency period of 5–50 years before becoming invasive.

Therapeutic management can range from no therapy (for elderly people in poor health), to superficial removal (dermabrasion, cryo-

therapy, radiotherapy, 5-fluorouracil) that occasionally results in recurrence, to surgical removal. It is estimated that 30% of lentigo maligna lesions develop into **lentigo maligna melanoma**. Lentigo maligna melanomas have diameters of 3–6 cm or more and typically have irregular pigmentation and papular or nodular components in areas where the melanoma has begun to invade.

Acral lentiginous melanoma is an aggressive tumor that occurs predominantly on the palms, soles, nail beds, and mucous membranes. Like other melanomas, acral lentiginous tumors can have irregular borders and vary in color, but even superficially invasive lesions have a much greater tendency to metastasize (Fig. 11-74).

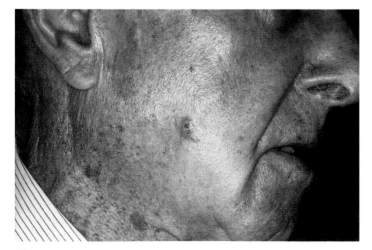

Figure 11-75

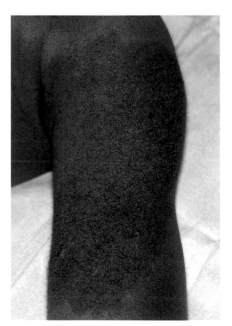

Figure 11-76

Primary melanomas are occasionally entirely unpigmented and are commonly of the nodular type. Often these **amelanotic melanomas** arise as small pink nodules within pigmented melanomas. Metastases of a pigmented melanoma may be amelanotic (Fig. 11-75).

Giant congenital melanocytic nevi are considered possible precursors to malignant melanoma and have a 2–30% chance of malignant degeneration. These lesions can cover large areas of the body (Fig. 11-76) including an entire arm, both buttocks ("bathing trunk" nevi), or the entire trunk. Early detection of melanomas that arise from giant

congenital nevi is difficult for a variety of reasons. The pigment pattern of giant congenital nevi may be irregular, making recognition of subtle malignant changes difficult. In addition, melanomas associated with giant congenital nevi can arise from dermal or subcutaneous tissues. Considering the risks of developing malignant melanoma, the physician must give careful consideration to early, full thickness, prophylactic removal of giant congenital melanocytic nevi. At least some cases of melanoma arise in small congenital melanocytic nevi, but the melanoma risk associated with these lesions is controversial.

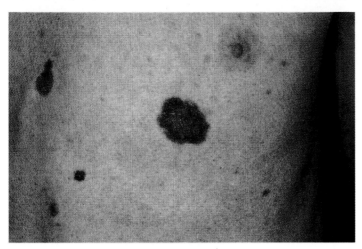

Figure 11-77

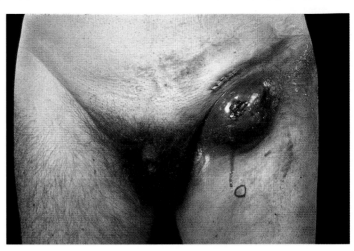

Figure 11-78

Dysplastic nevi are precursor lesions of malignant melanoma that have indistinct borders and some variegation of pigmentation (Fig. 11-77). The term dysplastic nevus syndrome, also known as familial melanoma, refers to patients that have multiple dysplastic nevi and two blood relatives with melanoma. Patients with this syndrome have a high risk of developing malignant melanoma and should undergo total skin examination every 3–6 months. Familial melanoma associated with dysplastic nevi is transmitted in an autosomal dominant manner and accounts for 10% of all melanoma patients. In the absence of a family history of melanoma, the significance of histopathologically diagnosed dysplastic nevi is controversial, since many normal individuals have such nevi. Nevertheless, the development of malignant melanoma within dysplastic nevi has been shown.

The prognosis of malignant melanoma is determined by the type of tumor and its thickness. If treated early, lentigo maligna melanoma is associated with long survival. In contrast, acral lentiginous melanoma has a 5-year mortality rate in excess of 80%. Of superficial spreading and nodular melanomas, thin tumors are easily cured by simple excision with adequate margins. Cure rates for lesions less than 0.76 mm thick approach 100%. Thicker melanomas unfortunately have a worse prognosis. The greater the depth at initial excision, the more likely a melanoma is to metastasize. For melanomas that have invaded subcutaneous fat, the 5-year mortality rate exceeds 50%.

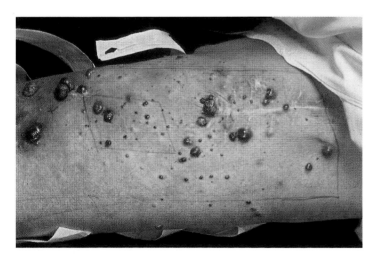

Figure 11-79

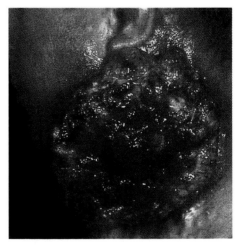

Figure 11-80

Melanomas can spread via lymphatics or by hematogenous dissemination. Metastasis to local nodes can result in massive enlargement of those lymph nodes. The blue–black pigmentation of the groin metastasis in Figure 11-78 allows easy identification of the primary tumor.

Hematogenous dissemination can give rise to widespread metastases. All the pigmented and amelanotic papules and nodules on the leg of the patient in Figure 11-79 proved to be metastatic melanoma.

Occasionally, primary or metastatic melanomas can be enormous. The ulcerated necrotic mass on the neck of the patient in Figure 11-80 was a melanoma.

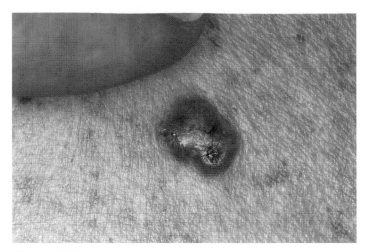

Figure 11-81

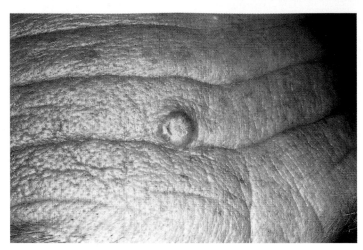

Figure 11-82

Basal cell carcinoma is the most common malignancy, with several hundred thousand new cases developing annually in the USA alone. This malignancy occurs in approximately one out of every seven Americans. Clinically, basal cell carcinomas have a number of different presentations. Most commonly, patients will complain of a sore that does not heal, or that keeps recurring in the same site. Early basal cell carcinomas often appear as crusted papules that bleed easily (Fig. 11-81). In males, the bearded part of the face is a commonly affected site. The malignancy is overlooked because the patient mistakenly thinks that

repeated irritation caused by shaving is responsible. Any sore, scab, ulcerated, or crusted skin lesion that does not heal within 3 weeks should be examined because of the possibility that it may be a basal cell carcinoma.

Before they ulcerate, basal cell carcinomas typically appear as translucent "pearly" papules with overlying telangiectases. They are dome-shaped in appearance and occasionally mistaken for intradermal nevi (Fig. 11-82). With time, the tumor enlarges and its surface erodes. The center of the tumor breaks down to form a "rodent ulcer"

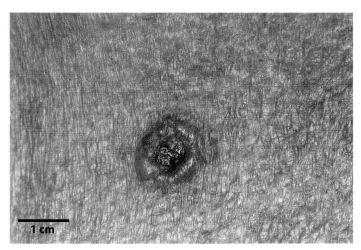

1 cm

Figure 11-83

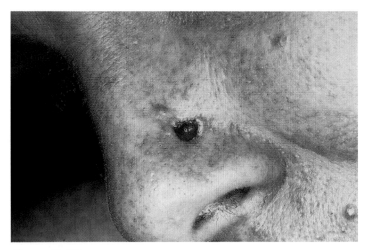

Figure 11-84

(Fig. 11-83), so named because of its resemblance to holes dug by rodents.

If untreated, basal cell carcinomas slowly progress. They can extend peripherally or invade the dermis and subcutaneous tissues, resulting in ulcers that can be sufficiently deep to perforate thin structures such as

the nose (Fig. 11-84). Basal cell carcinomas are most commonly found on sun-exposed parts of the body such as the face, bald portions of the scalp, the posterior neck, and the dorsal aspects of the hands and arms. Nevertheless, patients occasionally develop this malignancy on areas that are not sun-exposed, such as the buttocks.

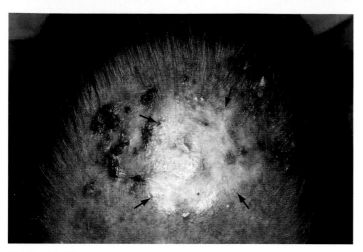

Figure 11-85

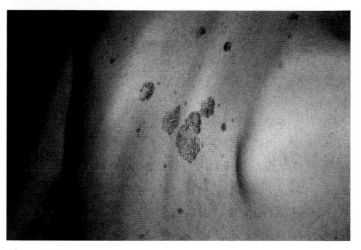

Figure 11-86

Several distinctive clinical and histologic variants of basal cell carcinoma exist. **Sclerosing basal cell carcinomas** are among the most destructive because they can attain a considerable size before diagnosis. They are white and resemble scars in appearance and consistency (Fig. 11-85). This variant has also been called "morpheaform" basal cell carcinoma because it feels indurated and tightly bound down. Unlike other basal cell carcinomas, the sclerosing variant may not ulcerate until late in its course. Histologically this variant is characterized by thin strands invading surrounding dermis, so the surgical margins must be examined carefully.

Superficial spreading basal cell carcinomas are annular erythematous plaques. They do not invade deeply but enlarge peripherally. The advancing border is slightly elevated and crusted, while the center is often flat, atrophic, and contains telangiectases. Multiple lesions commonly develop as shown on the back of a patient in Figure 11-86.

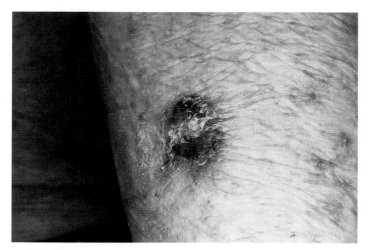

Figure 11-87

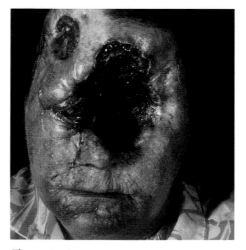

Figure 11-88

Pigmented basal cell carcinomas may develop, particularly in darkly pigmented patients. They contain variable amounts of pigmentation that appears as characteristic blue speckling within otherwise typical translucent papules that frequently ulcerate. In other patients, pigment may be so extensive that the basal cell carcinoma resembles a malignant melanoma (Fig. 11-87).

Basal cell carcinomas almost never metastasize, and there are only a few reports of dissemination to internal organs that are remote from the primary tumor. This neoplasm can be locally destructive and invasive, however, resulting in more than 1 000 deaths annually. The patient in Figure 11-88 had an aggressive basal cell carcinoma that ate through all layers of the skin, subcutaneous tissue, bone, and eye.

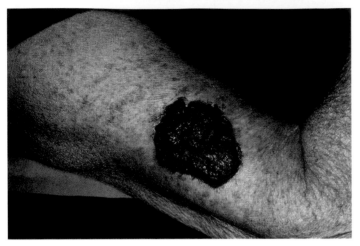

Figure 11-89

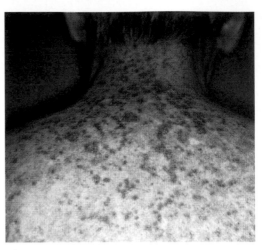

Figure 11-90

While **basal cell carcinomas** can be rapidly destructive and invasive, they can also grow slowly. Occasionally they increase minimally in size, over a long time. In other instances they may attain large sizes without impinging on critical structures. The patient in Figure 11-89 developed a large, exophytic, oozing, basal cell carcinoma that continued to grow over many years on the lateral aspect of the arm.

Squamous cell carcinoma represents the second most common type of cutaneous malignancy. The incidence of this tumor is markedly increased in fair-skinned patients with excessive sun-exposure. Sun-induced squamous cell carcinomas can arise in premalignant lesions called actinic keratoses. The latter premalignant lesions appear as red, scaly or crusted macules, or papules in areas of chronic sun exposure such as the face, scalp, dorsa of the hands, arms, and "V" of the neck and chest. Figure 11-90 shows numerous actinic keratoses appearing as erythematous macules on the back of a light-skinned patient who worked as a lifeguard for years.

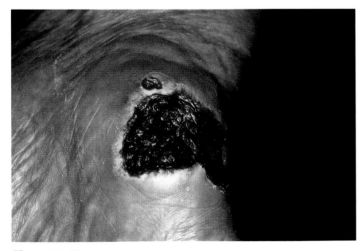

Figure 11-91

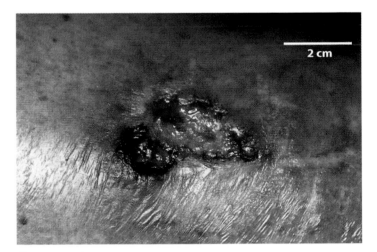

Figure 11-92

The appearance of squamous cell carcinomas can be variable. They occasionally arise as indistinct erythematous nodules, but eventually these become verrucous or papillomatous and ultimately ulcerate (Fig. 11-91). Sun-induced squamous cell carcinomas grow very slowly and, though locally invasive, there is little risk of metastasis in most patients.

By contrast, the squamous cell carcinomas that arise in scars, in skin treated with radiation, or mucous membranes such as the lip, perianal area, or genital skin, have a higher incidence of metastasis. Figure 11-92 shows a squamous cell carcinoma arising within a surgical scar on the leg. More commonly, these aggressive squamous cell carcinomas arise within scars caused by burns or radiation dermatitis.

NEOPLASTIC DISEASES **209**

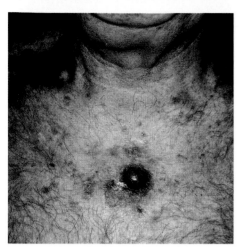

Figure 11-93

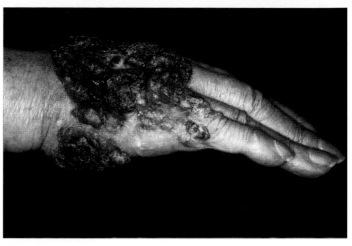

Figure 11-94

Squamous cell carcinomas are classically exophytic, meaning that they increase in elevation as well as depth while they grow. The patient in Figure 11-93 was on long-term immunosuppressive medication. As a result, he developed numerous squamous cell carcinomas, including the large presternal erythematous nodule shown.

In people who are immunosuppressed, squamous cell carcinomas can grow quickly and aggressively. Excision with a margin of normal skin is ideal but can be impractical in immunosuppressed patients, since they often develop numerous cutaneous malignancies. Alternative treatments such as curettage and desiccation or cryosurgery may therefore be necessary.

Figure 11-94 shows the hand of a patient with an invasive squamous cell carcinoma on both the dorsal and volar aspects. The tumor fortunately did not penetrate through the hand. Treatment with oral retinoids resulted in clinical resolution of the tumor. On discontinuation of the retinoid, however, the squamous cell carcinoma recurred.

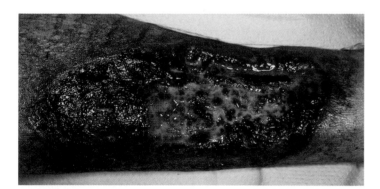

Figure 11-95A

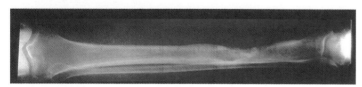

Figure 11-95B

The patient shown in Figure 11-95A had an extensive squamous cell carcinoma involving most of the leg. The tumor had been present for several years and invaded through the skin and subcutaneous tissues. Destruction of bone is shown in the radiograph in Figure 11-95B.

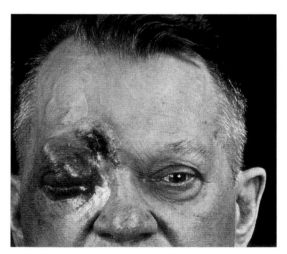

Figure 11-96

Figure 11-96 shows a squamous cell carcinoma invading the orbit. The patient presented with marked eyelid edema.

Squamous cell carcinomas can present as rock-hard nodules, fixed to underlying structures. The surface of the tumor may be smooth in some patients or ulcerated and crusted in others. The tumor often bleeds repeatedly.

Nonmetastasizing squamous cell carcinomas are increased in psoriasis patients treated with psoralen ultraviolet A (PUVA) for many years. These resemble sun-induced squamous cell carcinomas and are less invasive and destructive than squamous cell carcinomas arising in scars, chronic ulcers, or sites of radiation.

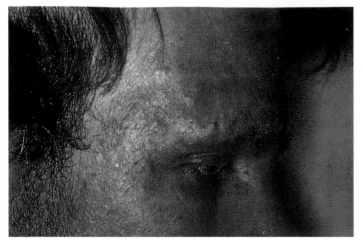

Figure 11-97

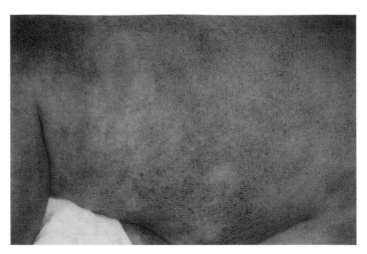

Figure 11-98

In addition to neoplasms that directly involve the skin, there are a number of dermatologic syndromes associated with internal malignancies. **Follicular mucinosis**, also called alopecia mucinosa, is characterized by follicular papules or indurated erythematous papules or plaques associated with hair loss in affected skin. Figure 11-97 shows loss of the lateral eyebrow in a patient with follicular mucinosis. This eruption can be associated with cutaneous T-cell lymphoma and occasionally may be the first clinical manifestation of malignancy, preceding diagnosis of the underlying neoplasm. In other people this histologically distinct condition is benign, self-limited, and is not associated with any malignancy.

Poikiloderma vasculare atrophicans is characterized by hypo- and hyperpigmented patches, atrophy, and telangiectasia (Fig. 11-98). The cutaneous atrophy results in shiny and occasionally wrinkled skin. The condition can range from a few small macules to large generalized patches involving most of the trunk and extremities. When extensive, the condition can be disfiguring. Pruritus may be severe in some patients but is absent in others. Poikiloderma vasculare atrophicans is often a precursor of cutaneous T-cell lymphoma, although not all patients develop this malignancy.

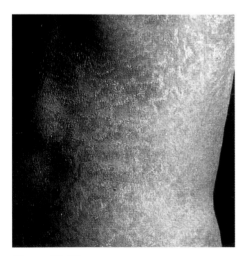

Figure 11-99

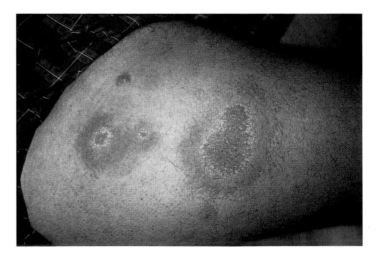

Figure 11-100

Erythema gyratum repens is a rare distinctive eruption characterized by concentric erythematous rings that give the skin a "woodgrain" pattern. The erythematous rings can enlarge and may be flat or elevated (Fig. 11-99). Most patients, though not all, have an underlying malignancy. Treatment of this may lead to resolution of erythema gyratum repens. Because of the frequency with which this condition is associated with underlying neoplasms, diagnosis of erythema gyratum repens should trigger a malignancy work-up.

Erythema annulare centrifugum begins with erythematous papules that gradually enlarge peripherally to form annular or polycyclic patches. The border of the annular rings may be elevated and indurated, resembling urticaria. Alternatively, the advancing erythematous border may have a "trailing scale" inside the ring (Fig. 11-100). In most cases of erythema annulare centrifugum the cause is unknown, but a number of cases have been associated with underlying malignancies such as Hodgkin disease, multiple myeloma, and lung cancer. Treatment of the malignancy has resulted in disappearance of the eruption, which can recur if the tumor recurs.

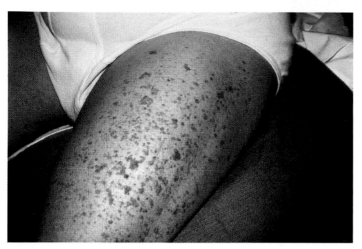

Figure 11-101

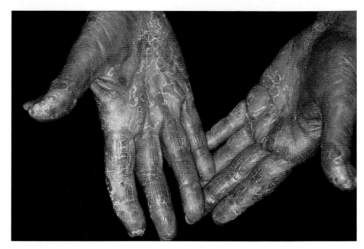

Figure 11-102

The **sign of Leser–Trélat** refers to the sudden development of hundreds of seborrheic keratoses associated with an underlying malignancy. Seborrheic keratoses are pigmented, hyperkeratotic, "stuck-on" papules that look like they could be easily scratched off with a fingernail (Fig. 11-101). The presence of a few seborrheic keratoses or the appearance of many in a patient with a familial tendency to develop them is common. Some have therefore expressed skepticism about a true association with underlying neoplasms. Nevertheless, the sign of Leser–Trélat has been associated with lymphomas, melanoma, and carcinomas of the lung, breast, colon, prostate, and stomach.

Bazex syndrome is a psoriasiform eruption that occurs in patients with tumors of the upper respiratory and digestive tracts. Carcinomas of the pharynx, tongue, larynx, tonsil, pyriform sinus, soft palette, esophagus, and lungs have been reported. Skin changes involve the hands, feet, ears, nose, elbows, knees, and cheeks. Hyperkeratosis of the palms and soles (Fig. 11-102) may be associated with dystrophic nails that are also psoriasiform.

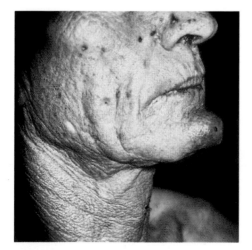

Figure 11-103

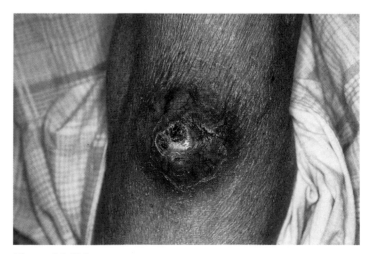

Figure 11-104

The **Muir–Torre syndrome**, first described in the 1960s, refers to an association between cutaneous sebaceous tumors with underlying malignancies. The sebaceous tumors include sebaceous adenomas, sebaceous hyperplasia, sebaceous epithelioma, and sebaceous carcinoma. Keratoacanthomas are present in some, but not all, patients. Colon cancers are the most commonly associated malignancy, although multiple neoplasms can be present. The patient in Figure 11-103 has

numerous scars where keratoacanthomas and sebaceous tumors had been removed. The tumor on the chin is a sebaceous carcinoma that metastasized to the parotid gland and mandible. The sebaceous carcinomas associated with this syndrome usually do not metastasize, as was the case for the sebaceous carcinoma of the leg of the patient in Figure 11-104. A colon cancer was subsequently discovered however.

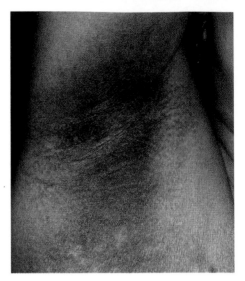

Figure 11-105

Acanthosis nigricans is a clinically distinctive disorder that has been associated with underlying malignancies. Skin lesions consist of gray–brown thickened plaques that on close inspection appear papillomatous. The axillae (Fig. 11-105), neck (Fig. 11-106), and groin are most commonly involved. In severely affected individuals the hands,

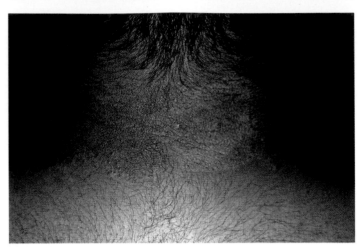

Figure 11-106

elbows, and even lips and eyelids can be affected. When associated with malignancy, acanthosis nigricans often develops suddenly and spreads rapidly. Almost all cases are associated with an underlying adenocarcinoma, and the primary tumor is usually intraabdominal. Most cases are associated with gastric carcinoma. Occasionally, acanthosis nigricans is the first manifestation of an underlying malignancy, and it will often clear upon treatment of the malignancy. A common benign

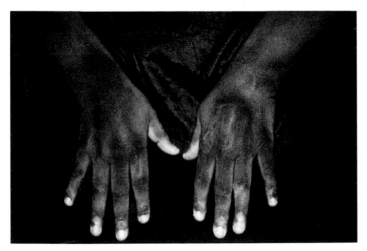

Figure 11-107

form of acanthosis nigricans is associated with obesity or with a number of endocrinopathies, including insulin-resistant diabetes, polycystic ovaries, Addison disease, pituitary tumors, and others. In addition, a number of medications such as nicotinic acid, steroids, and diethylstilbestrol can cause a benign form of acanthosis nigricans. Finally, occurrence of a transient form of acanthosis nigricans approximately

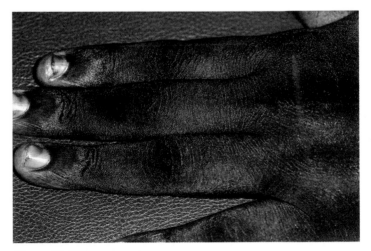

Figure 11-108

3 months after bone-marrow transplantation for lymphoblastic lymphoma, has been reported.

The patient shown in Figures 11-107 and 11-108 had generalized acanthosis nigricans, which prominently involved the dorsa of the wrists and hands (Fig. 11-107) with accentuation over joints, including the knuckles (Fig. 11-108).

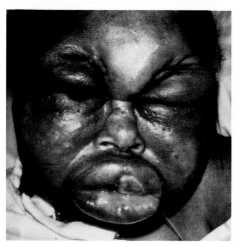

Figure 11-109

Profound edema of the skin and mucous membranes can occur in patients with the **superior vena cava syndrome**. This syndrome is caused by obstruction of the superior vena cava by tumor. The veins of the neck, chest, and upper extremities become prominently distended. Marked edema of the face, lips, and conjunctivae can occur. Any tumor invading the mediastinum can result in this syndrome. The patient in Figure 11-109 had an esophageal carcinoma.

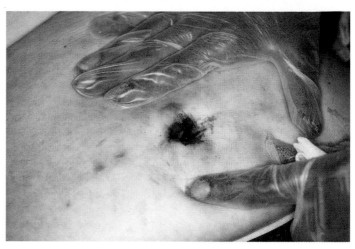

Figure 11-110

Sister Mary Joseph's nodule refers to metastatic subcutaneous nodules in the umbilicus (Fig. 11-110). This nodule is associated with intraperitoneal malignancy, particularly gastric adenocarcinoma. Cancers of the colon, ovary, and pancreas have also been associated with Sister Mary Joseph's nodule.

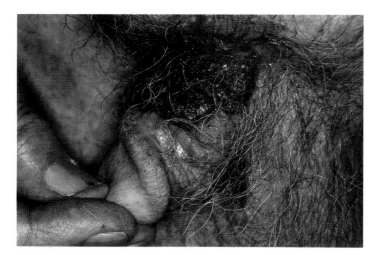

Figure 11-111

Extramammary Paget disease is a rare malignancy of the skin that occasionally results from intraepidermal extension of an adenocarcinoma of underlying secretory glands. The penis, scrotum, vulva, and perianal skin are most commonly affected, although the condition has arisen in axillae and periumbilical and presternal skin. Cutaneous lesions consists of sharply demarcated erythematous plaques that can be covered with scale, crust, or exudate (Fig. 11-111). Pruritus and pain can be present, and bleeding occurs later in the course of the disease. Patients are often misdiagnosed and treated for psoriasis, eczematous dermatoses, or fungal infections, until skin biopsy confirms the diagnosis of extramammary Paget disease.

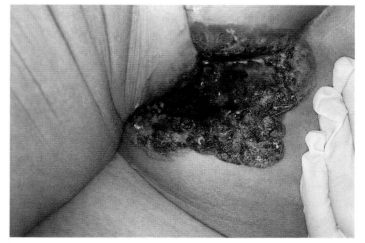

Figure 11-112

The patient in Figure 11-112 developed a sharply demarcated, erythematous, scaling plaque that was misdiagnosed as psoriasis of the perianal area. The condition failed to respond to topical corticosteroids and was finally biopsied long after its onset.

An associated primary adenocarcinoma of the rectum, urethra , or cervix should be sought. Renal cell carcinoma and prostate cancer have also been associated with extramammary Paget disease. Invasion of lymphatics by cancer cells can occur, and this disease unfortunately has a significant mortality. Removal by Mohs micrographic surgery can be curative, but recurrent rates are high because of the multifocal nature of the disease. Serum carcinoembryonic antigen (CEA) levels may be helpful in monitoring patients with extramammary Paget disease.

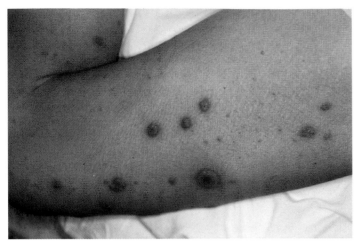

Figure 11-113

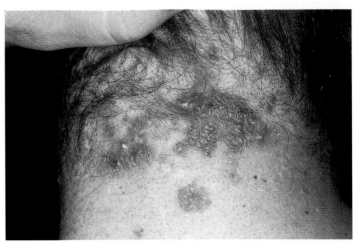

Figure 11-114

Sweet syndrome, also known as acute febrile neutrophilic dermatosis, is an uncommon disorder that usually follows an upper respiratory infection or other bacterial or viral illness. Approximately 20% of cases are associated with malignancies, especially AML and acute myelomonocytic leukemia. Patients present with the sudden onset of fever, leukocytosis and multiple, sharply demarcated, painful, erythematous papules and plaques (Fig. 11-113). Because the intense edema of the papillary dermis gives lesions a fluid-filled appearance, individual lesions may resemble vesicles or bullae. Occasionally, pustules develop on the surface of papules or plaques (Fig. 11-114). Lesions range up to several centimeters in diameter and may be few in number or widespread. The arms, neck, and face are most commonly involved but any part of the body can be affected, particularly when Sweet syndrome is associated with malignancy. Skin lesions usually precede the diagnosis of malignancy by months or years and recurrences of Sweet syndrome after treatment may signal tumor relapse.

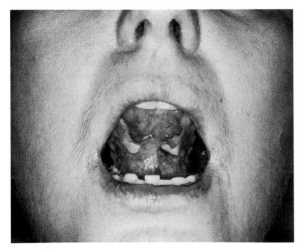

Figure 11-115

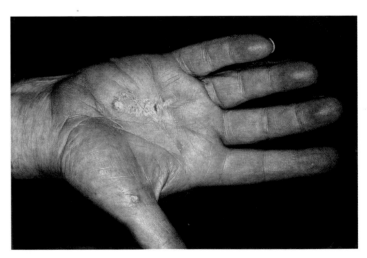

Figure 11-116

Paraneoplastic pemphigus is a recently described syndrome that has been associated with underlying malignancies, especially lymphomas and thymomas. Mucocutaneous lesions are characterized by oral erosions (Fig. 11-115) and variable skin lesions that may be vesicular, bullous, or crusted. On skin biopsy, direct immunofluorescence reveals epidermal cell-surface IgG, and circulating autoantibodies against desmoglein—especially desmoglein 3—can be found on indirect immunofluoresence of serum from most affected patients. Sera react with plakin family proteins including envoplakin and periplakin. The antibodies differ from those found with pemphigus vulgaris or pemphigus foliaceus.

Arsenical keratoses are verrucous, hyperkeratotic papules that occur most frequently on the palms and soles, but can also occur on other cutaneous surfaces. Lesions are often a few millimeters in diameter, but can become confluent to form hyperkeratotic plaques (Fig. 11-116). Some arsenical keratoses can be erythematous or pigmented. Arsenical keratoses result primarily from ingestion of arsenic in water from wells, particularly in parts of Asia where hundreds of thousands of people have been exposed to arsenic-contaminated wells. Arsenic is also present in pesticides and can be an occupational hazard to individuals exposed to them. Historically, arsenic was used in preparations such as Fowler solution for the treatment of asthma, atopic dermatitis, or psoriasis. While arsenical keratoses can develop into invasive squamous cell carcinoma, arsenic exposure has been associated with multiple superficial basal cell carcinomas and internal malignancies.

12 Dermatologic diseases and cutaneous drug reactions

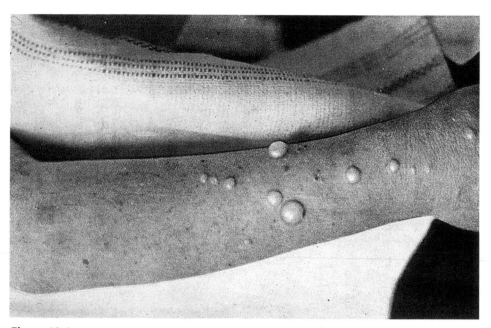

Figure 12-1

Pemphigus vulgaris is a non-contagious, chronic skin disease characterized by the formation of bullae in uninterrupted sequence, or more often in crops. Premonitory symptoms such as fever, chilliness, anorexia, and nausea, may be present for a day or two before the appearance of the first eruption or before each successive outbreak...The lesions appear as irregularly disseminated, pin-head-sized vesicles that develop in a few hours into tense, hemispherical bullae, one-half to three inches in diameter. The number varies from one or two to several hundred. The lesions show no predilection for particular regions nor any tendency to occur in groups. The bullae contain clear serum that becomes turbid or puriform in two or three days. Not until then does an inflammatory areola develop. Individual bullae persist two to eight days. They do not tend to burst, but dry to thin yellow crusts that fall off and leave light brown spots or no trace at all.

Rainforth SI. The stereoscopic skin clinic. New York: Medical Art Publishing; 1911.

The tense bullae shown in Figure 12-1 are more characteristic of bullous pemphigoid than of pemphigus vulgaris. Advances in immunofluorescence and immunoelectron microscopy have allowed the differentiation of many immunobullous disease. Undoubtedly, many bullous diseases were called pemphigus in the early part of the 20th century.

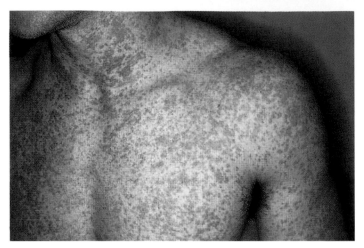

Figure 12-2

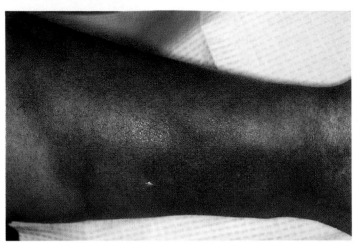

Figure 12-3

Cutaneous reactions to drugs constitute the most common complication of systemic therapy with up to 1 in every 50 hospitalized patients experiencing a suspected cutaneous drug reaction. Several kinds of drug rash occur, the most frequent being a **morbilliform** eruption, so named because of its similarity to the rash of measles. The rash consists of erythematous macules and papules (Fig. 12-2) that begin on the trunk or in sites of pressure and quickly become generalized. Pruritus is

common, and some patients develop an associated fever. This kind of rash usually begins within a week of treatment and lasts 5 days to 2 weeks. Figure 12-3 shows a patient whose rash was first misdiagnosed as contact dermatitis because it started under her surgical dressing. The next day the rash became generalized and was clearly attributed to penicillin that had been started 1 week earlier. Some drug reactions occur more than 2 weeks following cessation of drug therapy, particularly when the reactions are due to penicillins.

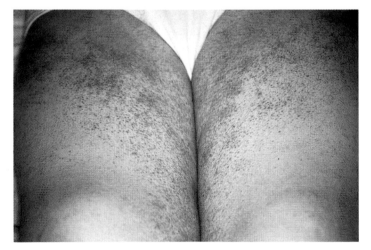

Figure 12-4

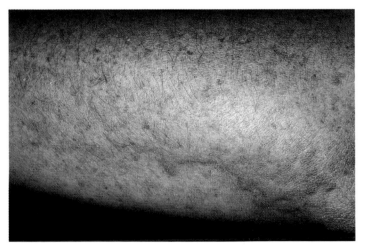

Figure 12-5

A morphologically similar reaction occurs in almost all patients with mononucleosis who are treated with ampicillin (Fig. 12-4). Unlike other drug allergies in which the rash occurs upon reexposure to the offending agent, the ampicillin rash of **mononucleosis** does not recur once the mononucleosis has resolved.

Amoxicillin is the most frequent cause of drug reaction, resulting in a rash in more than 5% of treated patients. Other drugs most frequently implicated in drug rashes include trimethoprim–sulfamethoxazole, other penicillins, and cephalosporins. Hypersensitivity eruptions also complicate transfusion of blood products in up to 1% of recipients.

Urticaria accounts for approximately a quarter of drug reactions. If IgE antibodies to the drug are present at the time of drug administration, urticaria develops within minutes of exposure. If antibodies are formed during the exposure, urticaria or angioedema can occur hours or days later. Skin lesions consist of pruritic erythematous wheals (Fig. 12-5) that last for a few hours. When swelling involves subcutaneous tissues, the condition is called **angioedema**. Urticaria and angioedema are occasionally associated with laryngeal edema, bronchospasm, or anaphylaxis with hypotension and shock.

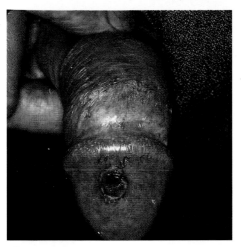

Figure 12-6

Figure 12-7

Fixed drug eruptions account for 10% of cutaneous drug reactions and present as one or a few well-demarcated erythematous patches that typically involve the genitals (Fig. 12-6), perianal area, face, hands, and feet. Lesions usually occur within 8 h of exposure and recur in the same sites on reexposure to the offending agent. The most common causes are tetracyclines, barbiturates, nonsteroidal antiinflammatory drugs, and sulfonamides. Dyes in pills and, rarely, foods may cause fixed drug eruptions. Phenolphthalein in laxatives is a common example of a dye that can cause this unusual reaction. Patients may complain of pain, itching, or burning, and occasionally the rash may blister (a "bullous fixed drug eruption") or become crusted. Fixed drug eruptions typically heal with hyperpigmentation that may persist for months or years (Fig. 12-7).

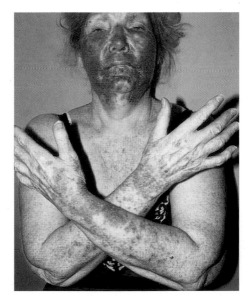

Figure 12-8

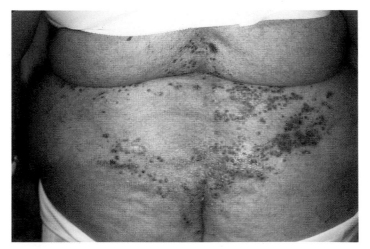

Figure 12-9

Several drugs are capable of producing **photosensitivity reactions** in sun-exposed skin. Some drugs, like tetracyclines or psoralens, cause dose-related phototoxic reactions in anyone given enough medication and sunlight. The resulting rash resembles sunburn and affects such areas as the face (Fig. 12-8), the neck and upper chest; it spares shaded areas of skin such as the submental region. In severe cases, bullous reactions can result.

An uncommon group of disorders that resembles lichen planus are called **lichenoid drug eruptions**. Scaling, pruritic, purple papules that are polygonal in shape are typical, but oozing or crusted papules can occur as well. Occasionally, a lichenoid drug eruption can develop into an exfoliative dermatitis. Skin lesions heal with residual pigmentation. Unlike lichen planus, in which lesions are concentrated on the genitals, hands, feet, and flexural aspects of the wrists, lichenoid drug eruptions can be generalized, symmetrically involving the trunk and extremities. Captopril, gold, and β-blockers are causes of this unusual drug reaction. The patient in Figure 12-9 developed lichenoid papules on the abdomen, back, and buttocks following administration of a calcium-channel blocker.

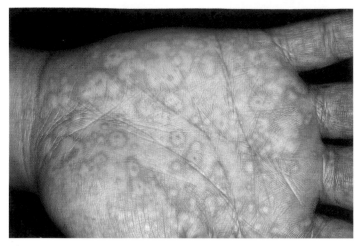

Figure 12-10

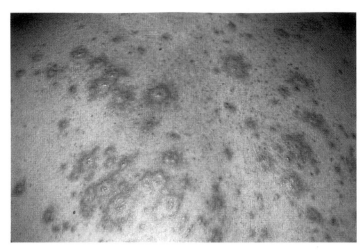

Figure 12-11

Erythema multiforme is occasionally caused by ingestion of drugs or it can follow an infection such as *Mycoplasma pneumonia*. Recurrent herpes simplex infection, which can be subclinical and therefore go unnoticed, is the most common cause of recurrent erythema multiforme. Erythema multiforme typically presents with very characteristic target-shaped lesions, created by alternating rings of erythema and pallor (Fig. 12-10). Lesions can be macular, papular, urticarial or, in some instances, vesicular. The latter condition has been termed **bullous**

erythema multiforme (Fig. 12-11). Lesions often begin on the distal extremities and symmetrical involvement of the palms and soles is common. Mucous membranes are occasionally affected, resulting in crusting of the lips, conjunctivitis, or genital symptoms. Sulfonamides, barbiturates, and penicillins are among the most common medications that cause erythema multiforme. This reaction occurs 1–15 days after exposure to the drug.

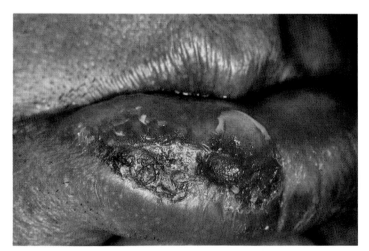

Figure 12-12

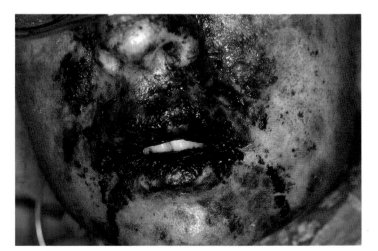

Figure 12-13

Stevens–Johnson syndrome is a severe form of erythema multiforme in which skin lesions are more extensive and mucous membranes are severely affected. Oral mucous membranes are eroded (Fig. 12-12) and often thickly crusted. Patients have severe pain upon eating. Involvement of the conjunctiva, cornea, and iris can endanger vision. Genital mucosal erosions and crusting can make walking and urination painful.

Associated systemic symptoms include fever, myalgias, and arthralgias. Like erythema multiforme, Stevens–Johnson syndrome can be caused by medications or infections. The patient in Figure 12-12 developed Stevens–Johnson syndrome on two occasions, each following an outbreak of genital herpes. Figure 12-13 shows a severely affected patient who developed Stevens–Johnson syndrome following ingestion of trimethoprim–sulfamethoxazole.

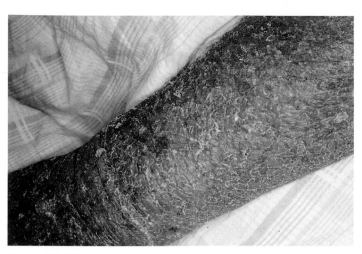

Figure 12-14

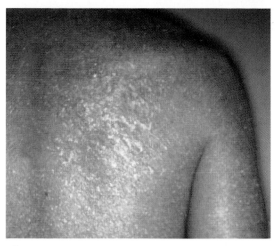

Figure 12-15

Exfoliative dermatitis is a severe, life-threatening disorder that has several diverse etiologies. Also called erythroderma or "red man's syndrome," the condition is characterized by severe generalized redness and scaling (Figs 12-14 and 12-15). The skin loses many of its protective functions, including the ability to protect against loss of body heat. Fever, chills, or hypothermia are common. Fluid loss through the skin can lead to hypotension and renal failure. Constant exfoliation leads to protein loss and hypoalbuminemia. Hypervolemia and edema result, and anemia develops in two-thirds of patients. All these factors, combined with cutaneous vasodilation, may result in high-output cardiac failure. The causes of exfoliative dermatitis include psoriasis and other skin disorders, malignancies, and drug reactions.

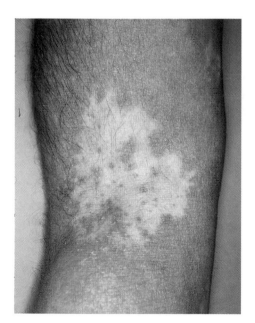

Figure 12-16

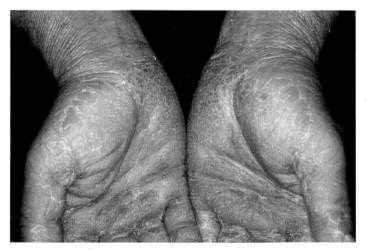

Figure 12-17

Pityriasis rubra pilaris, severe atopic dermatitis, or widespread contact dermatitis can give rise to the clinical picture of an erythroderma. A preceding history of psoriasis or atopic dermatitis may help identify the underlying causes in some patients. The presence of typical psoriatic plaques or characteristic findings such as islands of normal skin adjacent to involved skin in pityriasis rubra pilaris (Fig. 12-16) may be of diagnostic help. The malignancy most commonly associated with exfoliative dermatitis is cutaneous T-cell lymphoma, but Hodgkin disease and other lymphomas can lead to a generalized erythroderma as can other neoplasms. Numerous systemic medications have also been implicated in the pathogenesis of exfoliative dermatitis. Antibiotics, including sulfonamides, penicillins, and cephalosporins, and antimalarials are among the most common causes. Regardless of etiology, erythrodermas can involve the scalp resulting in alopecia, and nails become dystrophic or are shed entirely. Thick hyperkeratosis of palms and soles (Fig. 12-17) occurs in patients with psoriasis, pityriasis rubra pilaris, or Sézary syndrome. Lymphadenopathy and hepatomegaly are common findings, as are eosinophilia and elevated levels of IgE.

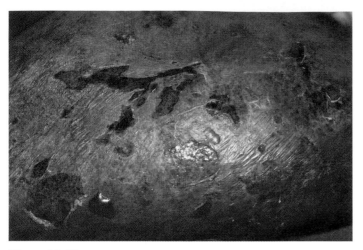

Figure 12-18

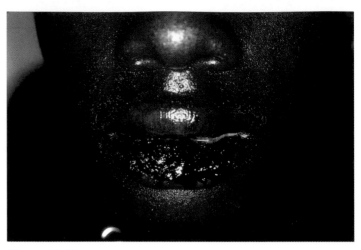

Figure 12-19

Toxic epidermal necrolysis is a severe cutaneous reaction most commonly triggered by exposure to drugs. Most cases begin within 2 weeks of administration of the responsible medication. Sulfonamides, nonsteroidal antiinflammatory drugs, phenytoin, and allopurinol are common causes. Skin lesions start with generalized erythema that may initially resemble a simple macular drug rash. One or 2 days later, patients form bullae over extensive areas of the body and slough skin in large pieces (Fig. 12-18). Patients may lose so much epidermis that most

of the body surface is replaced with weeping or crusted erosions. Painful mucous membranes may be covered with hemorrhagic crusts. Lips and oral mucosa are frequently involved, as shown in Figure 12-19. Involvement of the mucosal lining of the gastrointestinal tract occasionally leads to hemorrhage. Pneumonia may result from respiratory tract involvement. Fever and leukocytosis are common. Fluid and electrolyte imbalance, hypotension, and acute renal failure are frequent complications and many patients succumb to sepsis.

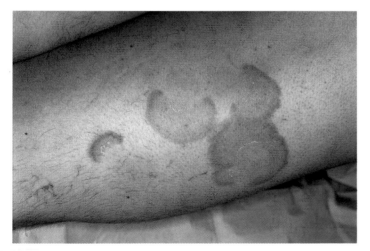

Figure 12-20

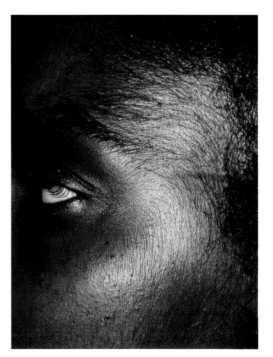

Figure 12-21

Erythema annulare centrifugum is a rare reaction pattern that has been attributed to antimalarials, cimetidine, and salicylates. Occasionally, the course of this eruption parallels that of an underlying malignancy or infection, but most often the etiology is unknown. Skin lesions are distinctive, beginning as small erythematous papules that enlarge peripherally by several millimeters daily. Eventually they form annular erythemas with central clearing. The leading red border may be followed by a characteristic inner rim of scaling (Fig. 12-20).

Hirsutism can be caused by numerous drugs, most notably cyclosporine, phenytoin, corticosteroids, and adrenocorticotropic hormone. Progesterones in oral contraceptives commonly result in a male pattern of hair growth with an increase in facial hair. Other drugs associated with increased hair growth include androgens such as testosterone, D-penicillamine, and diazoxide. The antihypertensive drug minoxidil occasionally results in dramatic hair growth, which has led to its use as a topical treatment for male pattern alopecia. The woman in Figure 12-21 developed striking hair growth on her forehead and malar areas after applying topical minoxidil to the scalp.

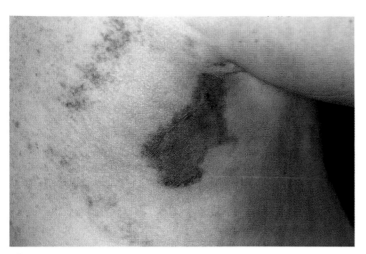

Figure 12-22

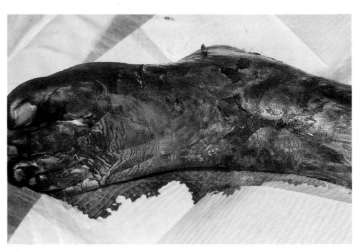

Figure 12-23

Coumarin necrosis, also known as warfarin necrosis, is a rare reaction that begins within 2 weeks of starting on systemic coumarin anticoagulants. This hemorrhagic infarct of the skin begins with pain, erythema, and swelling in the affected area. Petechiae may develop and may be followed by hemorrhagic vesicobullous lesions and, finally, by a characteristic black necrotic eschar (Fig. 12-22). The buttocks, breasts, abdomen, calves, and thighs are characteristic sites. Most patients are obese, postmenopausal women. Continuation of the coumarin anticoagulant does not lead to further necrosis.

Vasopressin, used to treated bleeding esophageal varices in patients with cirrhosis, acts by constricting blood vessels. Excessive vasoconstriction limits the blood supply to various organs. When cutaneous vessels are affected, necrosis of skin can result. Ischemia can develop at the site of the intravenous vasopressin infusion or at remote sites. Sloughing of the skin (Fig. 12-23), gangrene of digits, or necrotic eschars occasionally result.

A number of drugs cause specifically unique cutaneous reactions. Chronic treatment with **minocycline** has been associated with blue–

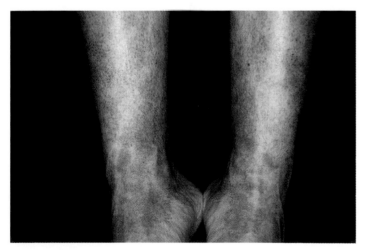

Figure 12-24

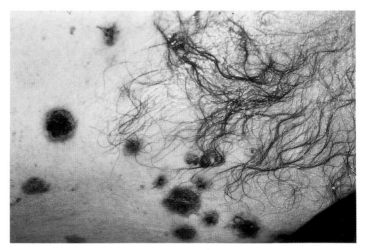

Figure 12-25

black pigmentation of soft tissues, specifically of the skin and thyroid gland. The color has been attributed to formation of a reactive metabolite that can polymerize to form black pigment. While minocycline can have antithyroid effects, these are seldom clinically significant. Some have suggested that localization of minocycline to areas of chronic venous stasis on the lower legs (Fig. 12-24) may be due to chelation of the minocycline or its metabolites with iron in the soft tissue of the legs. The color change is gradually reversible upon discontinuation of minocycline. Minocycline hyperpigmentation of the tongue has been treated successfully with the Q-switched ruby laser.

An unusual reaction to **vancomycin** leads to the development of scattered bullae and vesicles, which form crusts and erosions (Fig. 12-25). Histologic examination shows subepidermal bulla formation and, on immunofluorescence, biopsies taken from the edge of a bulla show linear deposition of IgA. More often, rapid intravenous administration of vancomycin also leads to arteriolar vasodilation and flushing. Similar reactions can occur with intravenous administration of theophylline, calcium, or doxorubicin. Flushing commonly occurs in patients treated with oral niacin.

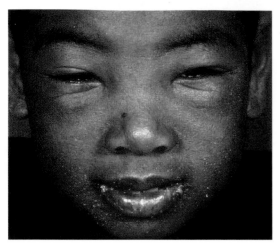

Figure 12-26

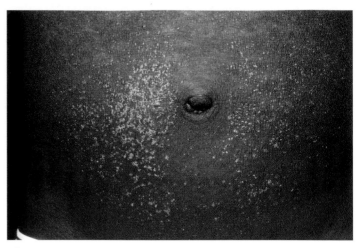

Figure 12-27

Dilantin hypersensitivity syndrome refers to an unusual systemic reaction to phenytoin and other hydantoin derivatives. The reaction usually begins 1–3 weeks after starting phenytoin, but delayed onset can occur. Patients develop fever, generalized lymphadenopathy, hepatosplenomegaly, and a cutaneous eruption. Facial edema with pronounced swelling of the eyelids is a characteristic feature (Fig. 12-26). Hepatitis, arthritis, nephritis, or pneumonitis can develop, and eosinophilia up to 40% is frequently found.

The systemic symptoms of the dilantin hypersensitivity syndrome occasionally mimic Hodgkin disease or non-Hodgkin lymphoma, but the skin lesions are more suggestive of a drug reaction. The most frequent cutaneous presentation of this syndrome consists of erythematous macules and papules followed by mild desquamation (Fig. 12-27). Vesicular lesions are occasionally reported, and some patients develop a toxic epidermal necrolysis-like picture. Histologic examination of skin biopsy specimens usually shows a nonspecific inflammatory infiltrate, but on rare occasions the histopathology may suggest a diagnosis of mycosis fungoides. Fortunately all symptoms resolve within 2 weeks of discontinuation of phenytoin.

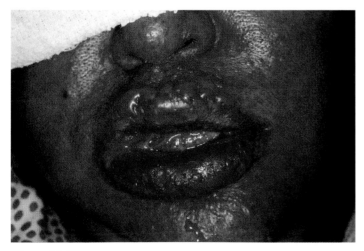

Figure 12-28

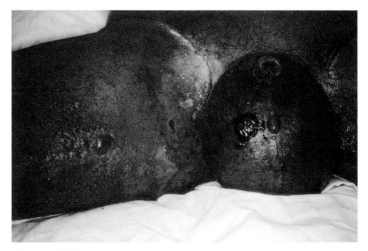

Figure 12-29

Following radiation therapy to the brain, an unusual form of Stevens–Johnson syndrome has been reported in patients with intracranial tumors. Many of the reported patients were being treated with phenytoin, leading to the suggestion that an alternative anticonvulsant be considered in patients scheduled for brain radiation therapy. Erythema begins on the scalp before spreading to the extremities. In severe cases, generalized erythema, formation of bullae, and sloughing occurs. Facial involvement with formation of bullae around the lips is shown in Figure 12-28.

Toxic epidermal necrolysis has been reported in a patient receiving whole-body electron beam radiation and doxorubicin. The patient shown in Figure 12-29 was treated with phenytoin and developed toxic epidermal necrolysis following whole-body irradiation. Widespread erythema was followed by edema, with dramatic swelling of the scrotum and formation of bullae. Localization of drug eruptions to sites of old sunburn or local radiation can also occur.

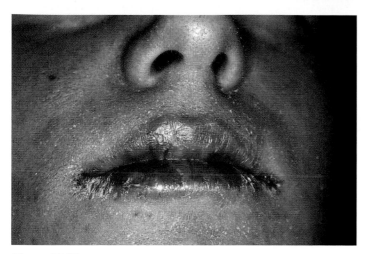

Figure 12-30

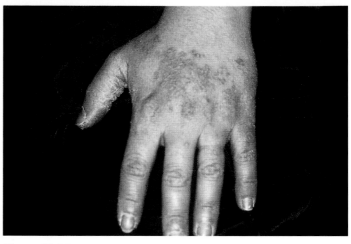

Figure 12-31

Retinoids have been used to treat a number of dermatologic conditions, including psoriasis, acne rosacea, and ichthyoses. More recently, a number of malignancies such as squamous cell carcinoma and mycosis fungoides have been shown to respond to this class of medication. Retinoids may also have a role in chemoprophylaxis of oropharyngeal squamous cell carcinomas and cutaneous basal cell carcinomas and squamous cell carcinomas.

Cheilitis is one of the earliest cutaneous reactions to oral isotretinoin (Fig. 12-30). Fissuring and cracking of the lips occur so predictably in patients on isotretinoin that their absence should suggest the patient is not taking an optimal dose. Isotretinoin and etretinate produce generalized dryness and desquamation. The palms and soles may shed large sheets of scale. Dryness of nasal mucous membranes can cause cracking and epistaxis. **Xerosis** of the skin leads to inflammation and fissuring especially on the hands (Fig. 12-31). Linear erythematous fissures often form a pattern called "eczema craquelé" because of its similarity to cracked porcelain.

Photosensitivity is another common reaction to systemic retinoids. Patients develop a typical sunburn reaction in sun-exposed sites even after only limited sun or ultraviolet exposure. This is particularly

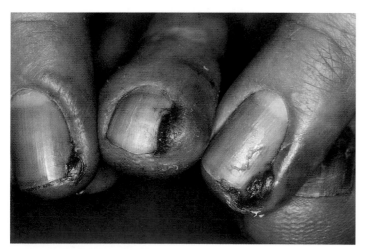

Figure 12-32

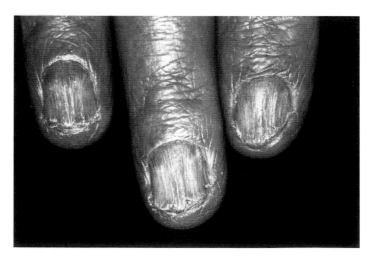

Figure 12-33

important for psoriasis patients being treated with ultraviolet photo-therapy, since addition of retinoids to their regimen can result in severe burns if their ultraviolet dose is not reduced.

Another unusual reaction seen in patients on oral retinoids is the development of **pyogenic granulomas** in skin adjacent to the fingernails and toenails (Fig. 12-32). These oozing, bleeding, painful papules resolve once the retinoid is discontinued.

Hair and nails are frequently affected in patients on oral retinoids and these effects are dose-related. At high doses, more than a third of patients on oral etretinate experience generalized **hair loss**. Alopecia is not limited to the scalp—patients even lose their eyebrows and eye lashes. Separation of the nail plate from the nail bed (onycholysis) occasionally occurs and some people lose the entire nail plate (onychomadesis) after starting on retinoids. Following several months of treatment on oral etretinate, patients form very thin nail plates (Fig. 12-33).

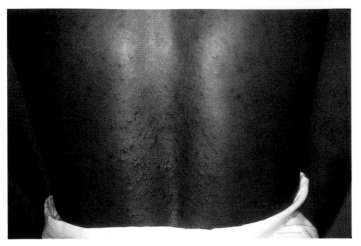

Figure 12-34

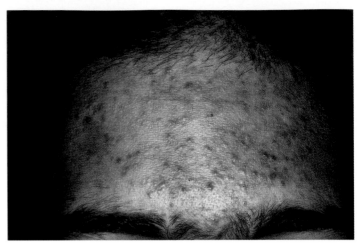

Figure 12-35

Acneiform eruptions are caused by a number of medications that result in inflammatory follicular reactions by nonallergic mechanisms. The patient in Figure 12-34 developed extensive follicular papules extending down to the lower back following treatment with **danazol**, a synthetic androgen. Drug-induced acneiform eruptions are characterized by the rapid onset of extensive papules or pustules in a distribution that may be unusual for acne vulgaris. For example, the lower back or distal arms may be affected. Comedones are either absent or are

minor components of most drug-induced acne. Isoniazid, phenytoin, phenobarbital, testosterone, iodides, bromides, lithium and vitamins B_2, B_6, and B_{12} can cause acneiform eruptions. Prolonged treatment with high doses of systemic steroids is one of the most common causes of an acneiform rash. Figure 12-35 shows a pustular eruption with postinflammatory hyperpigmentation in a patient receiving oral **steroids** for systemic lupus erythematosus.

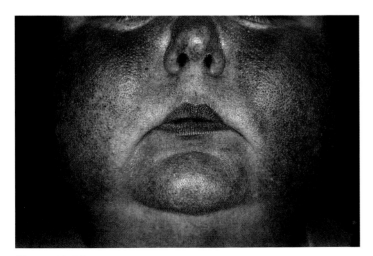

Figure 12-36

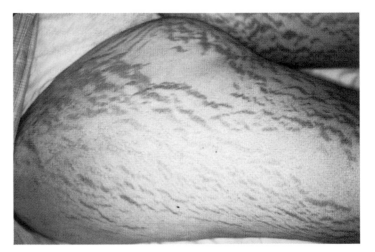

Figure 12-37

In addition to acneiform changes, Cushing syndrome resulting from excessive systemic corticosteroids has numerous cutaneous stigmata. Marked swelling of the face produces a characteristic **moon facies** (Fig. 12-36). Cutaneous atrophy causes skin to be thin, fragile, and easily lacerated. Vascular fragility leads to extensive purpura of extremities, and telangiectasia are easily seen through the thinned skin. **Striae distensae**, commonly known as stretch marks, are a frequent sequela of

long-term treatment with high-dose systemic corticosteroids and can also occur with excessive use of topical corticosteroids. These are commonly seen on the abdomen of women who are pregnant, in people who have rapid or extensive fluctuations in weight, or in weight lifters. People with Cushing disease also develop this irreversible sign of steroid excess. Striae begin as linear, red streaks (Fig. 12-37) which then fade to become yellow or skin-colored.

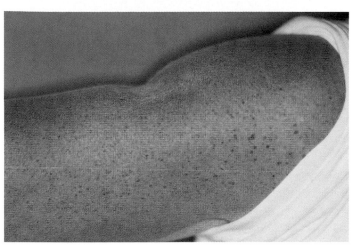

Figure 12-38

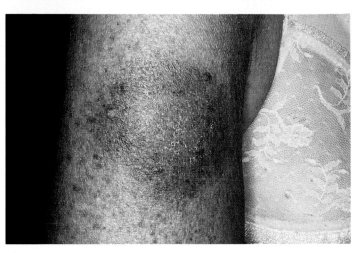

Figure 12-39

Lipoatrophy is a complication of injection of steroids as well as insulin. It most commonly develops following injection of crystalloid suspensions of corticosteroids, such as triamcinolone, into the subcutaneous fat. A poorly demarcated depression develops at the site of injection without overlying scar. The epidermis may appear normal but occasionally there is loss of pigment. This complication most frequently develops after intramuscular injections in the gluteal area or in the deltoid area of the arm (Fig. 12-38). The atrophy is reversible, but occasionally takes days to resolve.

Localized reactions to injection of vitamin K_1 (phytomenadione) are infrequently reported. Pruritus and erythema can develop at the site of injection (Fig. 12-39) and, over a period of months, the affected skin can become hyperpigmented. Local hypopigmentation with morphea-like induration and atrophy have also been reported following vitamin K_1 injection. Patch tests and intradermal skin tests with fat soluble vitamin K_1 in these patients reveals an allergic basis to the reaction. Most of the patients reported have had alcoholic liver disease, but cutaneous hypersensitivity to vitamin K_1 has also been reported in people with other hepatic disorders including primary biliary cirrhosis.

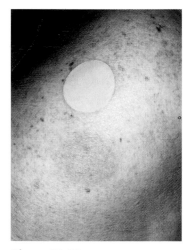

Figure 12-40

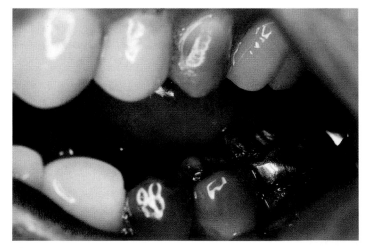

Figure 12-41

With the development of novel methods of drug administration, new kinds of cutaneous drug reactions are being seen. Percutaneous administration of drugs through medicated patches has led to the development of contact dermatitis. These reactions have been particularly problematic for people treated with nicotine patches. Over a third of them develop an irritant contact dermatitis at the site of application of the patch, and allergic contact sensitization occurs in approximately 2%. Transdermal patches containing nitrates have also result in an irritant contact dermatitis in those treated for angina. Areas of erythema that are exactly the same shape as the applied patch develop at the site of application (Fig. 12-40).

Tetracycline, one of the most common drugs in dermatologic therapy, rarely causes allergic cutaneous reactions, although phototoxic and monilial infections are common. Permanent yellow or brown discoloration of the teeth occurs if tetracyclines are administered to children under 8 years of age (Fig. 12-41). Similar changes occur in the teeth of children of women who inject tetracycline after the fourth month of pregnancy. Apart from the discoloration, tetracycline deposited in teeth results in enamel hypoplasia and increased susceptibility to dental caries.

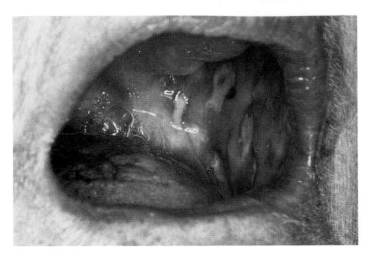

Figure 12-42

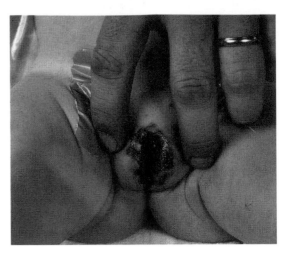

Figure 12-43

Chemotherapeutic agents target rapidly proliferating cells and cannot distinguish between malignant neoplasms and normal rapidly proliferating tissues such as hair, nails, and mucous membranes. It is therefore not surprising to find numerous mucocutaneous side effects of many chemotherapeutic regimens. Mucosal surfaces become inflamed approximately 5–10 days following administration of chemotherapy agents such as methotrexate, cyclophosphamide, 5-fluorouracil, and others. Painful erosions and painful ulcerations may follow over the ensuing days. The oral mucosa is most frequently involved (Fig. 12-42). **Oral ulcerations** may be discrete, resembling ordinary aphthae. Alternatively, more diffuse mucosal involvement may lead to extensive erosion or crust formation. Lips may be covered by a thick hemorrhagic crust and eating can be painful. Involvement of the vaginal (Fig. 12-43) and rectal mucosae often occurs. When rectal mucosa is involved, rectal bleeding and pain on defecation may develop.

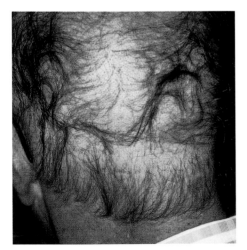

Figure 12-44

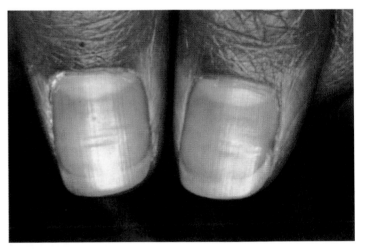

Figure 12-45

Diffuse **alopecia** (Fig. 12-44) is another side effect of many chemotherapeutic agents. Not surprisingly, hair loss affects anagen hairs, which are actively growing and account for more than 80% of scalp hairs. Hairs are lost diffusely, even from the temporal and occipital scalp, which are spared in male pattern alopecia. The degree of alopecia is affected by the amount and timing of chemotherapy and host susceptibility. Beard, eyebrows, eye lashes, axillary, and pubic hair can be lost but chemotherapy-related alopecia is completely reversible. Initially, regrowing hairs may be thinner and lighter.

Beau's lines are horizontal depressions of the nail that follow a sudden insult to the nail matrix from which the entire nail grows. Several weeks after each course of chemotherapy, these horizontal depressions may form in each of the nails. With successive courses, parallel lines form (Fig. 12-45). Beau's lines grow out distally as the nail grows, eventually growing out completely after approximately 6 months. Toenails can be affected and take somewhat longer to grow out.

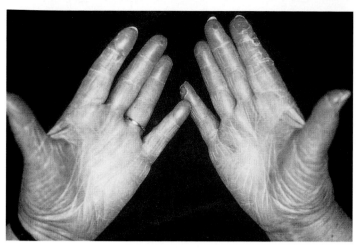

Figure 12-46

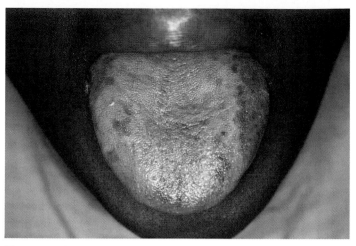

Figure 12-47

Desquamation of the palms and soles (Fig. 12-46) is a nonspecific reaction to several chemotherapeutic regimens and can also be seen in resolving drug eruptions, Kawasaki disease, scarlet fever, toxic shock syndrome, and other conditions. Diffuse scaling of volar skin may develop days to weeks after chemotherapy and can take up to 4 weeks to resolve. It has been suggested that subclinical inflammation caused by a cytotoxic effect of chemotherapy on proliferating epidermal cells is responsible for peeling of the palms and soles.

Several chemotherapy agents cause **hyperpigmentation** that may be striking in its extent or distribution. Skin, hair, nails, or mucous membranes may be affected. The patient in Figure 12-47, for example, developed well-demarcated areas of pigmentation on the tongue following treatment with **5-fluorouracil**. Diffuse or localized hyperpigmentation of the skin has been noted after treatment with bleomycin, 5-fluorouracil, doxorubicin, cyclophosphamide, busulfan, actinomycin D, and others. Hyperpigmentation of nail beds occa-

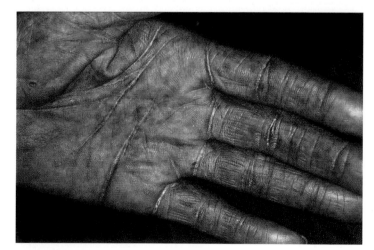

Figure 12-48

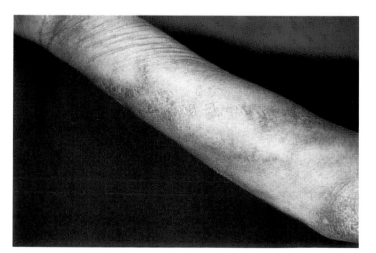

Figure 12-49

sionally gives the appearance of discolored nails. Pigmentation of pressure sites, such as the elbows is frequently reported after treatment with bleomycin. Addisonian pigmentation, which may be accentuated in sun-exposed sites and can also involve mucous membranes, follows treatment with **busulfan** in 5% of patients. Hyperpigmentation commonly affects the palms and soles, especially in creases (Fig. 12-48). Weight loss and diarrhea occur in patients with busulfan pigmentation.

Elevation of melanocyte-stimulating hormone or adrenocorticotropic hormone has been sought to explain the hyperpigmentation seen after chemotherapy but is seldom found. Postinflammatory hyperpigmentation following subclinical cutaneous inflammation caused by chemotherapy may explain some instances of skin darkening. Postinflammatory changes may play a role in the pigmentation that occurs over veins following intravenous infusion of 5-fluorouracil or bleomycin (Fig. 12-49).

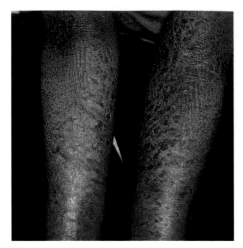

Figure 12-50

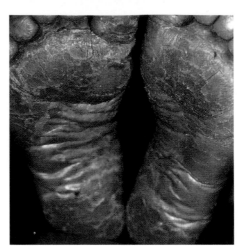

Figure 12-51

Ichthyosiform dermatoses are characterized by the shedding of large scales. Many forms, different inheritance patterns, and clinical presentations exist. A severe autosomal recessive form of ichthyosis called **lamellar ichthyosis** can be associated with systemic complications. Patients with classic lamellar ichthyosis develop large scales (Fig. 12-50) over the entire body. The scales have elevated edges and have been described as "plate-like" or "parchment-like." Large scales are often apparent on the face, and tautness of the face leads to ectropion and eclabium. Flexural involvement is characteristic and distinguishes lamellar ichthyosis from the more common ichthyosis vulgaris. Thick scaling of the palms and soles (Fig. 12-51) usually develops.

The ectropion that occurs makes patients prone to ocular infections, and breaks in the skin lead to cutaneous infection. Obstruction of sweat ducts interferes with normal sweating; consequently, patients lose one mechanism of temperature control and frequently develop fevers.

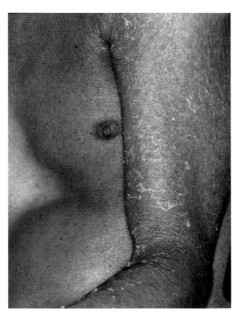

Figure 12-52

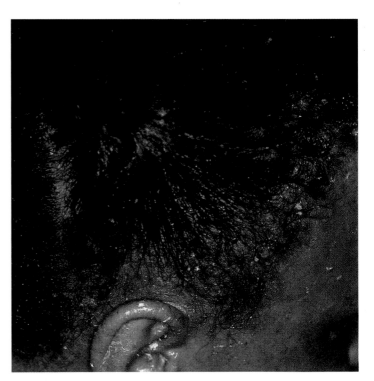

Figure 12-53

Some authorities have recognized a clinically and genetically distinct subtype of autosomal recessive ichthyosis that has been called **congenital ichthyosiform erythroderma**. Scales on the face and trunk are usually smaller than classic lamellar ichthyosis, and underlying erythroderma is usually seen (Fig. 12-52). As in classic lamellar ichthyosis, scales and skin markings are increased in the flexures. Large scales are usually present on the extensor surfaces of the legs. Palmar plantar keratoderma can occur, and ectropion is often present, but the severity of this disorder is much more variable than the uniformly severe cutaneous involvement in patients with classic lamellar ichthyosis. Thick scaling in the scalp (Fig. 12-53) can lead to secondary infection and scarring alopecia.

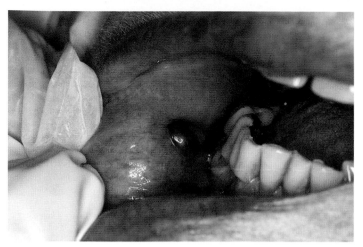

Figure 12-54A

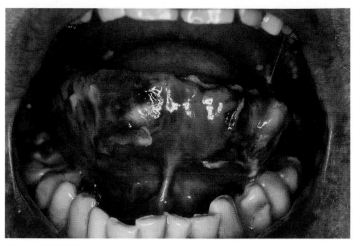

Figure 12-54B

Despite advances in therapy, **pemphigus vulgaris** remains one of the most dangerous dermatologic conditions. Pemphigus is an autoimmune disorder caused by IgG antibodies against the surface of epidermal and epithelial cells. In most patients, initial lesions occur on the oral mucosa months or years before the skin lesions. In the absence of skin lesions, painful oral erosions may be difficult to distinguish from ordinary aphthae but are more severe or occur more often. Occasionally, bullae can be seen on mucous membranes (Fig. 12-54A) but more often these break quickly to form erosions as shown on the tongue of a patient in Figure 12-54B. Less frequently, erosions can involve the pharynx, larynx, or esophagus, leading to hoarseness or dysphagia. Other mucous membranes such as the conjunctiva or anogenital mucosa can be involved as

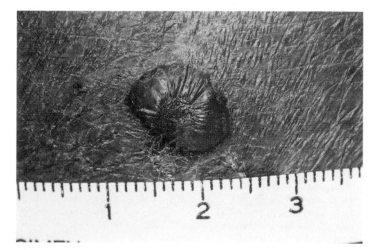

Figure 12-55

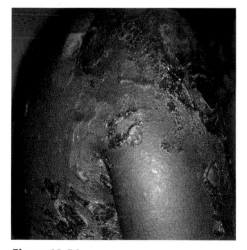

Figure 12-56

well. Skin lesions begin as flaccid blisters or bullae (Fig. 12-55) that are easily broken, leading to painful erosions. Blisters can occur anywhere on the body and spread peripherally when pressure is applied to them, a finding that is called the Nikolsky sign and occurs in a number of bullous conditions. Histologic examination reveals the bullae of pemphigus to be intraepidermal. Definitive diagnosis is made by direct immunofluorescence of perilesional skin and shows IgG antibodies on the cell surfaces of keratinocytes in the intercellular spaces of the epidermis. The latter finding can be shown in virtually all patients with pemphigus. Indirect immunofluorescence performed on serum from pemphigus patients reveals anti-cell surface antibodies in most patients. The antibody titer correlates with the severity of pemphigus in most, but not all, patients. Successful control of this disease may require high doses of systemic corticosteroids with up to 400 mg/day of prednisone. Alternatively, combining lower prednisone doses with immunosuppressive agents has been advocated. This condition used to be uniformly fatal but, with treatment, approximately 10% of patients succumb to the disease or to complications of its therapy. Sunlight or heat may exacerbate pemphigus. Figure 12-56 shows a patient whose condition first started after treatment with psoralen ultraviolet A (PUVA) was initiated for psoriasis.

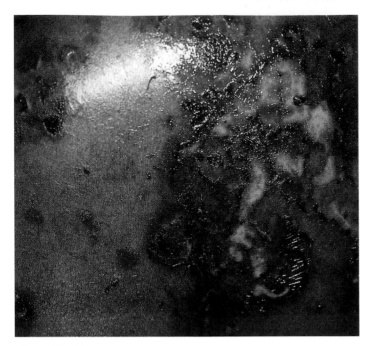

Figure 12-57

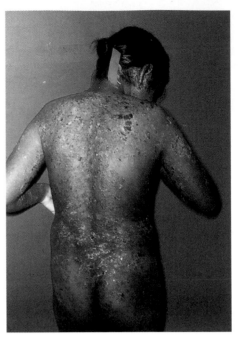

Figure 12-58

Several variants of pemphigus have been described. **Pemphigus foliaceus** refers to a very similar autoimmune condition caused by anti-cell surface antibodies, resulting in intraepidermal bulla formation in the superficial epidermis. Mucous membranes are often spared and bullae rapidly form crusts and are therefore not apparent. Initially, lesions may be confined to the face, scalp, and upper trunk (Fig. 12-57) but eventually they can become generalized.

Pemphigus erythematosus, also known as the **Senear–Usher syndrome**, resembles pemphigus foliaceus clinically and histologically, but patients may have circulating antinuclear antibodies. Crusted patches remain confined to the face, scalp, and upper trunk. Paraneoplastic pemphigus has been described in Chapter 11.

Fogo selvagem is a form of pemphigus foliaceus that is endemic to rural areas of Brazil. Most cases occur in children, adolescents, and young adults. The black fly, *Simulium pruinosum*, is thought to be a vector of this disease. Occurrence of the disorder in several members of the same family has led to the suggestion that there is a genetic predisposition to this condition. As in pemphigus foliaceus, the primary lesion is a bulla that arises in the superficial epidermis. Lesions present as crusts and erosions on the head, chest, and upper back (Fig. 12-58). Histologic and immunofluorescent findings are identical to those of pemphigus foliaceus.

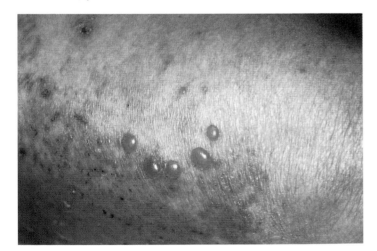

Figure 12-59

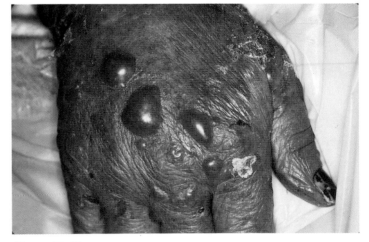

Figure 12-60

Bullous pemphigoid is another autoimmune bullous disease. Pemphigoid primarily affects elderly patients, with an average age of onset exceeding 60 years. The fully developed lesions of bullous

pemphigoid are tense bullae (Figs 12-59 and 12-60). These may be localized to the lower extremities or generalized, involving the trunk, head, and extremities. Eventually bullae break to form crusts and

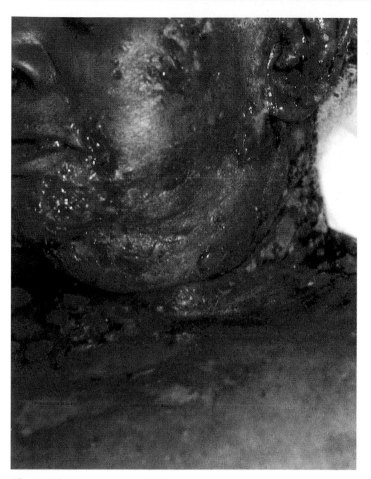

Figure 12-61

erosions (Fig. 12-61). Some patients may present with urticarial plaques, and still others may present with severe pruritus without any apparent skin lesions. The oral mucosa is involved in approximately 25% of patients, and other mucous membranes are spared.

Skin biopsy reveals a subepidermal bulla with a dermal infiltrate that typically includes eosinophils. On direct immunofluorescence there is a linear deposit of C3 and IgG. Indirect immunofluorescence reveals antibullous pemphigoid antibodies in the serum of approximately 75% of patients, but the titers of antibodies do not correlate with the severity of disease. Although bullous pemphigoid may be severe and even fatal, it has a better prognosis than pemphigus vulgaris. Bullous pemphigoid is often self-limited, resolving in some patients over a period of months to years.

Previous associations between bullous pemphigoid and internal malignancy are overstated. Pemphigoid affects an elderly population that has a higher incidence of malignancy even in the absence of this bullous disease.

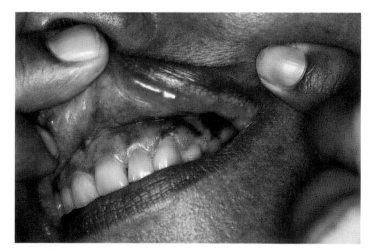

Figure 12-62

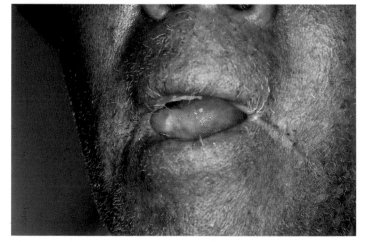

Figure 12-63

Cicatricial pemphigoid has immunopathologic features in common with bullous pemphigoid, but has an entirely different clinical course. Like pemphigoid, there is linear deposition of immunoglobulin and C3 at the basement membrane. Indirect immunofluorescence of sera is usually negative, however. In most people with cicatricial pemphigoid, lesions are limited to the mucous membranes and consist of bullae or erosions. The oral and conjunctival mucosae are most commonly involved but other mucous membranes can be affected too. Involvement of gingival mucosa is common (Fig. 12-62). Lesions heal with scarring (Fig. 12-63) and severe ocular involvement and blindness may occur. Some patients have skin lesions consisting of bullae or vesicles.

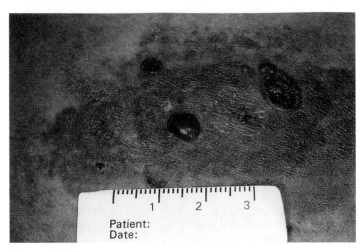

Figure 12-65

These can progress to form subepidermal vesicles and bullae and, eventually, erosions and crusts (Fig. 12-65). Symptoms often flare immediately after delivery and can persist for several months thereafter. There are rare reports of bullous lesions occurring in infants born to mothers with herpes gestationis.

On direct immunofluorescence of skin biopsy specimens, there is linear deposition of C3 along the basement membrane zone of lesional, perilesional, or normal appearing skin of patients with herpes gestationis. Indirect immunofluorescence of serum reveals an IgG anti-basement membrane zone antibody, but IgG is only detected in approximately one-third of skin biopsy specimens examined with direct immunofluorescence.

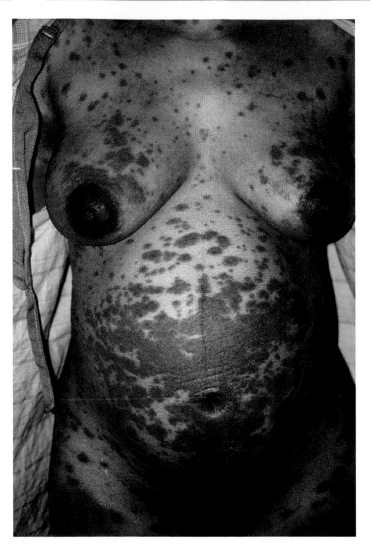

Figure 12-64

Herpes gestationis is a rare autoimmune bullous disease of pregnancy. Most cases begin between the fourth and seventh months of pregnancy but the condition can occur at any point during pregnancy or immediately postpartum. Skin lesions are severely pruritic and begin as erythematous papules or plaques that can be widespread (Fig. 12-64).

Index

Please note that tables are indicated by the letter *t*.

juvenile, 138t
pyoderma gangrenosum in, 70
rheumatoid nodules, 10
rheumatoid factor
in connective tissue disease, 160t
in essential mixed cryoglobulinemia, 19
in psoriatic arthritis, 22, 23t
in rheumatoid arthritis, 10
in rheumatoid vasculitis, 10
rheumatoid nodules, 10
rheumatoid vasculitis, 10
see also individual disorders (e.g. SLE)
Rhizopus, in mucormycosis, 161
rhus dermatitis, agammaglobulinemia in, 181
riboflavin deficiency in angular stomatitis, 61
rickettsial infection
in immunocompromised patient, 138t
Rickettsia akari, 157
rickettsialpox, 138t, 156t, 157
Rickettsia rickettsii, 156
Rocky Mountain spotted fever, 156
rifampin, in borderline leprosy, 149
Rochalimaea henselae, in bacillary angiomatosis, 172
Rocky Mountain spotted fever
in acute purpura associated with fever, 157t
clinical features, 156
atypical measles, similarity to, 161
Pseudomonas septicemia, similarity to, 145
in immunocompromised patient, 138t
rodent ulcer, in basal cell carcinoma, 206
roseola
erythema associated with fever, 160t
roseola infantum, 138t
roseola-like rash, in HIV infection, 176
RPR (rapid plasma reagin) test, in syphilis, 151
rubella (measles)
in acute purpura associated with fever, 157t
atypical, 161
Rocky Mountain spotted fever, similarity to, 161
in erythema associated with fever, 160t

S

saddle-nose deformity, in Wegener granulomatosis, 35
sagging skin, in cutis laxa, 38
salicylates, as cause of erythema annulare centrifugum, 220
see also aspirin
Salmonella infection, cause of Reiter syndrome, 23
sarcoid, cause of erythema nodosum, 32t
sarcoidosis
in Addison disease, 116
annular lesions in, 33
disease course, 31–32
erythema nodosum in, 31–32
ichthyosiform eruptions in, 34
lupus pernio in, 33
lymphadenopathy in, 33
noncaseating granulomatosis in, 31
papular lesions in, 32, 34
progressive pulmonary disease, 32
splenomegaly in, 33
sarcoma
in yellow nail syndrome, 40
see also Kaposi sarcoma

Sarcoptes scabiei var. *hominis*, 173
scabies
in AIDS, 173
scabicidal treatment, 173
scalded skin syndrome
toxic epidermal necrolysis, similarity to, 142
staphylococcal, 142
scaling of skin
in acquired ichthyosis, 178
in carcinoid syndrome, 80
in congenital ichthyosiform erythroderma, 228
in cutaneous T-cell lymphoma, 201
in exfoliative dermatitis, 199
in HIV infection, 177
in Norwegian scabies, 173
in papular eruptions of AIDS, 176
in pellagra, 76
in Sézary syndrome, 202
shedding in ichthyosiform dermatosis, 228
see also plaques; erythema
scalp symptoms
hair loss
in acrodermatitis enteropathica, 75
in hyperthyroidism, 114
congenital nevi, 131
tumors
in acute myeloid leukemia, 195
scarring alopecia in, 187
see also alopecia; hair abnormalities
scarlet fever, 144, 160t
Kawasaki disease, similarity to, 52
in immunocompromised patient, 138t
infectious diseases, 144
Pastia's lines, 52
scars and scarring
cribriform in pyoderma gangrenosum, 71
hypertrophic in dystrophic epidermolysis bullosa, 63
scarring alopecia
in discoid lupus erythematosus, 6
in scalp metastasis, 187
surgical
as site of breast carcinoma, 191
site of metastases, 187
as site of squamous cell carcinoma, 208
Schirmer test, for Sjögren syndrome, 13
sclera, in jaundice, 86
scleredema, 14–15
associated with benign monoclonal gammopathy, 15
in diabetes, 15, 119
hard skin, 15
skinfolds in, 15
sclerodactyly
in connective tissue disease, 14
in dermatomyositis, 9
in scleroderma, 11
scleroderma-like changes and syndrome
bleomycin-induced, 3
in carcinoid syndrome, 80
in graft-versus-host disease, 17
in livedo reticularis, 3
in progeria, 56
scleroderma (progressive systemic sclerosis)
antibodies in
anticentromere, 11
antinuclear, 4t, 13
calcinosis, 11, 12

congenital, 138t
CREST syndrome, 11
diffuse, 11, 12
eosinophilic fasciitis, similarity to, 14
morphea, 13
Parry–Romberg syndrome, 13
polymyositis, overlap with, 4t
in Raynaud phenomenon, 2, 3t, 11, 12
sclerodactyly, 11
Sjögren syndrome, 13
telangiectasia in, 11, 12
scleroderma sine scleroderma, 11
scleromyxedema (lichen myxedematosus), 15
sclerosing basal cell carcinoma, clinical features, 207
SCLE, *see* subacute cutaneous lupus erythematosus
scrofuloderma, in tuberculosis, 149
scoliosis
in Cowden disease, 67
in Hallermann–Streiff syndrome, 134
Sézary syndrome, in cutaneous T-cell lymphoma, 200, 202
seafood, in *Vibrio vulnificus* infection, 147
sebaceous carcinoma
association with Muir–Torre syndrome, 211
sebaceous (epidermoid) cyst formation, in Gardner syndrome, 65
sebaceous tumors, association with Muir–Torre syndrome, 211
seborrheic dermatitis
in AIDS, 177
Letterer–Siwe disease, similarity to, 37
differential diagnosis, 37, 73
in HIV infection, 177
in Parkinson's disease, 135
seborrheic keratoses, sign of Leser–Trélat in, 211
segmental neurofibromatosis, 125
seizures
in epidermal nevus syndrome, 133
in Hartnup disease, 64
in incontinentia pigmenti achromians, 127
in neurocutaneous melanosis, 131
in phakomatosis pigmentovascularis, 130
in Sturge–Weber syndrome, 128
in systemic lupus erythematosus, 5t
in tuberous sclerosis, 126
self-amputation, *see* autoamputation
Senear–Usher syndrome, *see* pemphigus erythematosus
sensory neuropathy, 134
sepsis and septicemia
in acute purpura associated with fever, 157t
in *Bacteroides* infection, 139
in cutaneous T-cell lymphoma, 202
in pustular psoriasis, 22
in Sézary syndrome, 202
in toxic epidermal necrolysis, 220
in *Vibrio vulnificus* infection, 147
septal panniculitis, diagnostic approach, 32t
serum sickness, from penicillin, 18
serum sickness-like prodrome, in viral hepatitis, 88
sexual abuse, in genital herpes, 154
sexually transmitted disease
chancroid, 153
genital herpes, 154–155
gonorrhea, 152
granuloma inguinale, 154
human papillomavirus infection, 189

in cutaneous T-cell lymphoma, 202
in dermatitis herpetiformis, 78
in large cell carcinoma of lung, 187
in noncaseating granulomatosis, 34
in scleroderma, 13
in Sjögren syndrome, 13
tongue disease and symptoms
in acanthosis nigricans, 120
in carcinoma of the oropharynx, 186
in Cronkhite–Canada syndrome, papillae, 68
drug-induced
hyperpigmentation due to 5-fluorouracil, 227
hyperpigmentation due to minocycline, 221
in dyskeratosis congenita, leukokeratosis, 103
in exfoliative dermatitis, 199
in glossitis, 85
in hereditary hemorrhagic telangiectasia, 81
in hypothyroidism, enlargement, 113
in Kawasaki disease, swelling, 52
in lipoid proteinosis, papules, 30
in macroglossia, indentations, 108
in Melkersson–Rosenthal syndrome, lingua plicata, 134
in oral hairy leukoplakia, 175
in pellagra, 76
in scarlet fever, 160t
squamous cell carcinoma, 188
strawberry tongue
in Kawasaki disease, 52
in toxic shock syndrome, 141
white, in scarlet fever, 144
telangiectasia, 2, 9, 81
in toxic shock syndrome, 141
in varicella, vesicles, 159
tonsillopharyngitis, in scarlet fever, 144
tooth abnormalities, *see* dentition abnormalities
tophi, in gout, 26
TORCHS acronym, 138t, 157t
toxic epidermal necrolysis, 142, 160t
bulla resemble graft-versus-host disease, 16
clinical features, 142
dilantin hypersensitivity syndrome, similarity to, 222
drug-induced
due to allopurinol, 220
due to doxorubicin and whole-body electron beam radiation, 222
due to NSAIDs, 220
due to phenytoin, 220
due to phenytoin and whole-body electron beam radiation, 222
due to sulfonamides, 220
scalded skin syndrome, similarity to, 142
toxic shock syndrome, 160t
in immunocompromised patient, 138t
Staphylococcus aureus in, 141
Toxoplasma antibodies, in acute purpura associated with fever, 157t
tracheostomy, for xanthoma disseminatum, 37
"tram line" streaks in skull radiographs, in Sturge–Weber syndrome, 129
transaminase
in graft-versus-host disease, 16
in graft-versus-host disease, 17
transdermal drug patches, as cause of contact dermatitis, 225
transplantation surgery, immunosuppressive therapy, 184

trauma, blunt, as cause of Raynaud phenomenon, 3t
tremulousness, in carcinoid syndrome, 79
Treponema pallidum, in syphilis, 150
triamcinolone
for annular sarcoid, 34
as cause of lipoatrophy, 225
trichilemmomas, in Cowden disease, 66
Trichophyton infection
after immunosuppressive therapy, 184
in septal panniculitis, 32t
trigeminal nerve
infection (nasociliary branch) in varicella, 159
in Sturge–Weber syndrome, 128
triglyceridemia, xanthoma, eruptive in, 48
trimethoprim–sulfamethoxazole
in AIDS, 178
in HIV-infected patients, reactions to, 178
in *Pneumocystis carinii* infection, 178
in Stevens–Johnson syndrome, 218
rash, as cause of, 216
Stevens–Johnson syndrome, as cause of, 218
L-tryptophan, drug-induced eosinophilia–myalgia, 14
tuberculosis (TB)
in Addison disease, 116
cause of erythema nodosum, 32
deficiency in pellagra, 77
diagnosis, 32
transport defect in Hartnup disease, 64
in yellow nail syndrome, 40
tuberculosis verrucosa, 137, 149
tuberous sclerosis, brain tubers, 126
tuberous xanthomas, in atherosclerosis, 46
tuboeruptive xanthoma, in hypertriglyceridemia, 48
tumor see neoplasms, carcinoma, 28
typhus (epidemic)
in acute purpura associated with fever, 157t
in immunocompromised patient, 138t
Tzanck smear
for diagnosis of herpes simplex virus infection, 155
in erythema multiforme, 160t
in herpes simplex infection, 168
in varicella, 159
vesicopustular eruptions associated with fever, 156t

U

ulcerative colitis, 69
erythema nodosum in, 69
in pyoderma gangrenosum, 71
relation to pyoderma gangrenosum, 69–70
ulcers
in acute myeloid leukemia, 194
in AIDS, crusted, 171
in basal cell carcinoma, rodent, 206
in blastomycosis, verrucous, 162
in breast carcinoma, 190
in classic Kaposi sarcoma, extremities 193
cutaneous
in actinomycosis, 147
in cutaneous leishmaniasis, 163
in eosinophilic pustular folliculitis, 176
genital

in Behçet disease, 19
in chancroid, 153
in genital herpes, 154–155
in granuloma inguinale, 154
in herpes simplex infection, 168
in syphilis, 150
in hyperoxaluria, 98
leg
in pyoderma gangrenosum, 71
in sickle-cell anemia, 101
in Werner syndrome, 57
in macroglossia, 108
mucosal
in AIDS-related Reiter syndrome, 177
in connective tissue disease, 160t
in *Mycobacterium haemophilum* infection, 172
in necrobiosis lipoidica diabeticorum, 118
neuropathic, 118, 149
oral
canker sores, similarity to, 19
due to chemotherapy, 226
due to cyclophosphamide treatment, 182
due to immunosuppressant therapy, 182
in AIDS-related Kaposi sarcoma, 175
in Behçet disease, 19
in Crohn's disease, 73
in cyclic neutropenia, 181
in histoplasmosis, 170
in pellagra, 76
in Reiter syndrome, 23t
in syphilis, 150
in systemic lupus erythematosus, 5t, 7
in papular eruptions of AIDS, 176
postoperative, peristomal, 82
in pyoderma gangrenosum, 70, 71
in Reiter syndrome, corneal, 24
in rheumatoid vasculitis, vasculitic, 10
in staphylococcal infection in AIDS, crusted, 171
in Stewart–Treves syndrome, 192
in syphilis, chancre, 150
in systemic lupus erythematosus, 5t, 6, 7
in T-cell lymphoma, 201–202
uremia
in Fabry disease, 95
petechiae formation, 101
in renal disease, 92
uremic frost, in renal failure, 91, 92
uremic pruritus, renal diseases, 92
urethritis, in Reiter syndrome, 25
uric acid crystals, in gout, 26
urinary casts
in Henoch–Schönlein purpura, 97
in systemic lupus erythematosus, 5t
urine analysis and examination
in acute purpura associated with fever, 157t
in congenital erythropoietic porphyria, 107
in dermatomyositis, 8
in jaundice, 86
in porphyria cutanea tarda, 105
in toxic shock syndrome, 160t
urolithiasis, in hyperoxaluria, 98
uroporphyrinogen metabolism, in porphyria, 105, 106
urostomy, 82
urticaria
allergic, similarity to urticarial vasculitis, 18
in allergic angioedema, 30
in bullous pemphigoid, 231